TMJ Internal Derangement & Arthrosis

Surgical Atlas

TMJ Internal Derangement & Arthrosis

Surgical Atlas

M. Franklin Dolwick, D.M.D., Ph.D.

Professor and Chairman,
Department of Oral and Maxillofacial Surgery,
University of Florida,
College of Dentistry,
Gainesville, Florida;
Diplomate, American Board of Oral and Maxillofacial Surgery

Bruce Sanders, D.D.S.

Adjunct Professor,
Section of Oral and Maxillofacial Surgery,
University of California, Los Angeles,
School of Dentistry,
Los Angeles, California;
Private practice, Santa Monica, California;
Diplomate, American Board of Oral and Maxillofacial Surgery

with **346** illustrations and **63** 4-color illustrations

Illustrations by **William M. Winn, Russell G. Jones,** *and* **Anne Irene Hurley**

The C. V. Mosby Company

ST. LOUIS • PRINCETON • TORONTO 1985

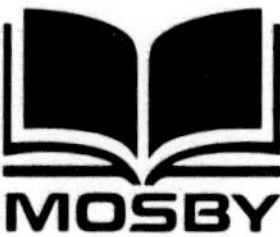

A TRADITION OF PUBLISHING EXCELLENCE

Editor: Darlene Warfel
Assistant Editor: Melba Steube
Editing Supervisor: Elaine Steinborn
Manuscript Editor: Carol Sullivan Wiseman
Book design: Jeanne Genz
Production: Carol O'Leary, Jeanne A. Gulledge

Printed in the United States of America

The C.V. Mosby Company
11830 Westline Industrial Drive, St. Louis, Missouri 63146

Library of Congress Cataloging in Publication Data

Dolwick, M. Franklin.
TMJ internal derangement and arthrosis.

Bibliography: p.
1. Temporomandibular joint—Surgery—Atlases.
2. Temporomandibular joint—Diseases—Atlases.
I. Sanders, Bruce, 1943- . II. Title. [DNLM:
1. Temporomandibular Joint—surgery—atlases.
2. Temporomandibular Joint Diseases—diagnosis—atlases.
WU 17 D665t]
RK470.D65 1985 617'.522 85-10627
ISBN 0-8016-1414-7

AC/W/W 9 8 7 6 5 4 3 2 01/B/050

Dedicated to my parents, Melvin C. and Elsie L. Dolwick, for their sacrifices, support, and love, which made my education possible.

M. Franklin Dolwick

Dedicated to the loving memory of my father, Mr. Leslie Sanders, and to the honored memory of my oral and maxillofacial surgery colleagues, Dr. John Ireland and Dr. Dennis Zielinski.

Bruce Sanders

PREFACE

During the last decade, rapid changes have occurred in the field of temporomandibular joint surgery. These changes have been stimulated by a renewed interest in internal joint derangements. The focus of interest has changed from the osseous tissues to the soft tissue structures of the joint. The accumulation of knowledge has been immense and is developing rapidly.

The development of TMJ arthrography has been the focal point of an increased understanding of articular disk function and dysfunction and has led to anatomic, pathologic, and clinical studies that have further clarified the subject. Concomitant with these developments, new surgical techniques for the correction of internal derangements have evolved. New techniques have been proposed, modified, and accepted, while others have been discarded. At the same time, some old techniques, such as meniscectomy, have become popular again.

The primary purpose of this book is to present, through photographs and illustrations, the information currently available in diagnosis and surgical management of internal derangements and arthrosis. Anatomic, clinical, and surgical photographs are used to demonstrate important features of internal derangements. Illustrations are used to clarify, emphasize, and highlight important points. A unique feature of the book is the inclusion of color photographs. It is our belief that color will give vitality to the photographs and convey a greater sense of appreciation of the tissues and the pathologic processes.

Each chapter has unique features, and no single chapter can be singled out as most important. The book begins with normal TMJ anatomy and pathology. These chapters establish the anatomic basis for understanding internal derangements and contrasting the pathologic conditions with the normal TMJ anatomy.

Chapters 3 and 4 discuss and illustrate clinical diagnosis and arthrography. Chapter 4 emphasizes interpretation of arthrograms by presenting photographs of the various diagnostic categories with illustrations. In Chapter 5, the surgical techniques used successfully by us in over 1000 cases during the past 10 years are demonstrated. No attempt has been made to include all currently used techniques. We recognize and acknowledge that other good techniques exist and are successfully used by other surgeons. It is our hope that the demonstrated surgical techniques will serve as a model for use by some surgeons and as a source of modification and improvement of techniques for others.

Chapter 6 discusses postoperative management and results. Complications and failure are discussed candidly in Chapter 7. Chapter 7 also includes several case reports illustrating complications, failures, and their management. The final chapter is a series of case reports demonstrating various diagnostic and treatment challenges. The book ends with an exhaustive reference list on TMJ internal derangements.

Presently the diagnosis and treatment of TMJ internal derangements and arthrosis has a scientific basis. The pathology has been documented, the diagnostic criteria have been established, and successful surgical treatment has been documented. Many scientists and clinicians have contributed to this accumulation of knowledge. No attempt will be made to individually name these people because the list is extensive and the possibility of oversight great. We wish to acknowledge their contributions and thank them for their tireless efforts.

Although much has been accomplished in the past decade, many questions remain unanswered. It is hoped this work will serve as a stimulus for continued research. It is also our sincere hope and desire that this work will contribute in some small way to the relief of pain and dysfunction in suffering TMJ patients.

M. Franklin Dolwick
Bruce Sanders

CONTENTS

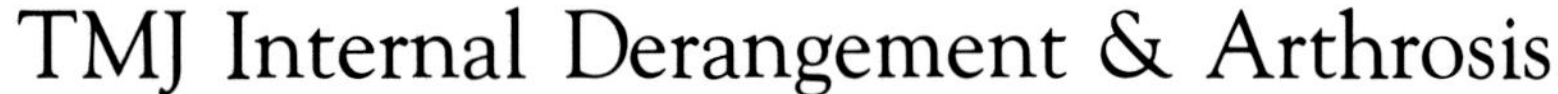

TMJ Internal Derangement & Arthrosis

Surgical Atlas

chapter 1

Anatomy

PLATE 1-1

The temporomandibular joint (TMJ) is the diarthrodial (freely movable) articulation between the condyle of the mandible and the squamous portion of the temporal bone. It is a true synovial joint and has much in common with other synovial joints of the body. It does, however, have several anatomic and functional characteristics that distinguish it from most other joints, including:

1. The articulating surfaces of the bones are covered by an avascular fibrous connective tissue that may contain a variable number of cartilage cells and thus can be designated *fibrocartilage*.
2. The two articulating complexes of bone carry teeth, whose shape and position influence the movements of the joint. It is the only joint with a rigid end-point of closure.
3. It has a bilateral articulation with the cranium, so the right and left temporomandibular articulations must function together.
4. The TMJ is a complex joint because each joint has an articular disc (meniscus) interposed between the condyle and the temporal bone.

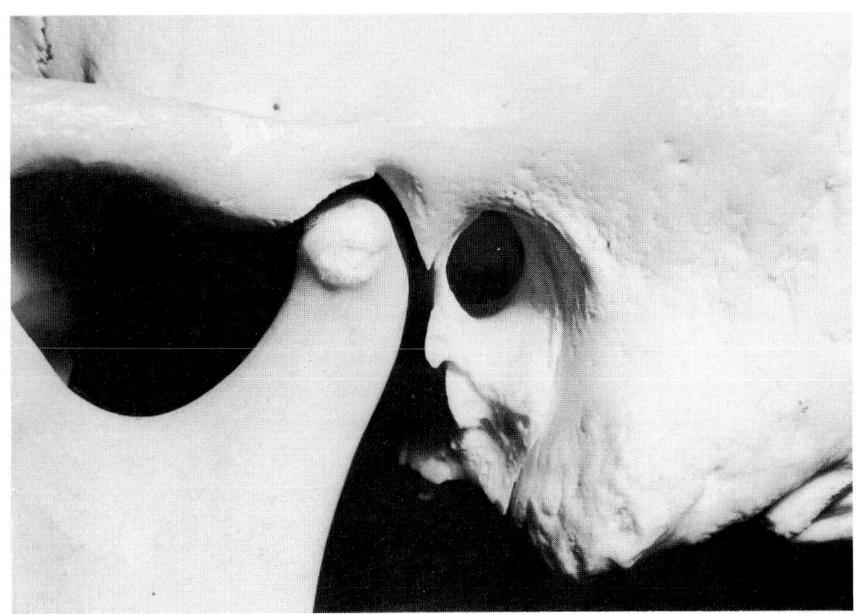

PREAURICULAR REGION

PLATE 1-2

A and **B** Several anatomic structures in the preauricular region are important when performing TMJ surgery. The region includes the parotid gland, superficial temporal vessels, and facial and auriculotemporal nerves.

The parotid gland lies below the zygomatic arch, below and in front of the external acoustic meatus, on the masseter muscle, and behind the ramus of the mandible. The superior pole of the parotid gland lies over the TMJ. The parotid gland is enclosed within a capsule derived from the investing layer of the deep cervical fascia.

The superficial temporal vessels emerge from the superior aspect of the gland and accompany the auriculotemporal nerve. The superficial temporal artery arises in the parotid gland, crosses the zygomatic arch, and divides into frontal and parietal branches. The superficial temporal vein lies superficial to the artery. The auriculotemporal nerve accompanies, and is posterior to, the superficial temporal artery. The terminal branches of the facial nerve emerge from the parotid gland and radiate forward in the face. The terminal branches vary in their arrangement but are commonly classified as temporal, zygomatic, buccal, marginal mandibular, and cervical. The location of the temporal branches is of particular importance during TMJ surgery, as these are the branches most likely to be encountered in the surgical field. The temporal nerve branches lie within a dense fusion of periosteum, temporal fascia, and superficial fascia at the level of the zygomatic arch. Al-Kayat and Bramley found that the nerve averaged 2.0 cm from the anterior concavity of the external auditory canal, but in individual cases the nerve approached as near as 0.8 cm and as far anteriorly as 3.5 cm. Protection of the nerve can be achieved by making an incision through the temporal fascia and periosteum down to the arch not more than 0.8 cm in front of the anterior border of the external auditory canal.

A

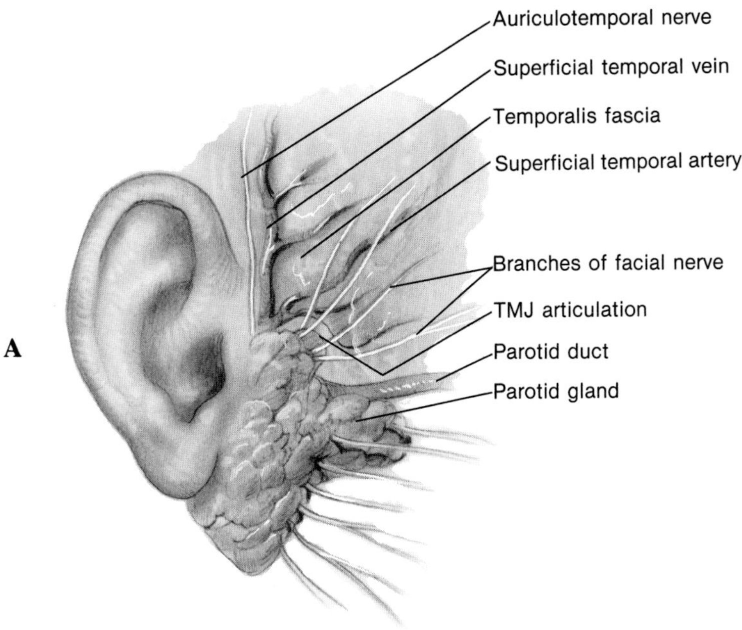
Auriculotemporal nerve
Superficial temporal vein
Temporalis fascia
Superficial temporal artery
Branches of facial nerve
TMJ articulation
Parotid duct
Parotid gland

B

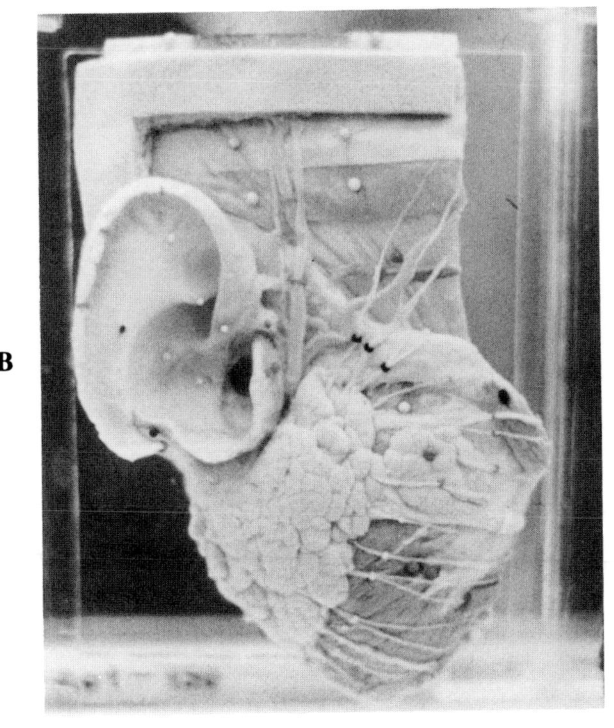

C and **D** The facial nerve exits the skull through the stylomastoid foramen. It enters the parotid gland, where it usually divides into two main trunks (temporofacial and cervicofacial), the branches of which variably anastomose with each other to form the parotid plexus. Anatomically the branches of the facial nerve divide the parotid gland into superficial and deep lobes. The facial nerve divides at a point between 1.5 and 2.8 cm below the lowest concavity of the bony external auditory canal, according to Al-Kayat and Bramley. These measurements can be used to identify the main trunk and, most importantly during TMJ surgery, to avoid it.

D courtesy J.E. Hausaman, Professor and Chairman, Department of Oral and Maxillofacial Surgery, Medizinische Hochschule Hannover, Hannover, Germany.

C

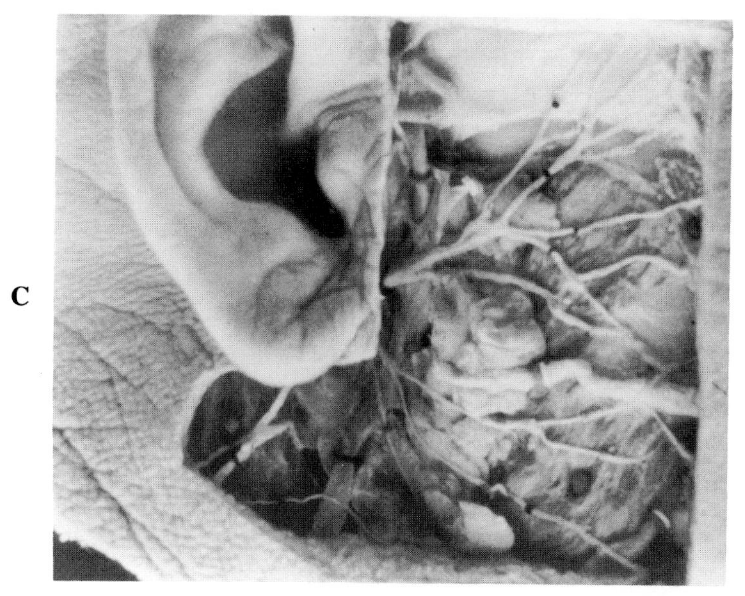

D

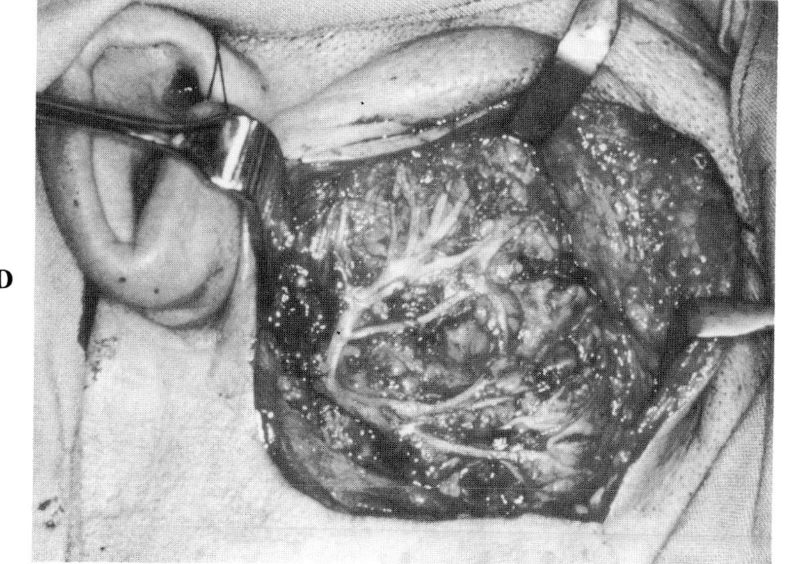

OSSEOUS ANATOMY

PLATE 1-3

A Each condyle of the mandible is elliptical, with its long axis oriented mediolaterally and at right angles to the plane of the mandibular ramus. The condyle measures about 20 mm mediolaterally and about one half this dimension anteroposteriorly, although these measurements vary widely from one individual to another (length 13 to 25 mm, breadth 5.5 to 16 mm).

B There is considerable variation in the angle at which the condyle relates to the ramus of the mandible. As a rule, the longitudinal axis of the condyles converge in a posterior direction. The angle this longitudinal axis makes with the frontal plane varies from 0 to 30 degrees. Thus lateral radiographs of the TMJ must be taken with an oblique projection to obtain an undistorted view of the condylar form and position. A submental vertex radiograph can be used to accurately determine this angle.

C and **D** The form of the condyle varies widely from one individual to another. The superior outline in the mediolateral plane is rounded or convex (about 60%) but occasionally flat or straight (20% to 30%). Other shapes, such as angular or round, are rare.

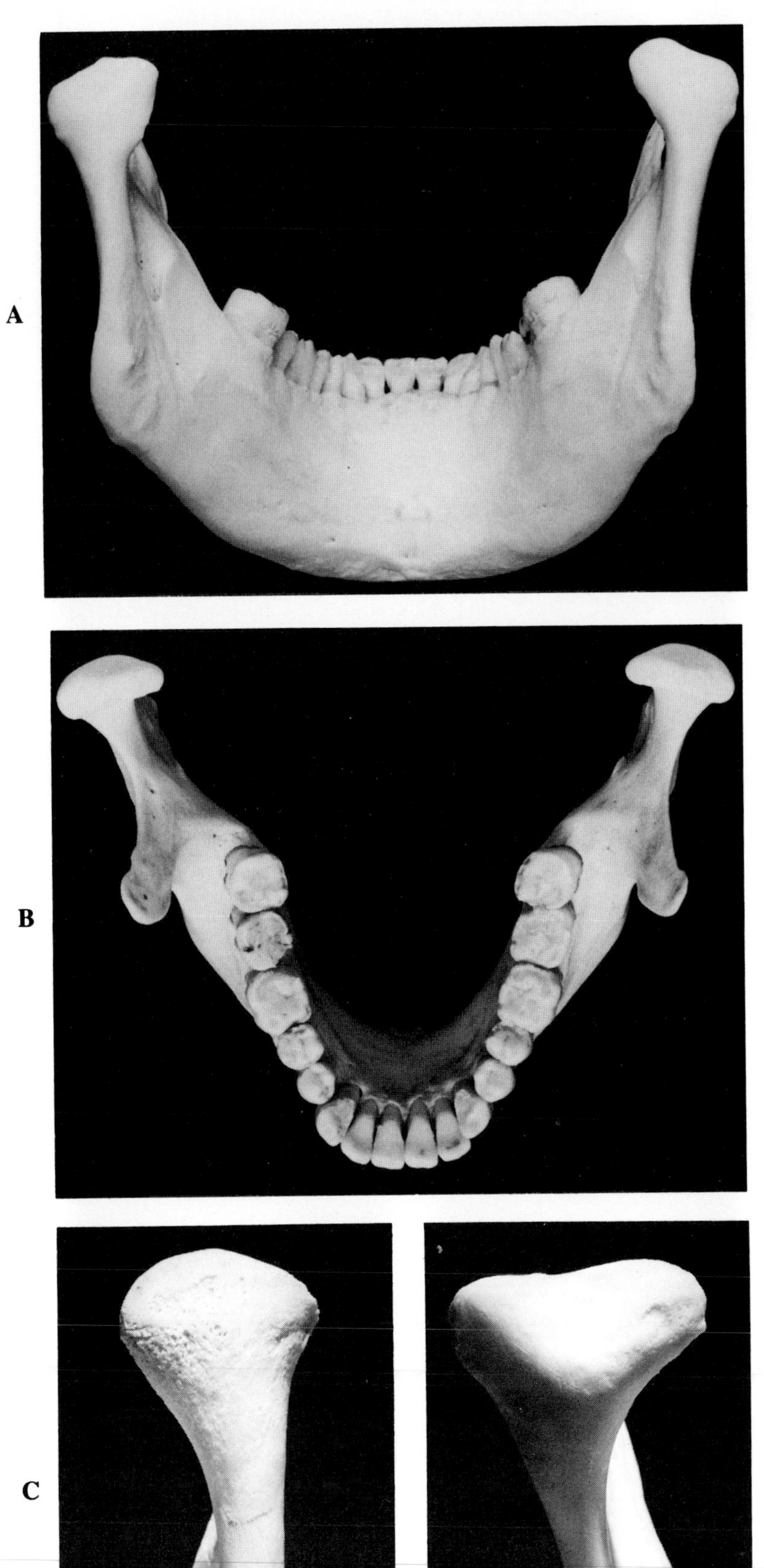
A
B
C
D

PLATE 1-4

The articulating surface of the temporal bone is anterior to the tympanic bone and comprises the concave articular fossa and convex articular eminence. A thin region of the squamous temporal bone forms the roof of the articular fossa and separates the TMJ from the middle cranial fossa. The articular surface of the fossa is largely oval and wider mediolaterally than anteroposteriorly, on the average 23 and 19 mm, respectively.

The anterior wall of the glenoid fossa is formed by the posterior slope of the articular eminence of the temporal bone. The articular eminence is strongly convex anteroposteriorly and somewhat concave mediolaterally. The medial and lateral borders of the articular eminence are sometimes accentuated by bone ridges. A prominent lateral bony ridge may obstruct access into the upper joint space. The anterior boundary of the articular eminence is indistinct, continuing into the infratemporal surface of the temporal bone. The foramen spinosum is located at the medial aspect of the articular eminence. Injury to the middle meningeal artery may be a source of major hemorrhage after articular eminectomy. The posterior wall of the glenoid fossa is formed by the tympanic plate of the temporal bone. The tympanic plate separates the TMJ from the bony part of the external auditory canal.

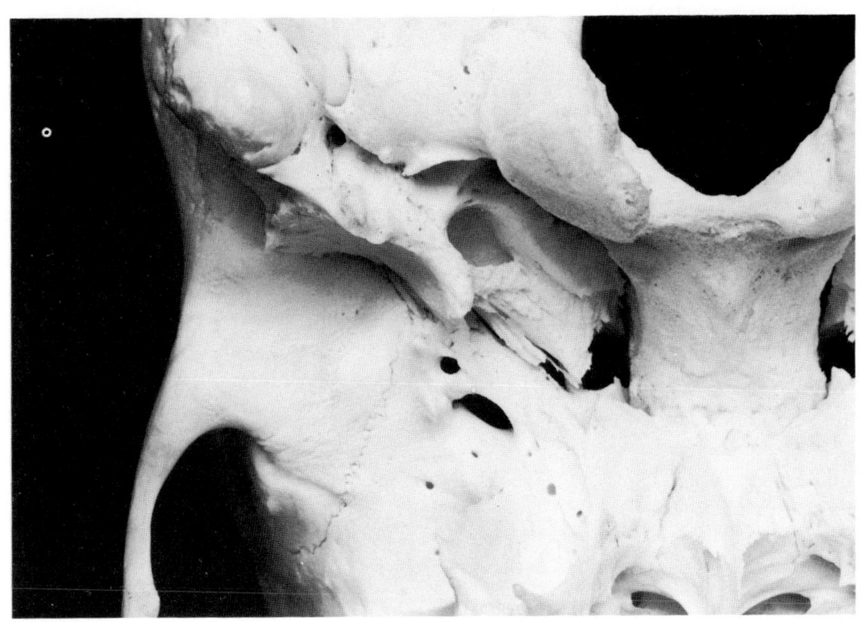

SOFT TISSUE ANATOMY

PLATE 1-5

A The TMJ is an encapsulated articulation. The capsule defines the anatomic and functional boundaries of the TMJ. The thin, loose fibrous capsule surrounds the articular surface of the condyle and blends with the periosteum of the mandibular neck.

On the temporal bone the articular capsule completely surrounds the articular surfaces of the eminence and fossa. Anteriorly the capsule is attached in front of the crest of the articular eminence, and laterally it adheres to the edge of the eminence and fossa. Posteriorly, it extends medially along the anterior lip of the squamotympanic and petrotympanic fissures. Its medial attachment runs along the spheno-squamosal suture.

The tympanic plate separates the TMJ from the bony part of the external auditory canal. The middle ear structures are located at the posteromedial aspect of the mandibular fossa.

A

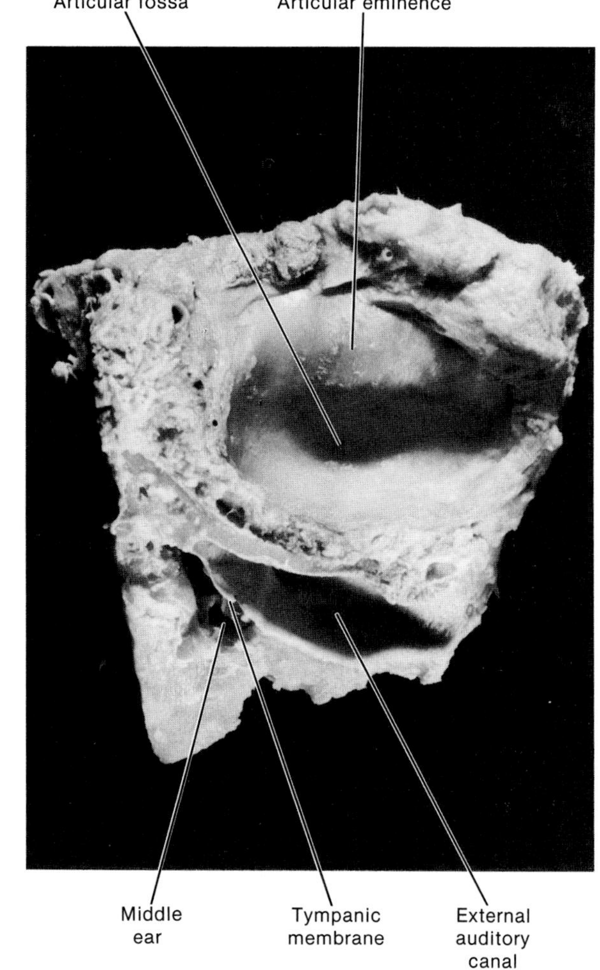

B and **C** The articular capsule is strongly reinforced laterally by the temporomandibular (lateral) ligament, which is composed of a superficial fan-shaped layer of obliquely oriented connective tissue fibers and a deeper, narrow band of fibers that run more horizontally. The ligament attaches broadly to the outer surface of the root of the zygomatic arch and coverges downward and backward to attach to the back of the condyle below and behind its lateral pole.

The principal biomechanical function of the temporomandibular ligament, acting singly or with its controlateral mate, is to "check" or limit movements of the condyle-disc complex. It is by far the most important ligament associated with the TMJ. A primary function of this ligament is to limit retrusion of the condyle against retrocondylar structures, for example, posterior disc attachment tissues. This ligament prevents the condyle disc complex from being displaced away from the articular eminence and limits the anterior movement of the condyle.

C courtesy P.A. Neff, Professor and Chairman, Department of Occlusion, Georgetown University, Washington, D.C.

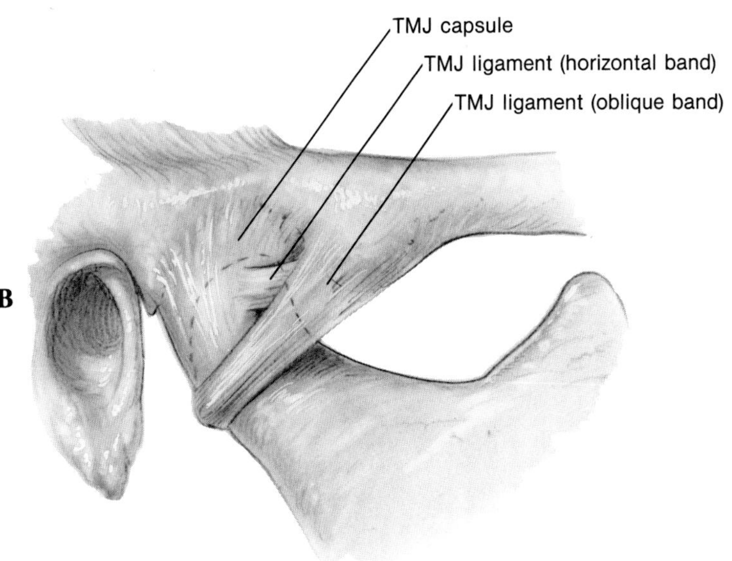

B

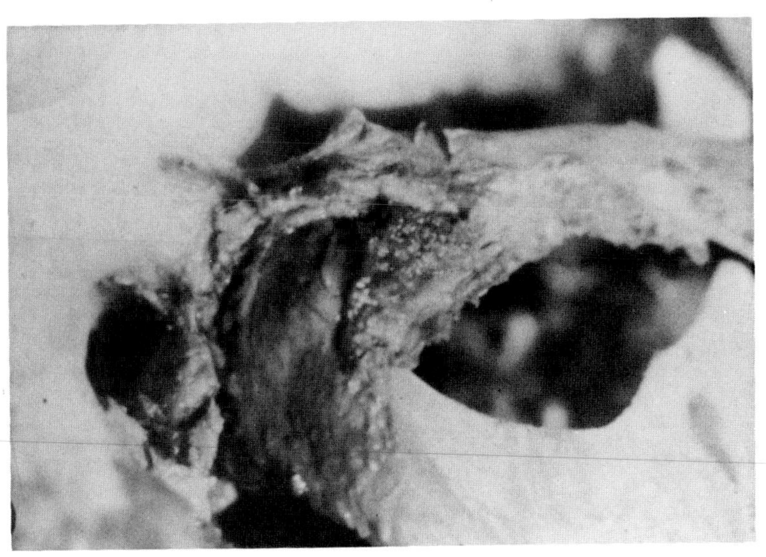

C

PLATE 1-6

A to **D** The articular disc is a firm but flexible structure with a specialized shape and function. Rees divided the disc into three regions: posterior band, intermediate zone, and anterior band. The central zone is considerably thinner (1 mm) than the posterior and anterior bands. The posterior band is generally thicker (3 mm) than the anterior band (2 mm). The upper surface of the disc adapts to the contours of the fossa and eminence of the temporal bone, and the lower surface of the disc adapts to the contour of the mandibular condyle.

Posteriorly the disc is contiguous with the loosely organized posterior attachment tissues (bilaminar zone, retrodiscal pad). The posterior attachment tissues are attached to the tympanic plate of the temporal bone posterosuperiorly and to the neck of the condyle posteroinferiorly.

Anteriorly the disc is contiguous with the capsule and the fascia of the superior head of the lateral pterygoid muscle. The superior head of the lateral pterygoid muscle may have some fibers inserting directly into the disc anteromedially.

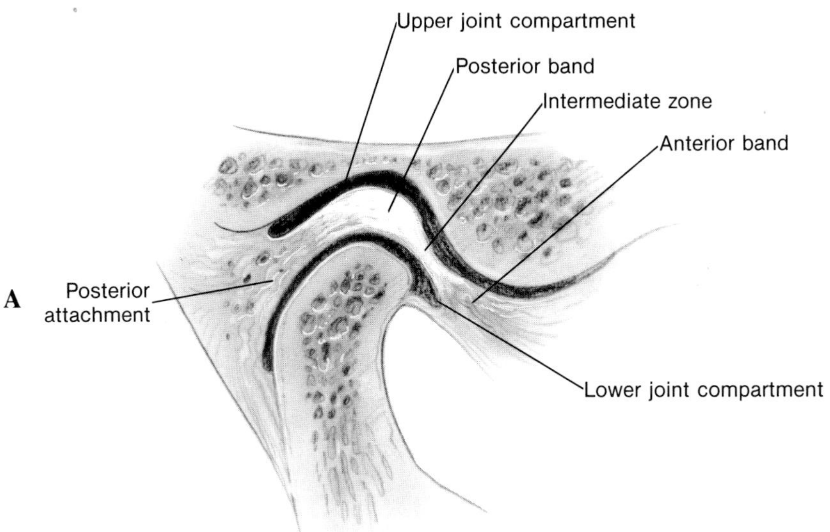

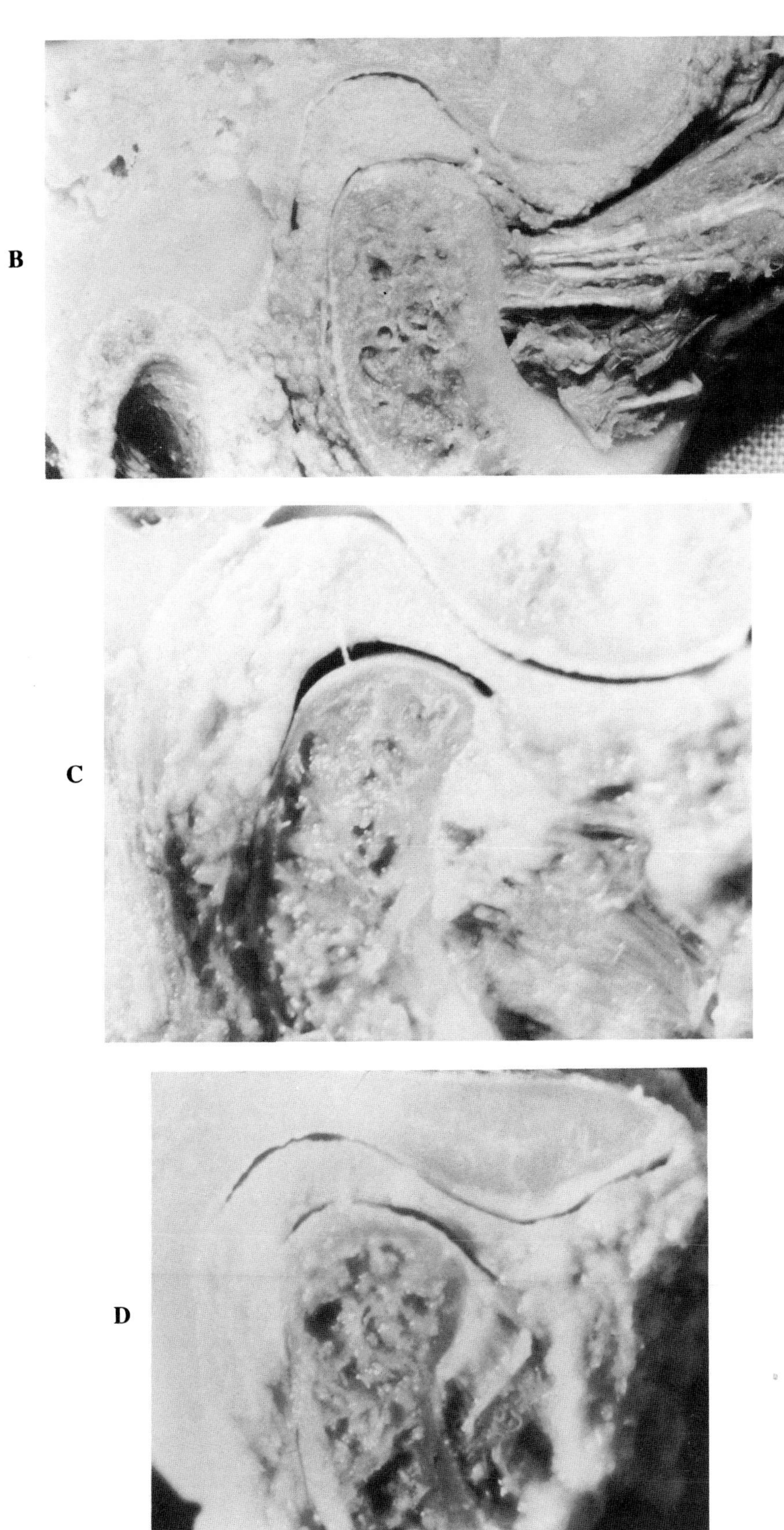
B
C
D

E and **F** The articular disc is firmly and independently attached to the condyle at its medial and lateral poles. It is not directly attached to the temporal bone. Thus the disc will move with the condyles as the latter translates in relation to the articular eminence.

E

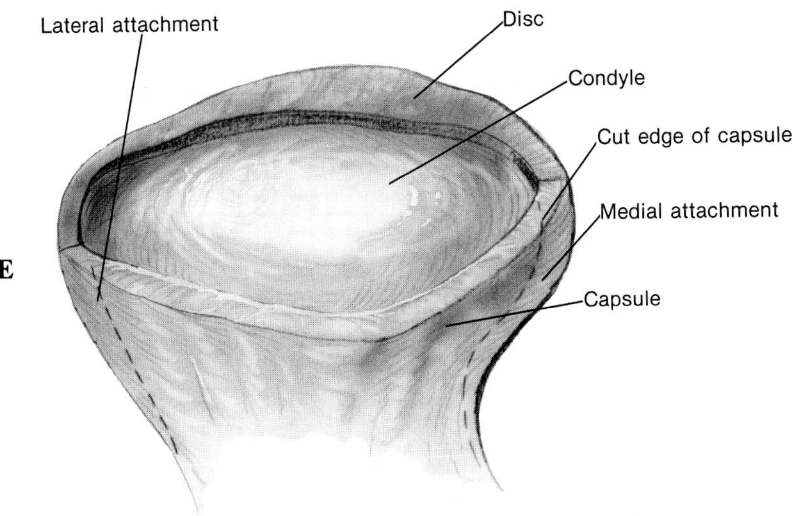

F

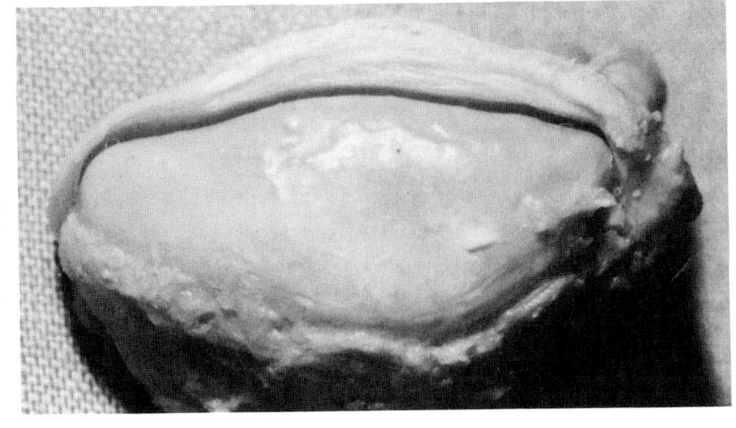

G Lateral view of the disc-condyle complex showing the parts of the disc in relation to the condyle. The articular disc and its posterior attachment tissues merge with the capsule around their periphery.

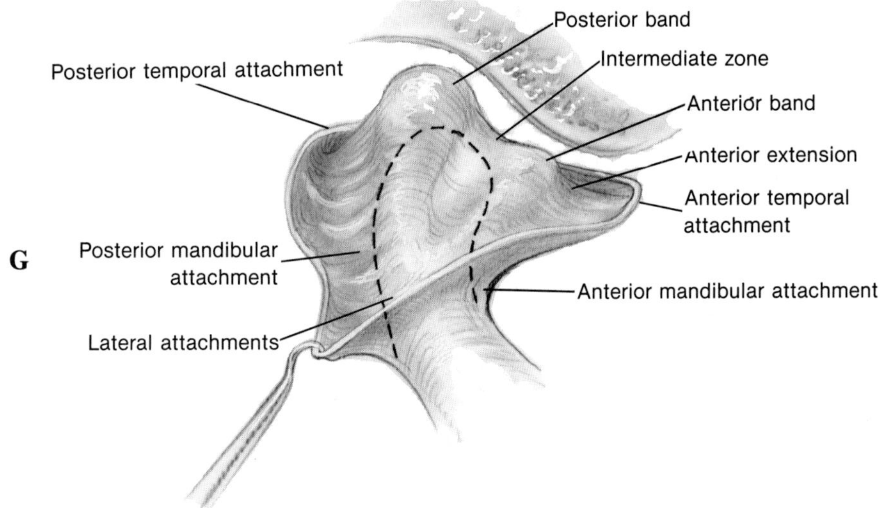

PLATE 1-7

Histologically the articular disc is composed of dense fibrous connective tissue. The fibers in the intermediate zone of the disc take a predominantly anteroposterior course and interlace with transversely oriented fibers in the thickened posterior and anterior bands. The articular disc is avascular and noninnervated, with possible exceptions around its periphery. The articular disc is designed to transmit the forces generated through the condyle to the articular eminence.

The posterior attachment tissues of the disc are described as having superior and inferior strata. The superior stratum consists of a loosely organized meshwork of elastic and collagen fibers, fat, and blood vessels. A substantial venous plexus is present. The inferior stratum consists of a fairly compact, inelastic sheet of collagen fibers that attach to the posterior surface of the condyle. The posterior attachment tissues are highly innervated by the auriculotemporal nerve. Histologic examination of this tissue reveals that it is not designed for loading.

The articular surfaces of the condyle and eminence are covered by dense fibrous connective tissue also. This connective tissue layer is thickest on the anterior and superior surfaces of the condyle and on the posterior slope and crest of the articular eminence.

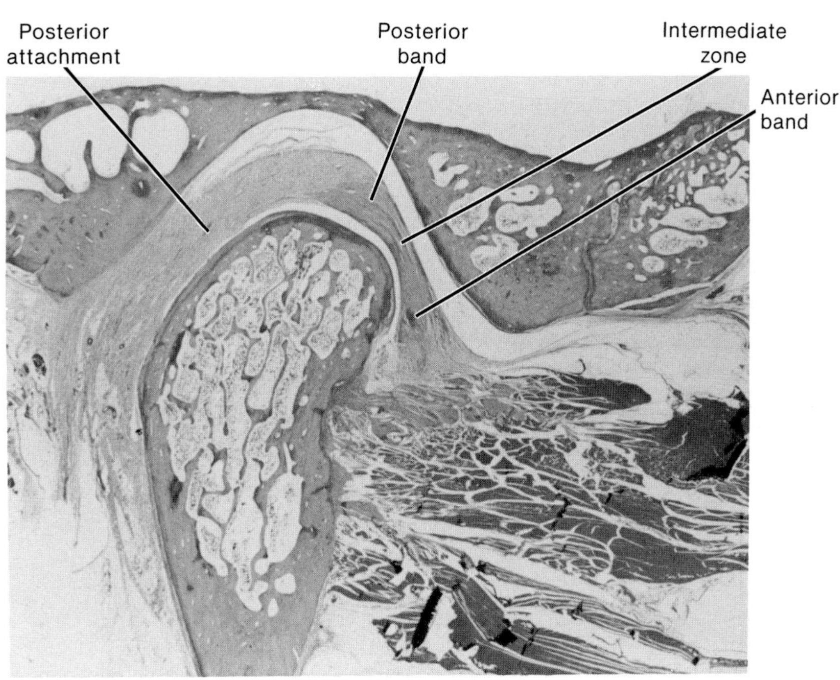
Posterior attachment
Posterior band
Intermediate zone
Anterior band

PLATE 1-8

A and **B** The disc and its attachments divide the joint space into separate superior and inferior spaces. In the sagittal plane the upper joint space is contiguous with the glenoid fossa and the articular eminence. It generally extends to the greatest curvature of the articular eminence. The upper joint space always extends farther anteriorly than the lower joint space. The lower joint is contiguous with the condyle and extends only slightly anterior to the condyle along the superior aspect of the superior head of the lateral pterygoid muscle.

A

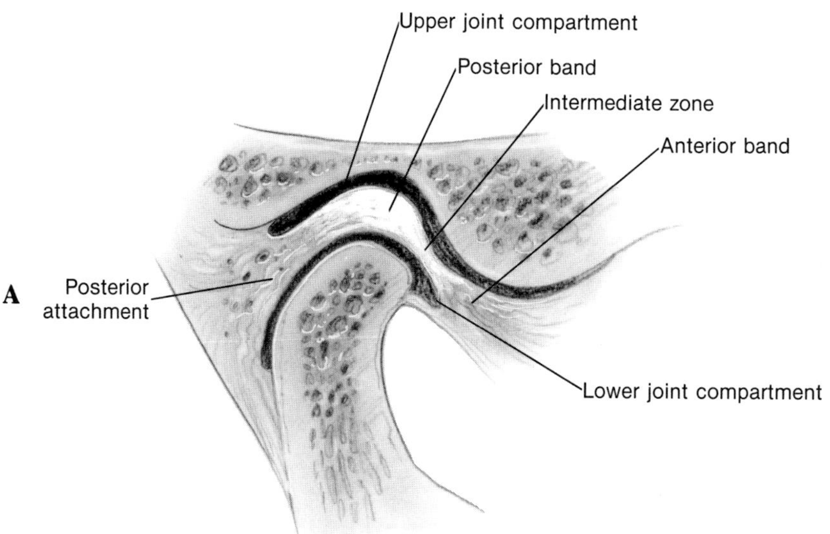

B

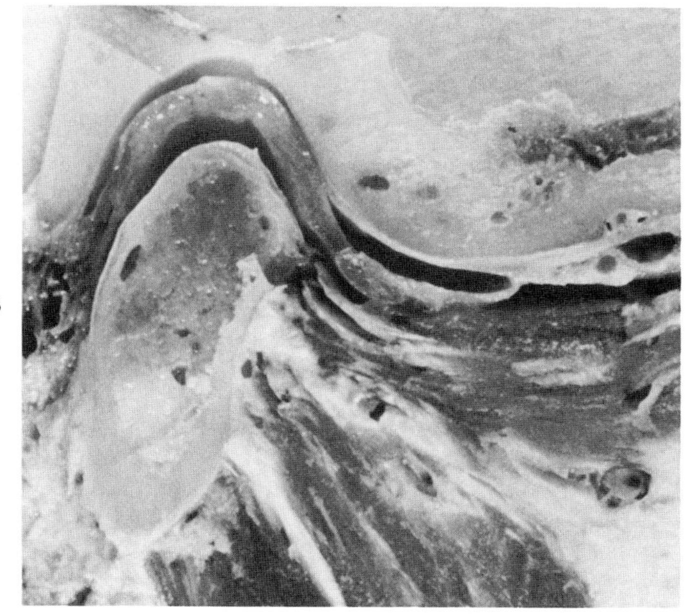

C and **D** In the frontal plane the upper joint space overlaps the lower joint space.

The lower joint space is smaller and more tightly reinforced by the disc attachments, whereas the upper joint space is larger and not as well reinforced. Both joint spaces have relatively small capacities. The volume of the upper joint space is about 1 ml, and the volume of the lower joint space is about 0.5 ml.

C

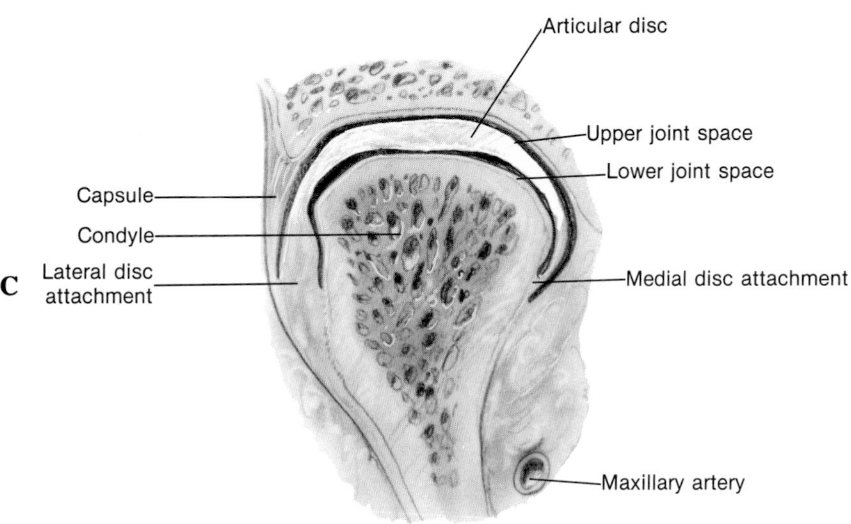

D

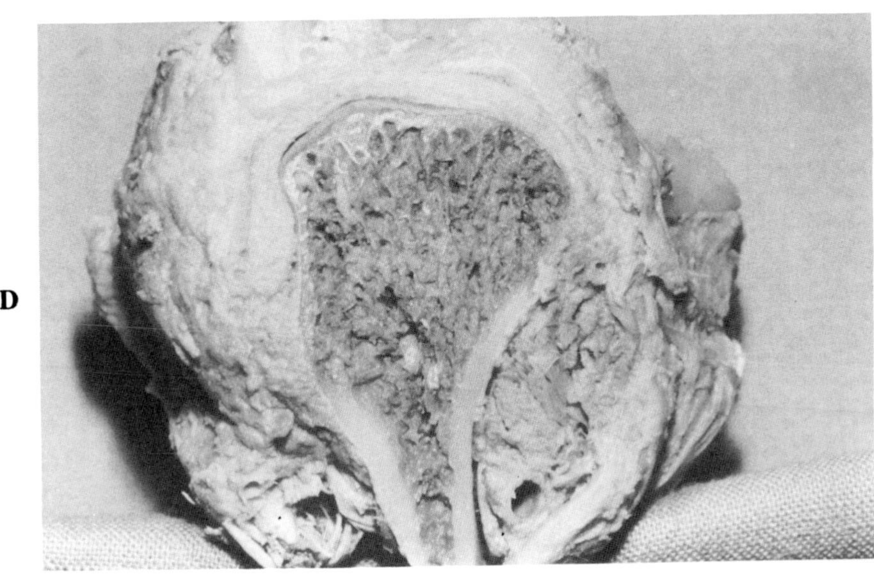

FUNCTIONAL ANATOMY

The TMJ is a combined hinge-glide articulation of the mandibular condyle with the mandibular fossa and articular eminence of the temporal bone. The muscles of mastication and the suprahyoid muscles act bilaterally to produce three types of movement: rotation, translation, and a combination of rotation and translation movement of the condyles. Rotation and some slight translation take place in the lower joint space between the condyle and the articular disc. Translation of the condyle-disc complex takes place in the upper joint space.

PLATE 1-9

A and **B** In the closed-mouth position the thick posterior band of the disc envelops the superior portion of the condyle. The intermediate zone and anterior band lie between the condyle and the posterior slope of the articular eminence.

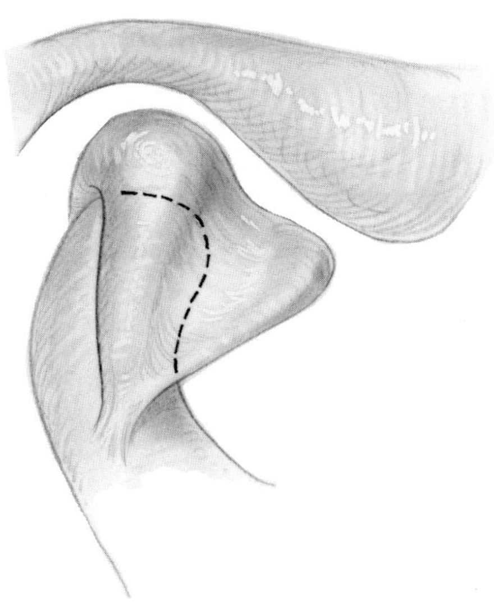

B

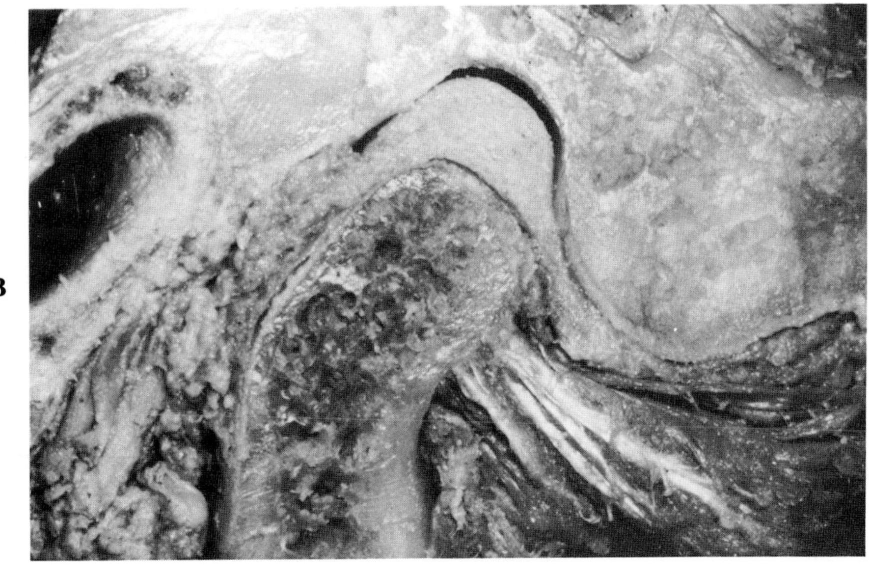

C and **D** During opening the posterior band assumes a more posterior relationship to the condyle as condylar rotation occurs. The intermediate zone becomes the articulating surface between the condyle and articular eminence. This condyle-disc relationship is maintained during most jaw movements.

C

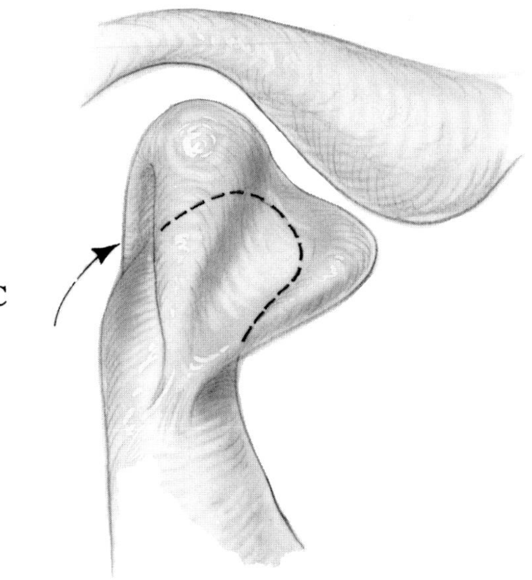

D

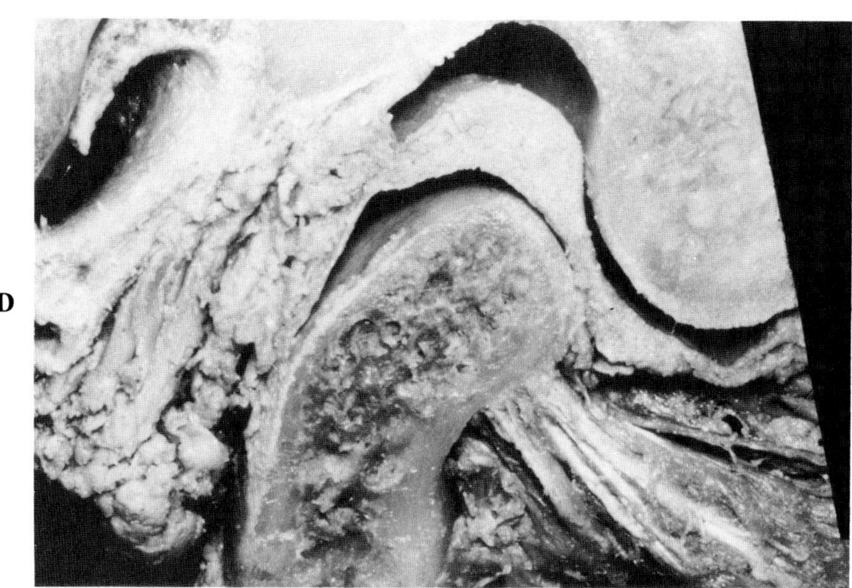

E and **F** During maximum opening of the mandible the condyle may rotate under the anterior band of the disc. The vascular posterior attachment tissues fill with blood to occupy the space created as the condyles move anteriorly from the mandibular fossa. During closure, or retrusion, of the mandible, the blood-filled posterior attachment tissues empty as the condyles return to the fossa.

E

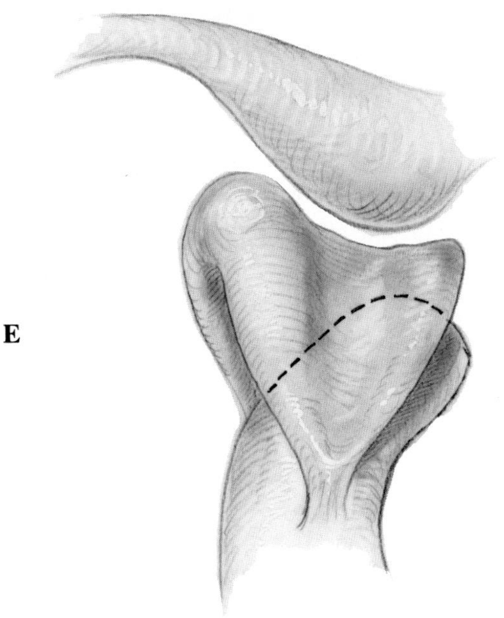

F

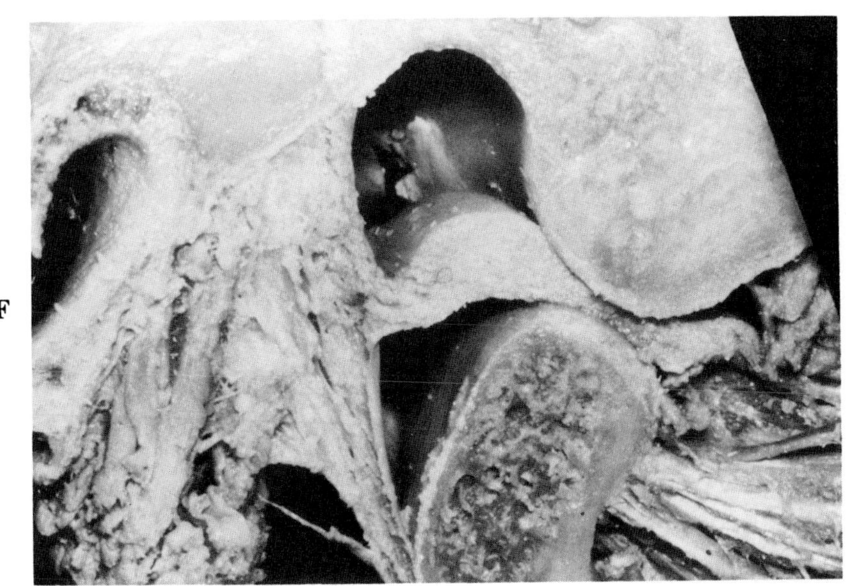

The mechanism(s) responsible for movement of the disc with the condyle has (have) not been determined. The superior head of the lateral pterygoid muscle has been shown to be inactive during the opening phase of the mandible. Additionally, the superior head of the lateral pterygoid has most of its insertion into the condyle and not into the disc. These evidences make the superior head of the lateral pterygoid an unlikely source responsible for movement of the disc.

Perhaps the forward movement is a result of shear force generated by the condylar head pressing on the thickened anterior band of the disc. Additional forces pulling the disc forward might result from the tight lateral and medial attachments of the disc to the condyle.

Retrusive movement of the disc during mandibular closure (retrusion) may be caused by the shear force generated on the posterior band of the disc and the forces pulling the disc backward as a result of its tight attachments to the condyle. Additionally, the elastic tissue recoil of the posterior attachment tissues may contribute to the posterior movement of the disc.

The principal functions of the disc are as follows:

1. Load distribution by adapting incongruous surfaces (condyle and eminence) to each other in the various functional positions of the mandible
2. Prevention of wear on the articular surfaces

chapter 2

Pathology

The term *internal derangements of the TMJ* alludes to any disturbance between the articulating components within the joint proper. In the last few years, however, it has been adapted mainly for changes in the disc-condyle relationship. The disc is most commonly displaced anteromedially. It often produces pain and/or functional disturbances in the masticatory system.

PREVALENCE

Little is known about the prevalence of disc displacement. Some authors (McCarty, 1979; Farrar and McCarty, 1979) maintain that it is extremely common, whereas others believe it is rare. In a recent autopsy study of young adults, Solberg et al. found disc displacement in 11.6% of the TMJs and noted it to be present more commonly in women. In another study of adult cadavers by Westesson and Rohlin (1984), disc displacement was found in 56% of the TMJs. Thus the prevalence of disc displacement appears to increase with age.

Buckley and Dolwick (1985) have reported a prevalence of 25% internal derangements and 15% internal derangement combined with a muscle disorder in the University of Texas Health Science Center at San Antonio TMJ clinic group of patients; and Clark (personal communication, 1983) reported a prevalence of 35% internal derangement patients in the UCLA TMJ clinic. Although neither patient group represents a random TMJ population, both do demonstrate that internal derangement is common in patient groups.

DEVELOPMENT

Convincing evidence exists demonstrating the reality of disc displacement. These evidences include clinical, anatomic, radiographic, and surgical findings. It has been shown that the TMJ disc is displaced anteromedially and that the displaced disc can mechanically interfere with jaw movement. Westesson and Rohlin (1984), studying adult cadaver TMJs, have shown a progression of internal derangements that includes not only changes in disc position but also in disc configuration. A progression from oblique disc position with biconcave disc or disc of even thickness to complete displacement with biconvex disc configuration was shown. The most advanced form of internal derangement showed perforation of the disc and/or its attachment tissues. The occurrence of osteoarthrosis was observed to increase with more advanced disc displacement and changes in disc configuration. Discs of even thickness were associated with osteoarthrosis in 50% compared to 90% for biconvex discs.

Plates 2-1 through 2-6 illustrate the progression of internal derangement.

PLATE 2-1

A and **B** This example of an early stage of internal derangement demonstrates the anterior position of the disc's posterior band. The disc overlies more of the lateral pterygoid muscle than normal, and the lower joint space is increased in length anteriorly. The disc is more uniform in thickness, which is reflected in a more uniform-appearing lower joint space. The upper joint space appears normal.

The posterior attachment tissues are very thin and appear to be compressed between the condyle and the tympanic plate of the temporal bone. The articular surfaces of the condyle and eminence appear normal.

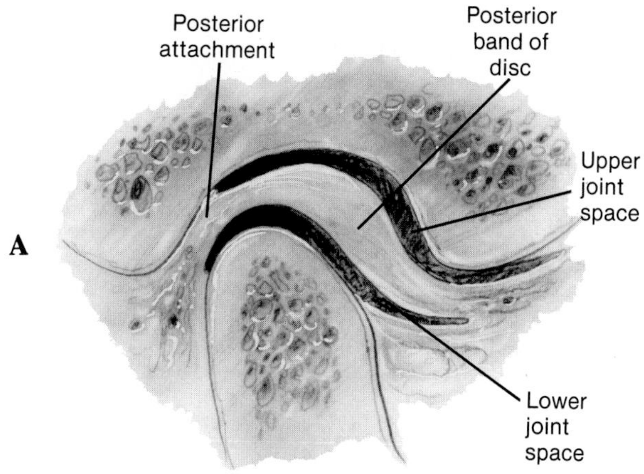

A

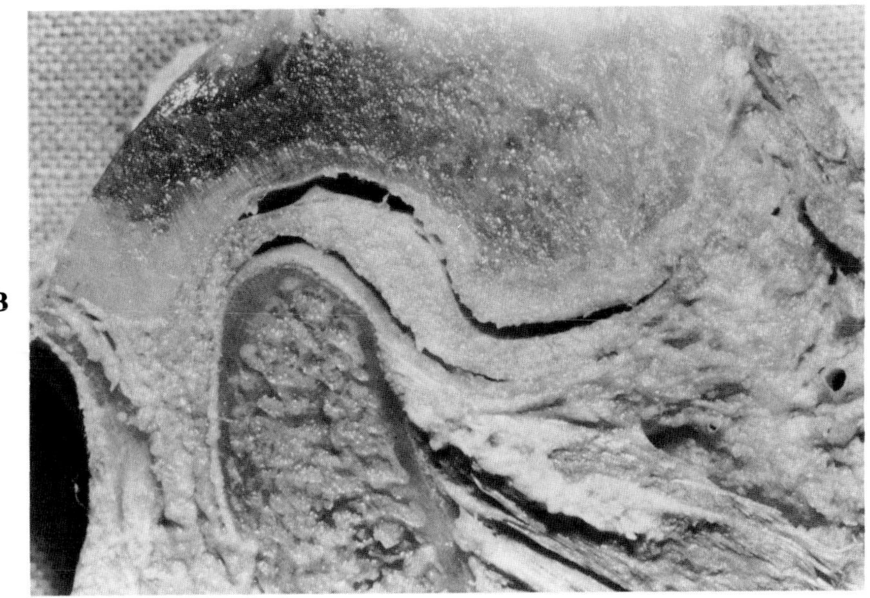

B

PLATE 2-2

A and **B** This specimen demonstrates classic disc displacement. The posterior band of the disc lies anterior to the condyle, the intermediate zone lies below the summit of the articular eminence, and the anterior band is adjacent to the anterior slope of the eminence. The disc overlies more of the lateral pterygoid muscle than normal. The upper joint space appears normal, and the length of the lower joint space is increased anteriorly. Note the concavity in the lower joint space produced by the posterior band. Also note the convexity produced by the intermediate area. These are important landmarks when interpreting TMJ arthrograms.

The condyle articulates against the vascular, innervated posterior attachment tissues that have been stretched over its articular surface. The tissue immediately behind the posterior band appears quite dense, in fact, of density similar to the disc. This probably represents adaptation of the posterior attachment tissues to the increased functional load placed on them.

At this level the articular surfaces of the condyle and eminence appear normal. Functionally one can imagine how this disc could interfere mechanically with condylar translation. As the condyle moves anteriorly it will strike the posterior band of the disc, which resists condylar movement.

B courtesy William K. Solberg and Tore L. Hansson, TMJ Laboratory, Dental Research Institute, University of California, Los Angeles.

A

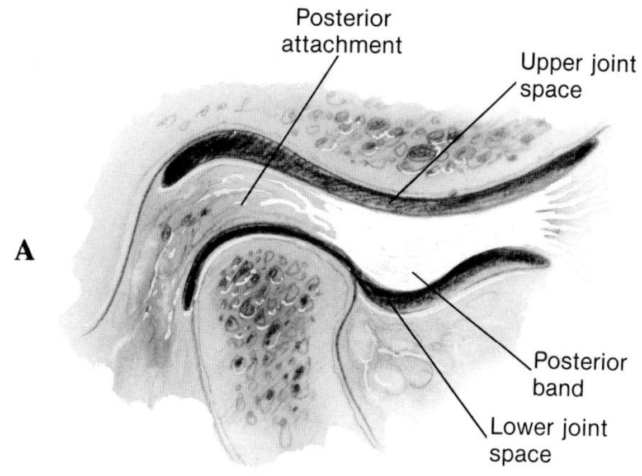
Posterior
attachment
Upper joint
space
Posterior
band
Lower joint
space

B

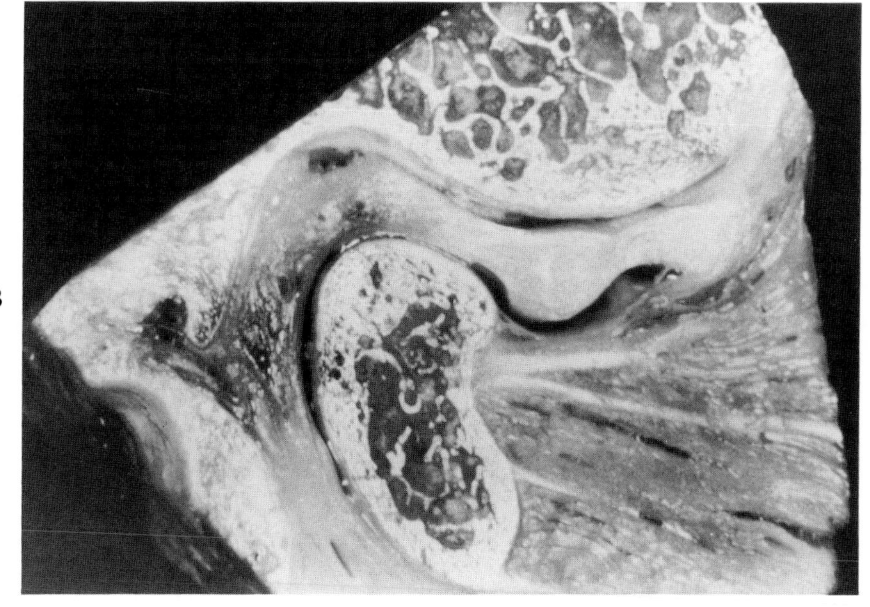

PLATE 2-3

A and **B** This specimen demonstrates significant anterior displacement and deformity of the articular disc. The posterior band of the disc is very thick and is positioned in front of the condyle. The intermediate area is deformed and very narrow. The anterior band is quite small.

The posterior attachment tissues just behind the posterior band of the disc appear very dense, in fact, similar in density to the disc tissues. This probably represents adaptation of those tissues to the increased load placed on them as a result of the disc displacement.

The articular surfaces of the condyle and eminence appear normal.

A

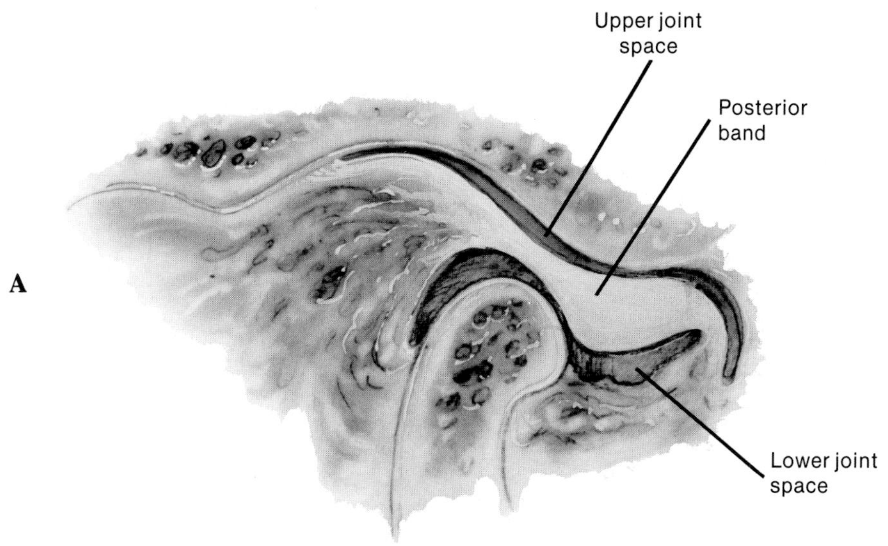

B

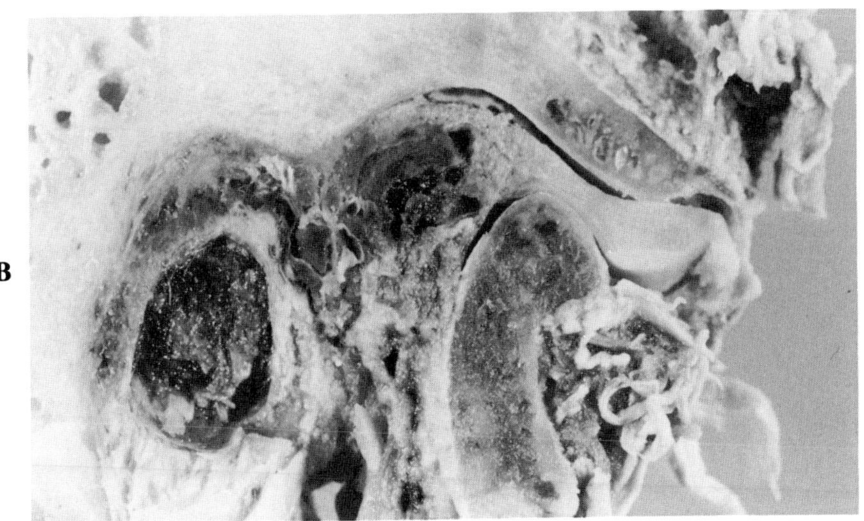

PLATE 2-4

A and **B** This specimen is similar to that in Plate 2-3, **A,** but shows a more advanced stage of internal derangement. The posterior band is quite thick and located in front of the condyle. The intermediate area is deformed and very narrow. The anterior band is indistinct. The lower joint space extends anteriorly and appears highly concave. The upper joint space appears normal.

The posterior attachment tissues appear very dense, again indicative of adaptation. The articular surface of the condyle has a deviation on its superior surface, however. The articular connective tissue appears intact, and there is considerable anterior lipping of the condyle. The articular surface of the eminence appears flattened, but the articular connective tissue is intact. Note the large air cell within the eminence. Extensions of the mastoid air cells are occasionally seen in the eminence. Obviously this can be a problem during eminectomy or eminence recontouring procedures.

A

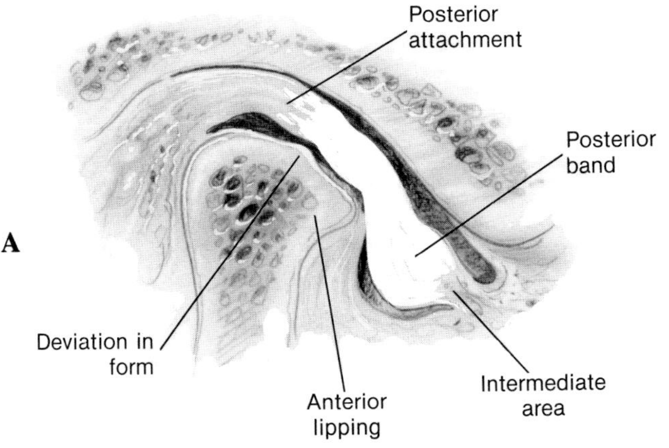

B

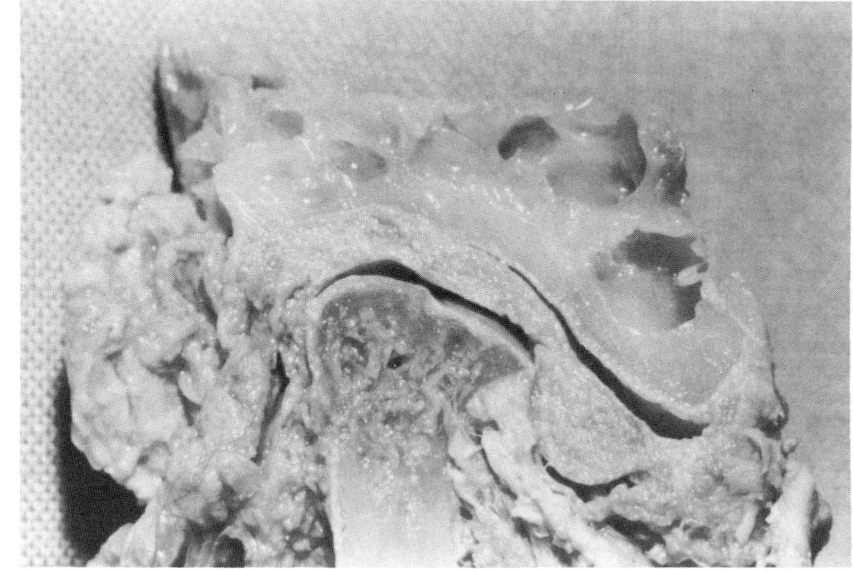

C and **D** The articular disc is anterior to the condyle. The posterior band is thick, and the disc is folded downward through the intermediate area. The posterior attachment tissue is very thin behind the posterior band of the disc and is almost perforated.

The lower joint space appears concave and extends anteriorly. The upper joint space is also abnormal, reflecting the downward flexure of the disc. The joint space between the condyle and posterior slope of the eminence is quite narrow.

The articular surfaces are normal on gross examination, although the subarticular bone does appear dense and sclerotic.

C

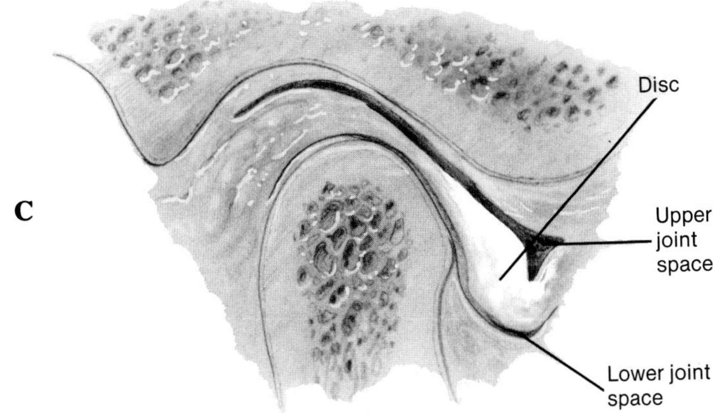

D

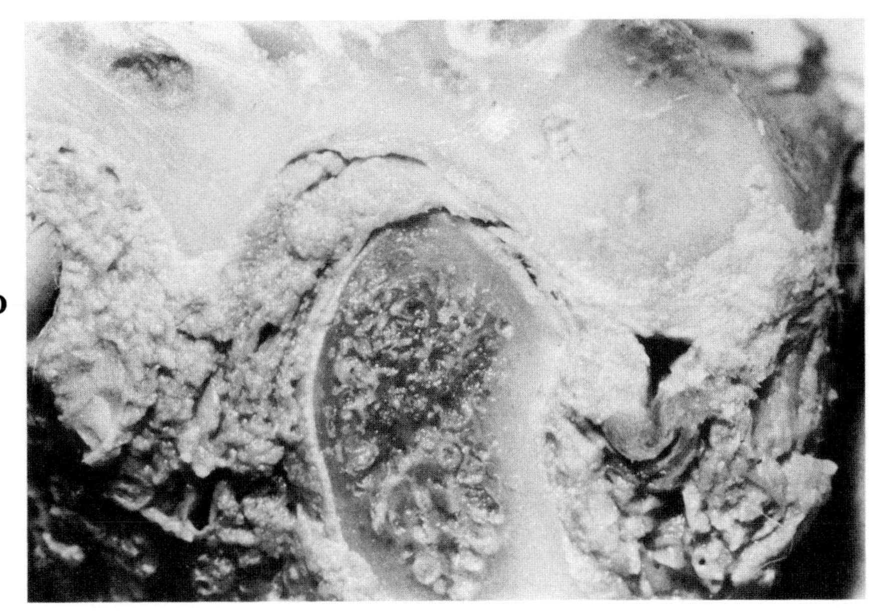

PLATE 2-5

A and **B** In the most advanced stages the disc and/or attachment tissue perforates. In this specimen the posterior attachment tissue is very thin immediately behind the disc and is perforated laterally behind the disc. Most perforations occur in the lateral aspect of the disc and/or its attachments. The disc is markedly deformed and almost biconvex. Only a slight crease remains as evidence of the intermediate area.

A

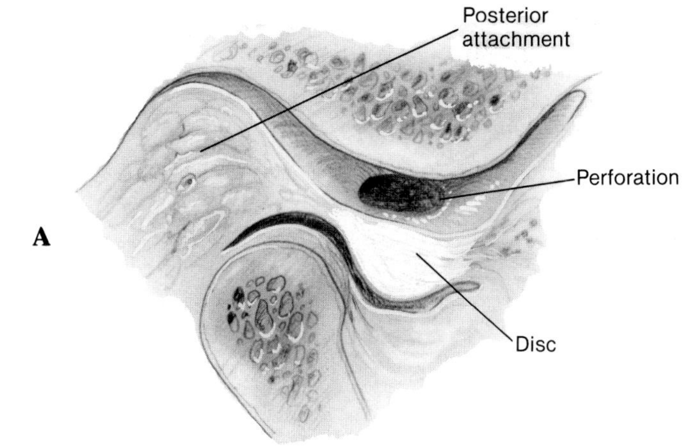

B

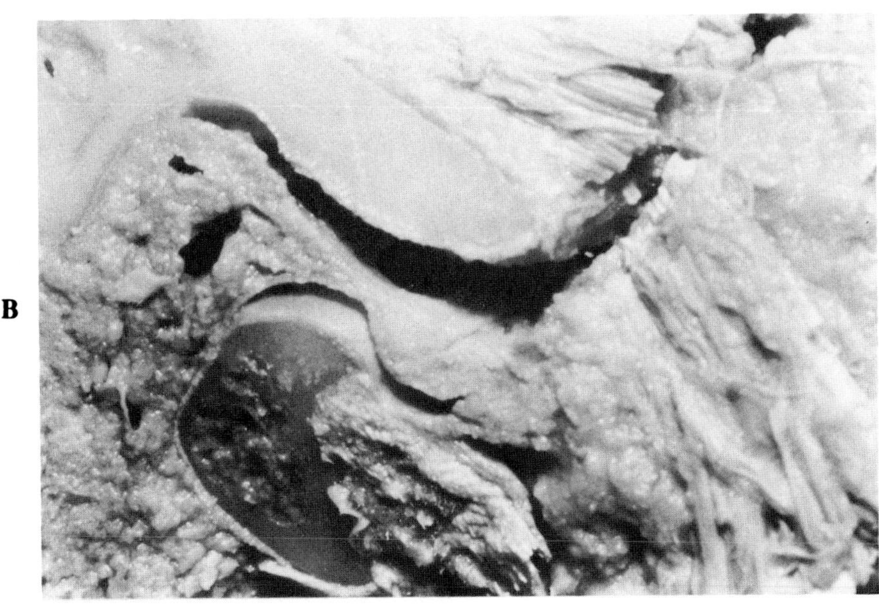

C and **D** This specimen demonstrates complete perforation and detachment of the disc. The disc is biconvex and located in front of the condyle.

The articular surface of the condyle is smooth but does have considerable anterior lapping. The articular surface of the eminence is flattened, and the articular connective tissue is disrupted. The joint space between the condyle and eminence is very narrow. This joint illustrates advanced osteoarthrosis of the eminence and beginning osteoarthrosis of the condyle. Generally significant osteoarthrosis is present with perforations. Perforated joints are usually crepitant during movement.

E Advanced internal derangement and osteoarthrosis are demonstrated by this specimen. This disc is located anteriorly and is biconvex in shape. The posterior attachment tissue is perforated behind the disc.

The condyle and articular eminence show severe alterations with disruption of the articular connective tissue. The joint space is very narrow between the condyle and eminence. This joint would undoubtedly have had crepitus during function.

E courtesy C.A. Helms, University of California, San Francisco.

Because the TMJ is most commonly viewed sagittally, disc displacement can be thought to exist only anteriorly. The disc displacement is, however, generally anteromedial, with the greatest amount occurring along the lateral aspect of the joint.

C

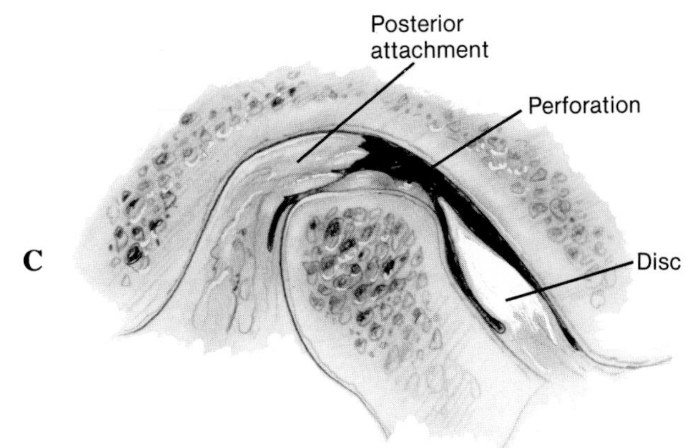

D

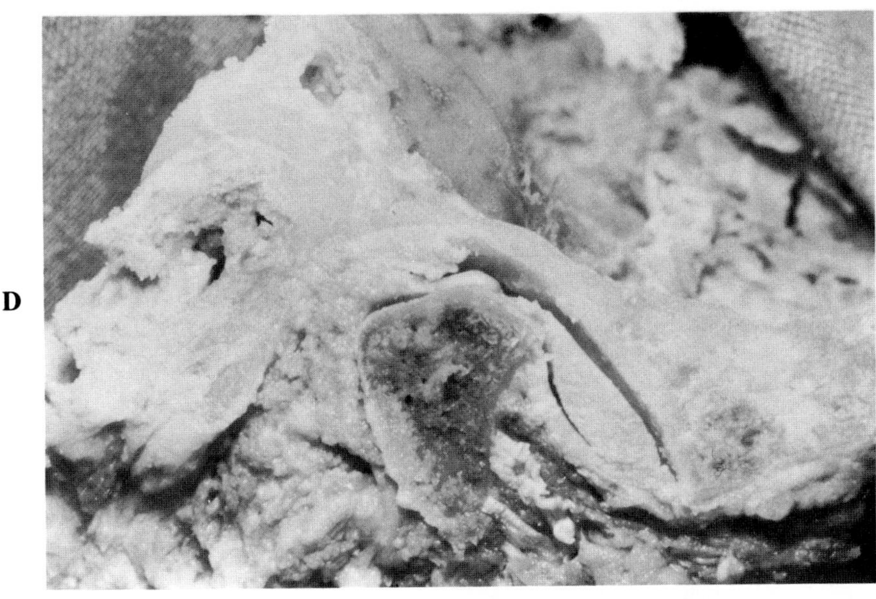

E

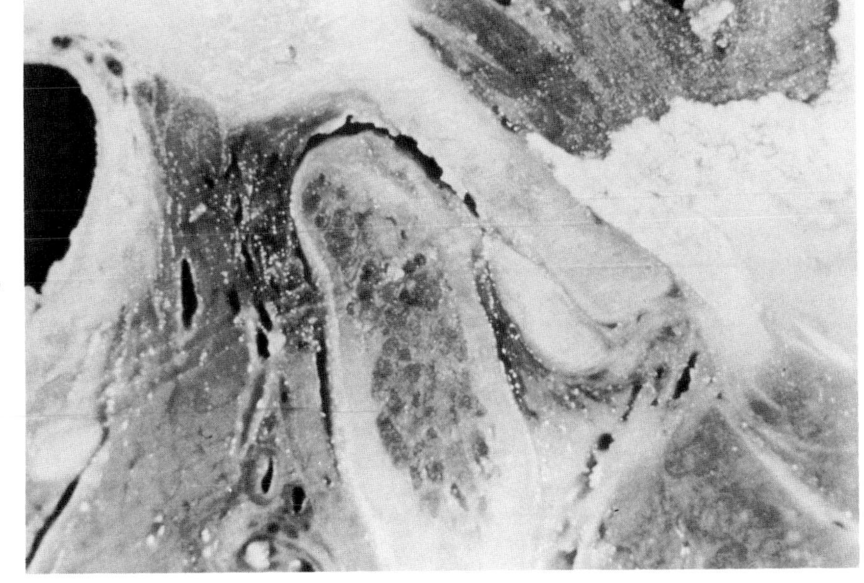

PLATE 2-6

A This frontal view of the condyle-disc complex demonstrates the disc's anteromedial displacement. From the anterior aspect one can see a perforation along the lateral disc attachment, with the disc positioned anteromedially. Dividing the disc mediolaterally demonstrates more clearly its medial position.

B This specimen shows anteromedial disc displacement with a perforation of the lateral disc attachment. Note the thick ridge along the medial aspect of the condyle-disc complex. This thick disc ridge is associated with a prominent deviation of the medial aspect of the articular eminence.

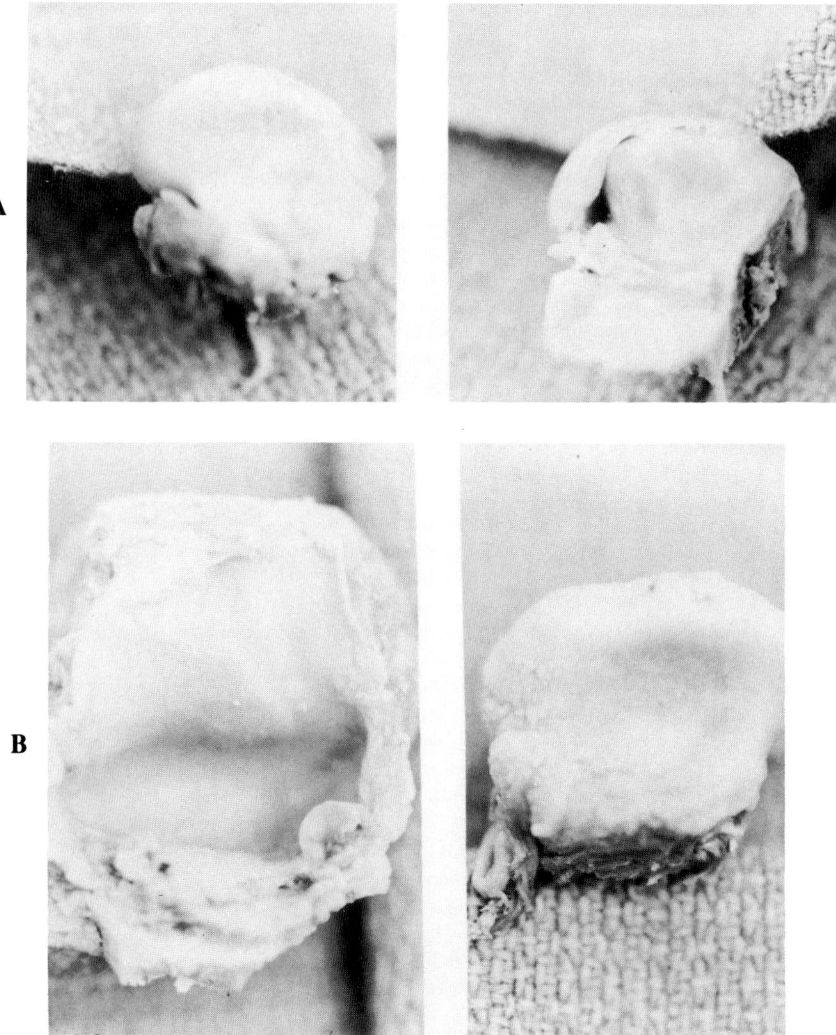

PATHOPHYSIOLOGY

The exact pathophysiology of internal derangements has not been elucidated. The following sequence of pathologic progression, however, has been proposed based on the available clinical, surgical, and anatomic evidence.

The initial pathologic condition develops in the lateral disc attachment to the condyle and causes a loose condyle-disc relationship so that this complex does not function harmoniously. The lateral aspect of the disc rotates anteromedially, resulting in oblique or partial disc displacement. As the lateral and posterior attachment tissues become further stretched, the disc is further displaced anteriorly until it is completely in front of the condyle from lateral to medial position—complete disc displacement. In the final stages the attachment tissues become thinned and may perforate.

Simultaneously with disc displacement, changes are occurring in the morphology and histology of the disc, attachment tissues, and articular surfaces of the condyle and eminence. The disc changes from a biconcave to a biconvex configuration and from dense connective tissue to fibrocartilage. In some severe cases there may be calcifications within the disc.

The posterior or lateral attachment tissues become denser and thinner, eventually perforating. As these and attachment tissue changes are occurring, progressive and regressive remodeling changes take place in the condyle and articular eminence. If the regressive remodeling becomes severe, breakdown of the articular surfaces occurs and results in osteoarthrosis. This generally occurs after perforation of the disc and/or attachment tissues.

Plate 2-7 demonstrates the clinical progression of internal derangement. Only the upper joint space has been opened by reflecting the capsule laterally; the disc and its attachments have not been disturbed.

PLATE 2-7

A The initial pathologic change occurs in the lateral disc attachment to the condyle. The lateral attachment tissue is very *red,* indicative of increased vascularity. The lateral aspect of the disc is slightly displaced anteromedially. This patient had painful reciprocal clicking, with the opening click occurring at 10 mm.

B This case demonstrates partial (oblique) disc displacement. The lateral aspect of the disc is displaced anteromedially, and the posterior attachment tissue is stretched across the condyle on its lateral aspect. This patient had painful reciprocal clicking, with the opening click occurring at 20 mm.

C As the process progresses, the disc may become completely displaced, as shown here. The posterior attachment tissue is stretched completely across the condyle. This patient had painful reciprocal clicking, with the opening click occurring at 35 mm. The patient also had intermittent locking.

D This case is similar to the previous case (**C**) except the disc is displaced further anteriorly. The patient had painful closed-lock but was occasionally able to reduce the disc by manipulating her mandible.

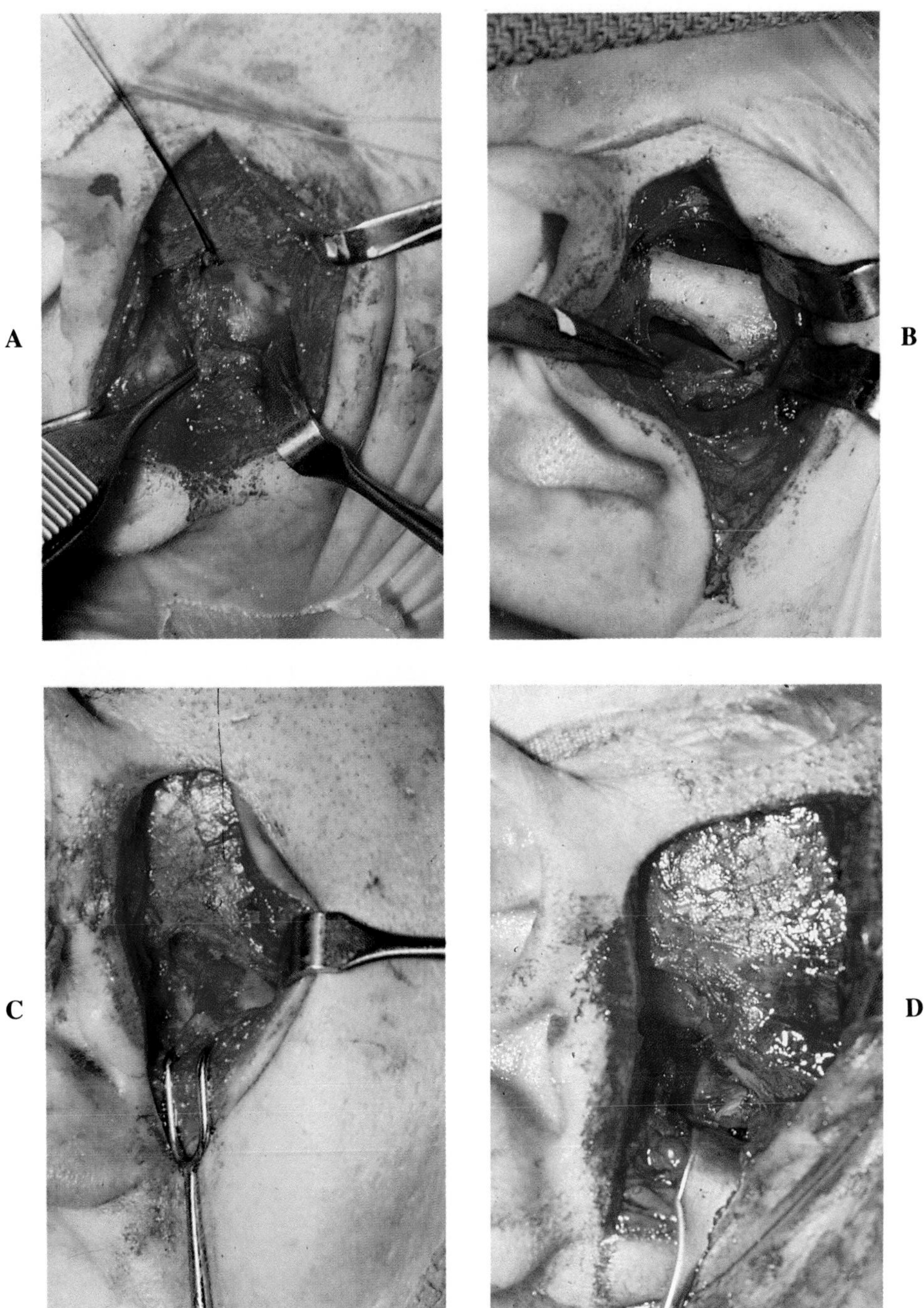
A
B
C
D

E The disc is completely displaced anteriorly under the articular eminence. The condyle articulates only with soft, vascular, innervated posterior attachment tissue. The patient had had a painful closed-lock for about 3 months with a previous history of clicking and intermittent locking.

F A large perforation exists at the junction of the posterior attachment tissue and the articular disc. Although not obvious in this picture, the articular surfaces of the condyle and eminence were devoid of the connective tissue surface adjacent to the perforation. The patient had painful crepitus.

G A large perforation involving most of the disc and its attachment tissues is shown here. The articular surfaces of the condyle demonstrated severe osteoarthrosis. The patient had painful crepitus.

E

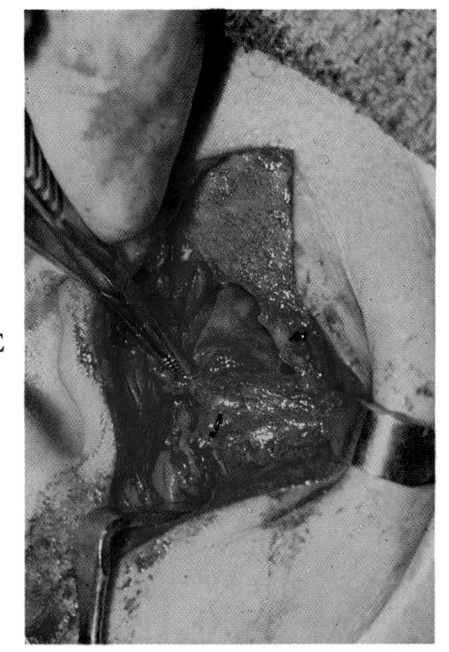

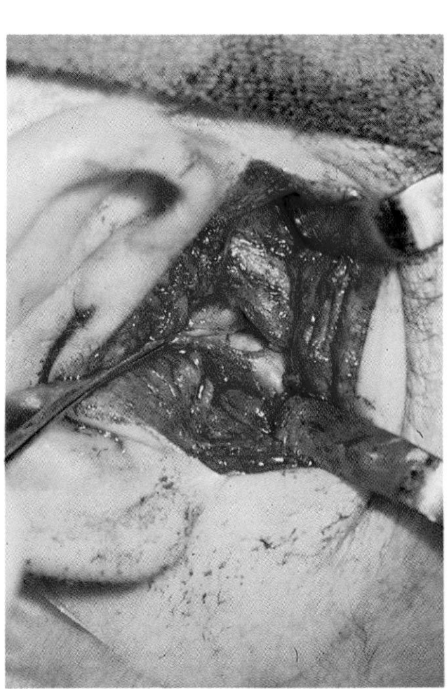

F

G

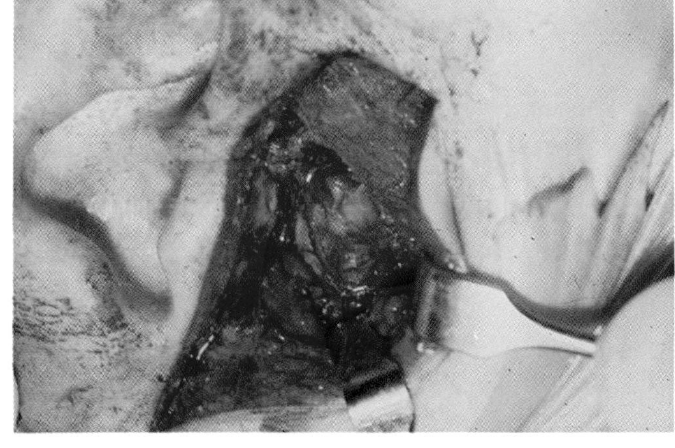

PLATE 2-8

A This case demonstrates changes in disc morphology associated with internal derangement. The posterior band is very thick, and the intermediate zone is very deformed and narrow. This disc must be reshaped to a more normal contour if it is not removed.

B The posterior band of this disc is very thick, causing a prominent ridge the condyle would hit during translation. The tissue immediately behind the posterior band appears very dense, probably reflecting adaptation of the posterior attachment tissue. This disc must also be reshaped if it is not removed.

A

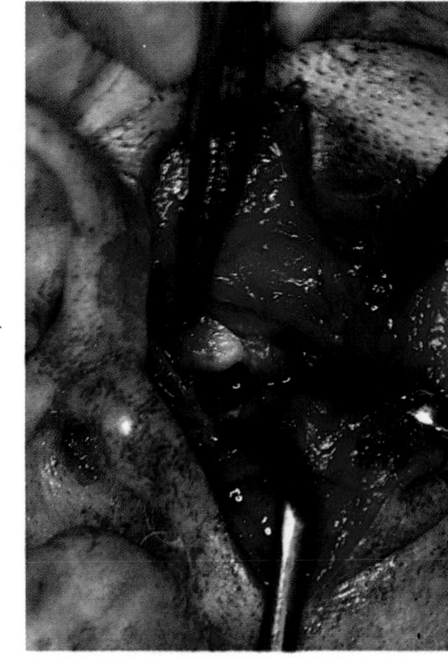

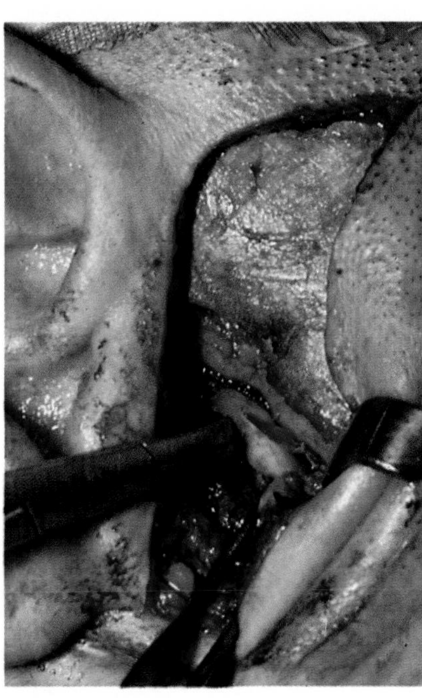

B

PLATE 2-9

A The removed disc, inferior surface, demonstrates a thick posterior band, a narrow central articulating zone, and thin anterior band. This disc had undergone fibrosis anteriorly and could not be repositioned. Its severe alteration also precluded its use.

B Removed disc, inferior surface, demonstrating a thick biconvex configuration. The disc had undergone fibrosis anteriorly and could not be repositioned.

C This removed disc demonstrates a large perforation involving both disc and posterior attachment tissue. It could not be repaired because of its size and also because the remaining disc tissue had undergone fibrosis anteriorly.

D Because of the large perforation involving the posterior and lateral disc attachments as well as the posterior band and intermediate zones of this disc, repair was impossible.

A courtesy Doran E. Ryan, D.D.S., M.S., Medical College of Wisconsin, Milwaukee, Wisconsin.

A

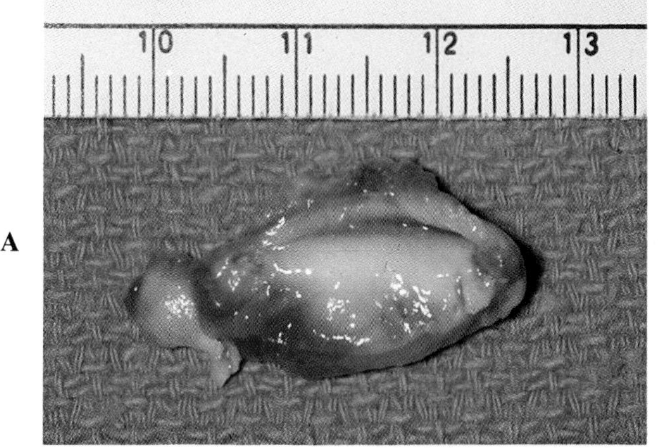

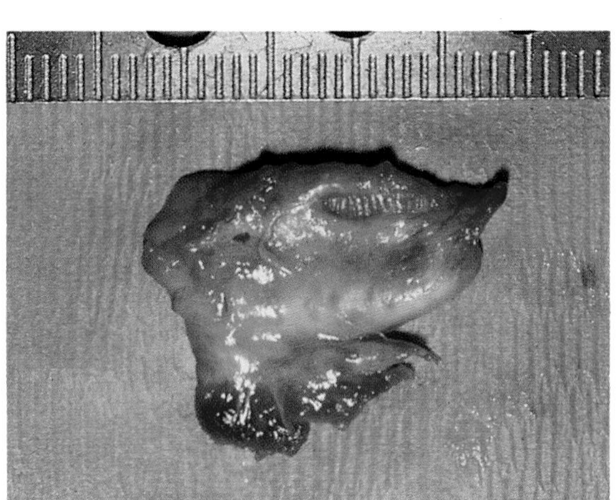

B

C

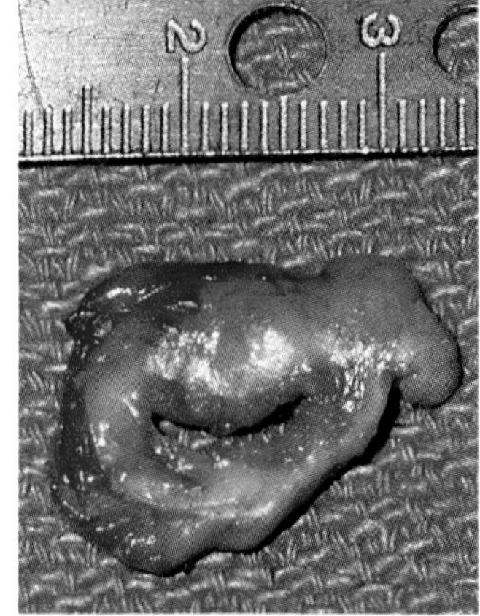

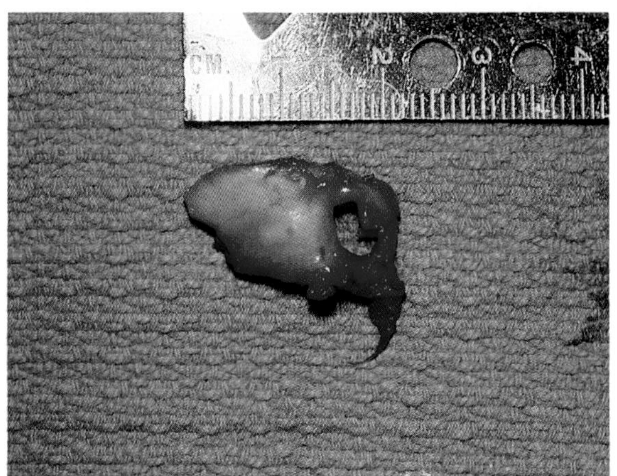

D

Abnormal Function—Disc Displacement with Reduction

The initial mandibular dysfunction is characterized by reciprocal clicking of the TMJ, which refers to an open click followed by a closing click.

PLATE 2-10

A In the closed-mouth position the thick posterior band is located anterior to the condyle.

B As the condyle translates forward it pushes against the posterior band of the disc instead of rotating under the intermediate zone. The disc is pushed anterior to the condyle and functions as a mechanical obstruction to movement. When sufficient tension develops in the attachment tissues to overcome the force of the condyle pushing the disc forward, the opening click occurs and the disc reduces to a normal relationship with the condyle. The noise occurs as the condyle strikes the articular eminence. The closing occurs as the disc becomes anteriorly displaced during closure.

C The disc is in a normal relationship to the condyle after the opening click.

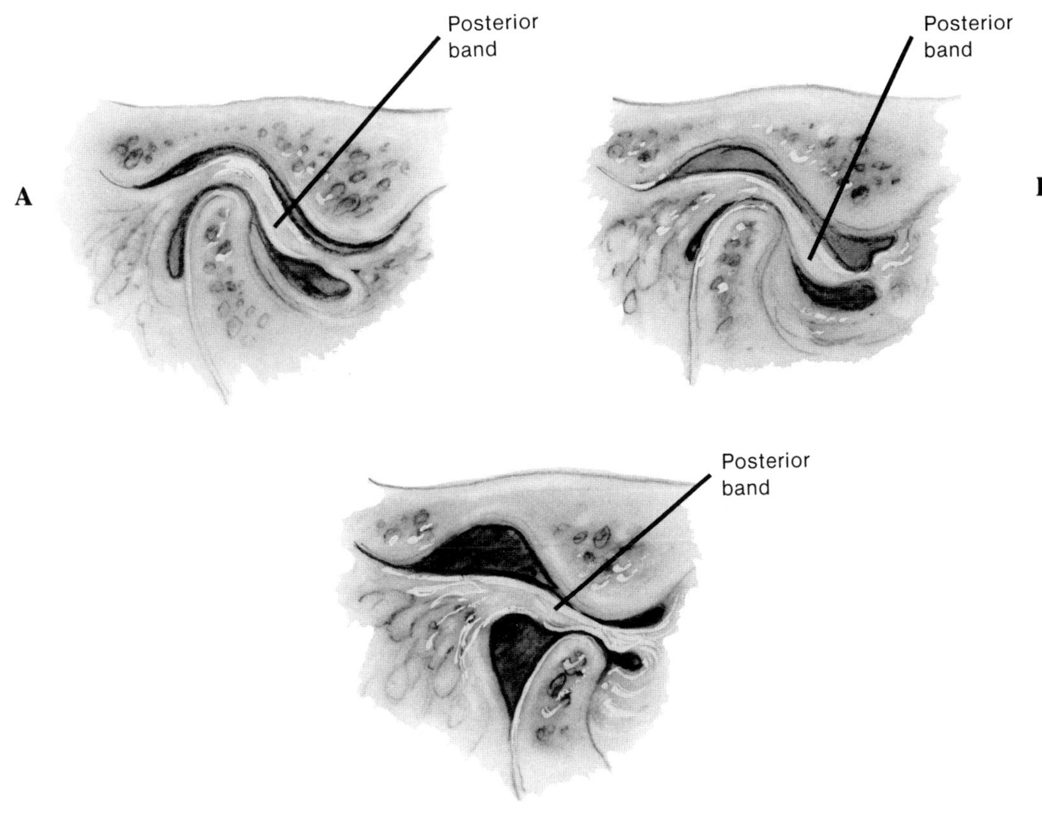

Abnormal Function—Disc Displacement without Reduction (Closed-lock)

Disc displacement without reduction (closed-lock) is a more advanced form of internal derangement than disc displacement with reduction. There is usually no joint noise, but the condition is almost always preceded by a period of reciprocal clicking.

PLATE 2-11

A In the closed-mouth position the thick posterior band is located anterior to the condyle.

B During opening, the condyle pushes against the posterior band of the disc. The disc mechanically obstructs movement and does not return to a normal relationship with the condyle at any jaw position.

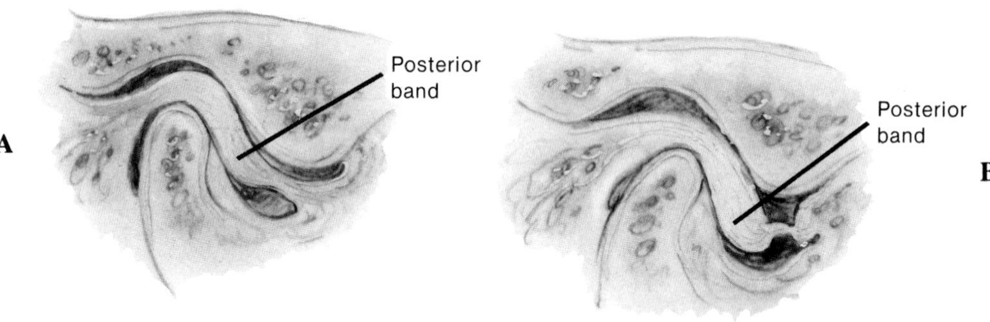

Abnormal Function—Disc Displacement with Perforation

The most advanced form of internal derangement is disc displacement with perforation. It is manifested by crepitus and osteoarthrosis and is usually preceded by periods of reciprocal clicking and closed-lock. The crepitus is caused by the rough articular surfaces functioning against each other.

PLATE 2-12

Disc displacement with perforation can be seen here.

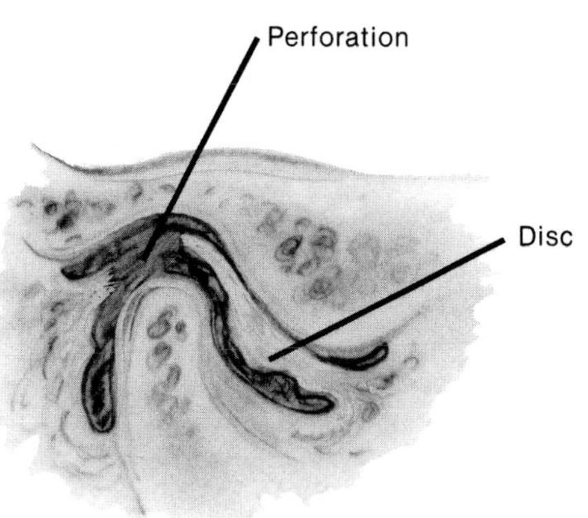

ETIOLOGY

The causes of internal derangement have as yet been only speculated. Acute anterior disc displacement may be caused by macrotrauma to the mandible (through accident, extraction of teeth, intubation, etc.). Chronic disc displacement may be caused by microtrauma, such as that resulting from loss of posterior teeth, or occlusal contacts, resulting in posterior displacement of the mandibular condyle. Muscle hyperactivity disorders (for example, bruxism) have also been proposed as etiologic factors. It would seem that the combination of a muscle hyperactivity disorder with distal deflective occlusal contacts may be especially damaging to the joint structures.

chapter 3

Diagnosis

Diagnosis is defined as the art of distinguishing one disease from another. An accurate diagnosis is of prime importance if appropriate treatment modalities are to be used with a high degree of success. It will be shown later that failure to make an accurate diagnosis is one of the most common causes of poor surgical results. The major diagnostic challenge is to distinguish those patients whose signs and symptoms are caused by TMJ internal derangement from those whose disturbances are caused by muscular disorders, that is, myofascial pain and dysfunction syndrome, muscle hyperactivity, or bruxism. Furthermore, it must be recognized that internal derangements and muscular disorders frequently occur together.

Diagnosis of TMJ internal derangement is made by a thorough evaluation of the masticatory system. This evaluation should include the following parts:

1. History
2. Physical examination
3. Routine radiographs
4. Special diagnostic procedures

HISTORY

PLATE 3-1

The history may very well be the most important part of the patient evaluation. It has been said, *"Listen to the patient, doctor; she is telling you the diagnosis."* The purpose of the history is to furnish clues for diagnosis. During the interview it is important to assess the patient's reliability as a historian. Are symptoms or significance exaggerated? If so, the patient will tend to exaggerate treatment effects. Is the problem accurately described in well-defined terms or is the patient vague as to where and what the problem is? Patients who clearly describe their problem do better than patients who are vague.

The history begins with the *chief complaint(s).* This should be a statement of the patient's reason(s) for seeking consultation and/or treatment. The patient with an internal derangement will generally have a chief complaint related to pain and dysfunction of the masticatory system. The chief complaint often serves as an important clue with which to begin making a diagnosis. It also serves as a reminder for the physician as to why the patient sought care.

The *history of the present illness* should be comprehensive, including an accurate description of the patient's symptoms, symptom chronology, how the illness affects the patient, previous treatments, and the patient's response to those treatments. Specifically the history should include location of the pain, duration of the pain, character of the pain, joint noise, range of movement, related discomforts, patient characteristics.

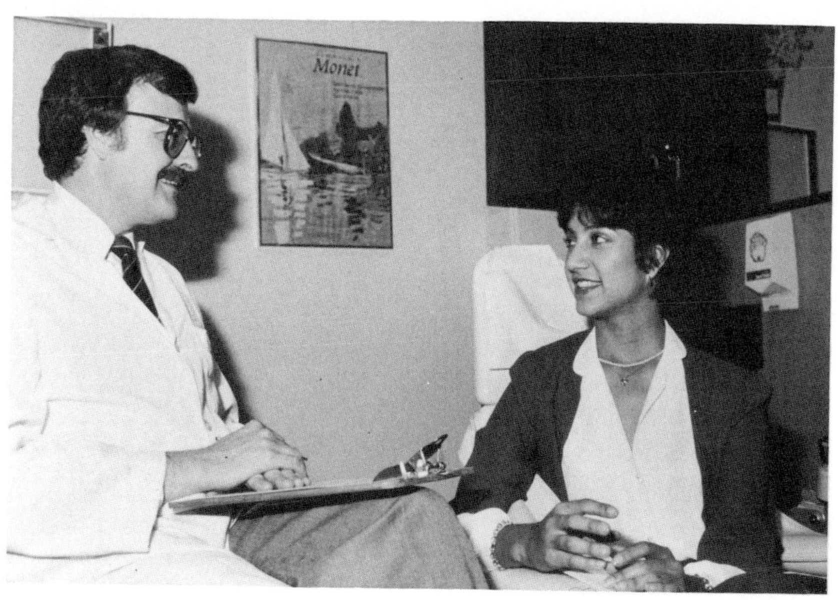
Monet

Location of the Pain

PLATE 3-2

The patient should be asked to identify the location of the most severe pain. Patients with joint derangements usually identify the joint area as the location of the most severe pain, *a,* whereas patients with muscle disorder describe diffuse areas, often following muscle distributions, *b*. Patients with symptoms of both disorders will usually describe the major component as worse. For example, in some patients the joint derangement is the primary component, with muscle symptoms being secondary. These patients will describe the joint symptoms as worse than the muscle symptoms. The opposite would be true for patients in whom the muscle component predominates.

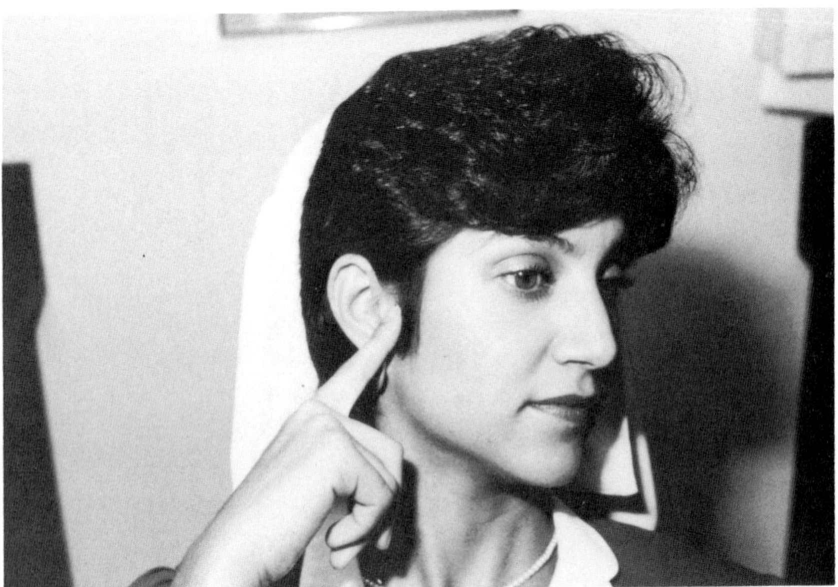

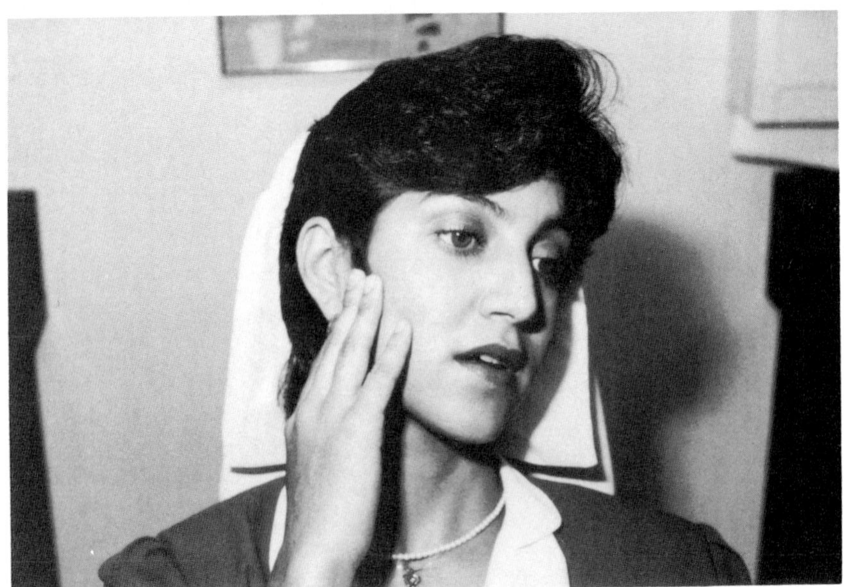

Duration of the Pain

How long the patient has had the pain should be determined. Generally, the more acute the symptoms, the more likely the problem can be managed with simple therapies; conversely, the more chronic the problem, the more difficult it will be to resolve. The patient should be asked when and how the problem began and what could have caused the problem—specifically, acute trauma, dental treatment, etc. Frequently the patient will not have any idea. A history of trauma directly related to the onset of symptoms may identify the etiology.

Character of the Pain

Joint derangements are characterized by constant pain. The pain may fluctuate in intensity but generally is present at all times. Joint pain usually decreases with rest and therefore would be expected to be less in the mornings. Conversely, joint pain is aggravated by function and hurts more with jaw usage. Rarely are patients with joint disorder completely free of pain.

Muscular disorders are characterized by intermittent pain that may vary in intensity. A most significant finding is pain that is worse in the morning. This indicates noctural muscle activity, specifically, bruxism. Muscular disorders are frequently cyclic, with periods in which the patient may be free of pain.

Joint Noise

The patient should be questioned regarding the presence of joint noises now or in the past. Patients with internal derangement almost always have or have had joint noises. The noise has two ways of presenting: clicking and crepitus.

If the patient has clicking, it should be determined *when* the jaw clicks—all the time, only in the morning, when eating, etc. Clicking that occurs only on awakening is usually related to nocturnal bruxism; clicking that occurs when eating may be related to occlusal disharmony.

It should also be determined whether the click is painful or not. Patients with internal derangement frequently experience increased pain before the click and decreased pain afterward. It is important to determine if the noise is changing, that is, occurring more or less frequently, occurring later during opening, becoming louder, or changing type of sound. Changing joint noise may indicate the presence of an active etiologic factor and progression of the disorder.

Crepitus is generally considered to represent advanced disease and occurs as a result of movement across irregular surfaces. Patients with internal derangement typically report having had clicking of the TMJ, then a period of no joint noise, and finally a grating or grinding noise. Frequently crepitus will indicate a perforation of the disc or its attachments, especially when degenerative changes are observed in the radiographs.

Range of Motion

Limited range of movement can be in at least two forms, which usually occur together: limited opening and limited lateral movement. When the disc is anteriorly displaced and does not reduce to a normal position during opening, the patient will have limited opening (closed-lock). The closed-lock condition may be either intermittent or permanent. Patients with intermittent closed-lock usually report that the jaw suddenly "catches" or "gets stuck." If pain is present, it generally is reported to be worse during the closed-lock condition. Patients may be able to "unlock" the jaw by relaxing the masticatory muscles or by moving the mandible in some manner. Some patients will have to apply pressure, usually over the lateral aspect of the condyle, to unlock the jaw. Intermittent locking may occur at any time but seems to occur most frequently on awakening and during eating. Closed-lock present on awakening is a clue to the presence of night bruxism. The frequency of locking and the length of time the mandible stays locked should be determined, as should whether or not the intermittent locking is progressive, that is, locking is occurring more frequently and lasting longer.

Permanent closed-lock is usually preceded by a period of progressive clicking and intermittent locking. Katzberg et al. reported that 29 of 31 patients with arthrographically proven closed-lock had a history of intermittent locking. When questioned, patients frequently explained that they could not open because "something is stuck in the joint."

Limited opening occurring because of a muscular disorder does not usually appear suddenly. Patients describe a tight feeling as opposed to the sensation of the jaw being stuck.

Related Discomforts

Tooth pain or *sore teeth,* assuming odontogenic pathology has been excluded, indicates bruxism. Patients should be questioned as to whether or not they grind or clench their teeth at night or during the day. Many patients will not know, but others will be aware of grinding or clenching their teeth. Patient awareness generally indicates a high level of bruxism.

Headaches are a common complaint of patients both with and without TMJ disorder. Farrar and McCarty have reported that retroorbital headaches are the most common symptom of internal derangement. Those patients with internal derangement frequently complain of headaches on the affected side, but no specific diagnostic pattern has been documented. Empirically, headaches associated with internal derangement seem to be more vascular in quality than muscular headaches, which are reported as squeezing or bandlike. Since headaches are such a common complaint, one should not assume that internal derangement is the cause unless more specific diagnostic evidence is present. One should inquire as to a relationship between the headaches and the jaw problem, for example, whether the headache is precipitated by jaw use.

Earaches are a common complaint and include ear pain, tinnitus, and occasionally dizziness. As with headaches, a complaint of earache is not specifically diagnostic. Ear pathology should be considered and ruled out before assuming that an earache may be TMJ related.

Neckaches and shoulder pain are frequently reported by patients with TMJ disorder. Again, these complaints are not specifically diagnostic but do reflect a more generalized muscular disorder.

Patient Characteristics

It is important to determine *how the problem affects the patient.* What does the problem keep the patient from doing? Most patients with TMJ disorder report the inability to eat a normal diet and some interference with jaw usage, for example, during talking. Most patients do not have their whole life, marriage, job, etc. disrupted by the problem. When patients report total disability, other factors, such as poor family relationships or job problems, may be involved.

Patients should be questioned about stress, and many will report being under considerable stress and being anxious. Although stress may or may not cause the problem, it certainly affects the patient's response to the problem and its treatment. Patients should also be questioned about significant life events, such as death in the family, divorce, or sickness. Again, the presence of major significant life events affects the patient's response to illness and its treatment. Generally, during times of major life events caution should be exercised in starting irreversible therapies.

During the history, patients should be observed for signs and symptoms of *depression,* including loss of interest in family, job, sex, or even life. Depression may also be indicated by uncleanliness in dress or personal hygiene. Again, depression markedly affects a patient's response to illness and its treatment.

Previous treatments and their outcome should be determined. Patients must be asked about drug usage. Most patients with TMJ disorder do not regularly require narcotic medications; individuals taking narcotics regularly generally have complex problems and will need comprehensive management of both the TMJ and the drug problem. The effect of sedative drugs such as diazepam (Valium) should be carefully assessed. If a sedative, particularly one taken at night, significantly reduces the pain, a muscular disorder is more likely.

Other previous treatments such as splints, occlusal adjustment, physical therapy, and surgery should be carefully assessed as to how they were done and what their outcome was. Generally the more treatments a patient has had, the more difficult the problem is to manage. Physicians who have previously treated a patient should be contacted; this can obviously provide valuable insight to the patient's problem.

History Form

The question always arises as to the need for a comprehensive history questionnaire. We believe a questionnaire is valuable in terms of documenting the patient's history. It should not be used as a substitute for the interview. The form used in our clinic is presented on p. 58.

HISTORY

1. Name ______________________ Age ________
   Address ______________________
2. Referred by ______________________
3. Describe your problem: ______________________
   ____
4. Which side hurts? Right ________ Left ________ Both ________
5. For how long? ______________________
6. Is the pain constant or intermittent? ______________________
7. Is the pain worse in morning, afternoon, evening? ______________
8. Does it hurt to move your jaw ________? To chew ________?
9. On the figures below please outline where your pain is.

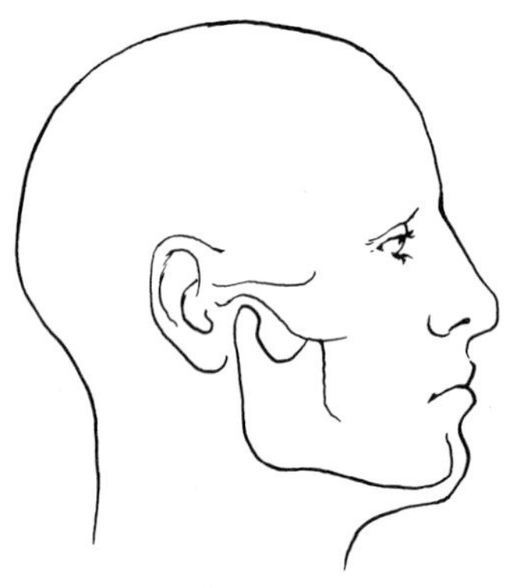

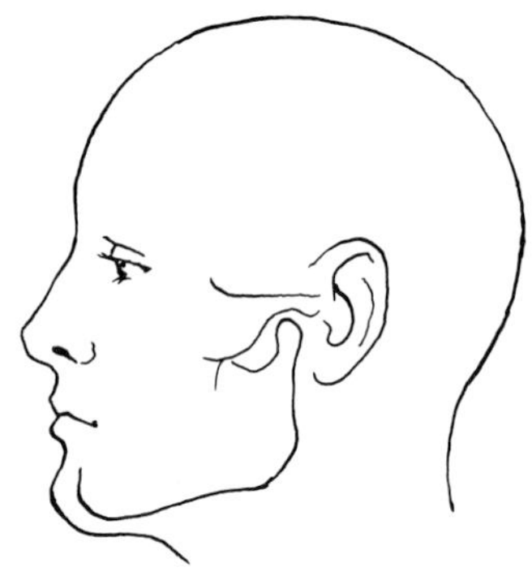

10. Does your jaw make noise?
    Clicking ________ Grinding ________ Other ________
    When? ________ For how long? ______________
11. Has your jaw ever locked open? ________ Closed? ________
    When? ______________ How often? ______________
12. If your jaw does not make noise or lock now, has it ever in the past? __
    Describe: ______________________
    ____
    ____
13. Do you have?
    a. Headaches ________
    b. Neckaches ________
    c. Shoulder pain ________
    d. Ear pain ________

HISTORY—cont'd

e. Ringing in the ears ________
f. Dizziness ________
g. Change in hearing ________

14. Do you grind or clench your teeth? ________
    At night ________ During the day ________
15. Do you have sore or sensitive teeth? ________
16. Do you have trouble getting to sleep? ________
    Do you sleep well? ________
17. Do you consider yourself to be under a lot of stress? ______________
    Are you nervous or anxious about anything? ________
18. Have you ever had a nervous stomach, ulcers, skin disease? ________
19. Do you have or have you ever had arthritis? ________
20. Does your pain keep you from doing anything? ________
    If yes, what? ____
    ____
21. Can you remember any injury to your jaw? ________
    If yes, describe: ____________________________________
    ____
22. Do you take medications for the pain? ________
    If yes, what? ____
23. Do you take medications for relaxation? ________
    If yes, what? ____
    ____
24. Have you had any treatments for your problem? ________
    If yes, what kind? ____________________________________
    a. Bite splint ________
    b. Medication ________
    c. Physical therapy ________
    d. Counseling ________
    e. Occlusal adjustment ________
    f. Orthodontics ________
    g. Surgery ________
    h. Other ____

PHYSICAL EXAMINATION

The physical examination should evaluate the entire masticatory system, including the following:

1. Articular (joint)
2. Muscular
3. Dental
4. Cervical

Articular Examination

The articular examination should evaluate the following: joint tenderness, joint noise, and range of motion.

PLATE 3-3

Both TMJs should be palpated for the presence of *joint tenderness* and they should be palpated both laterally, **A** and **B**, and through the external auditory canal *(EAC)*, **C** and **D**. Generally, tenderness arising intraarticularly will be manifested laterally over the joint and also through the EAC. Although it will be highly subjective, some estimate of the degree of tenderness should be made, characterizing it as mild, moderate, or severe.

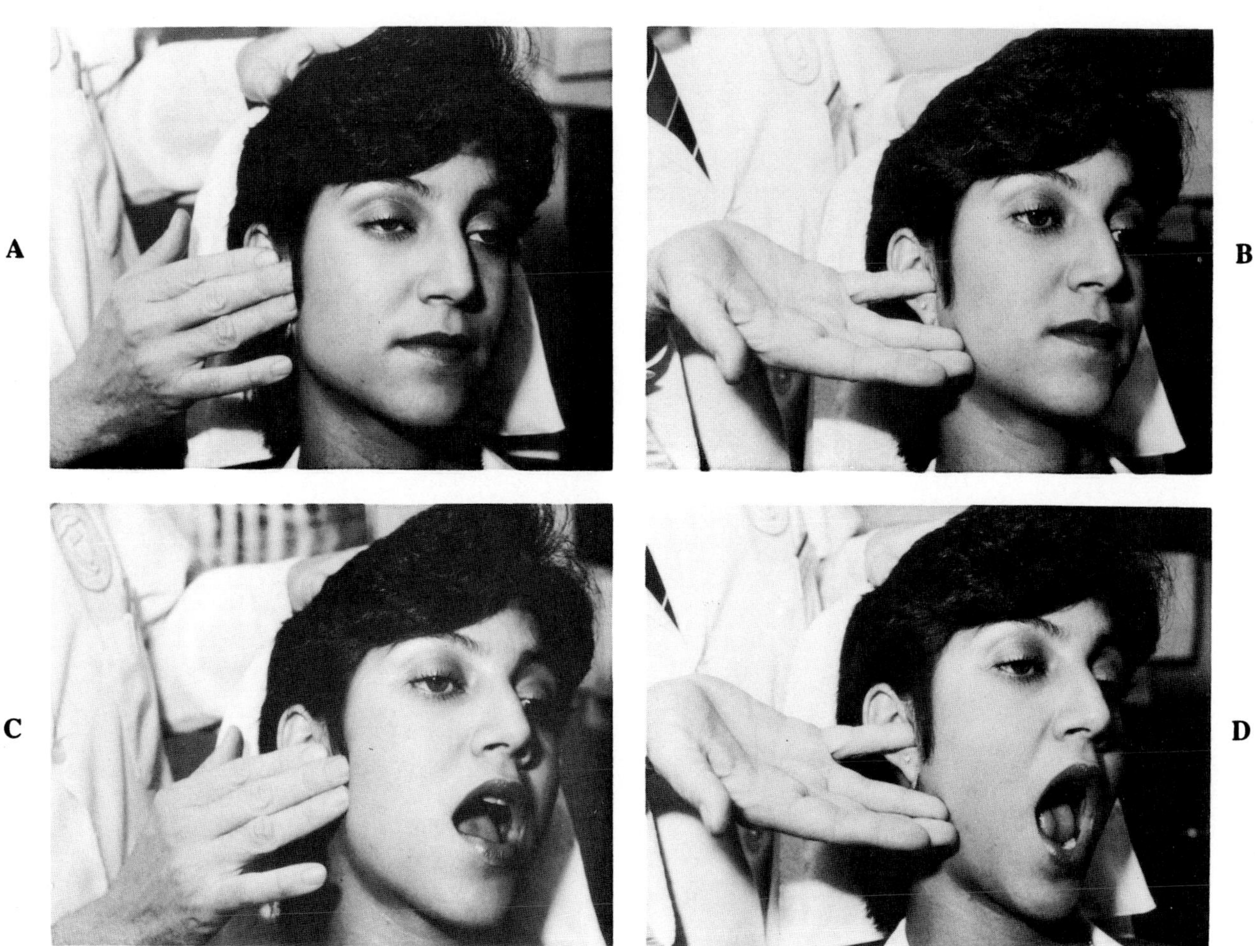
A
B
C
D

PLATE 3-4

The *mandibular range of motion* should be determined. Normal mandibular range of movement is about 50 mm vertically, **A,** 10 mm protrusively **B,** and 10 mm laterally, **C** and **D.** The normal movement is straight and symmetric.

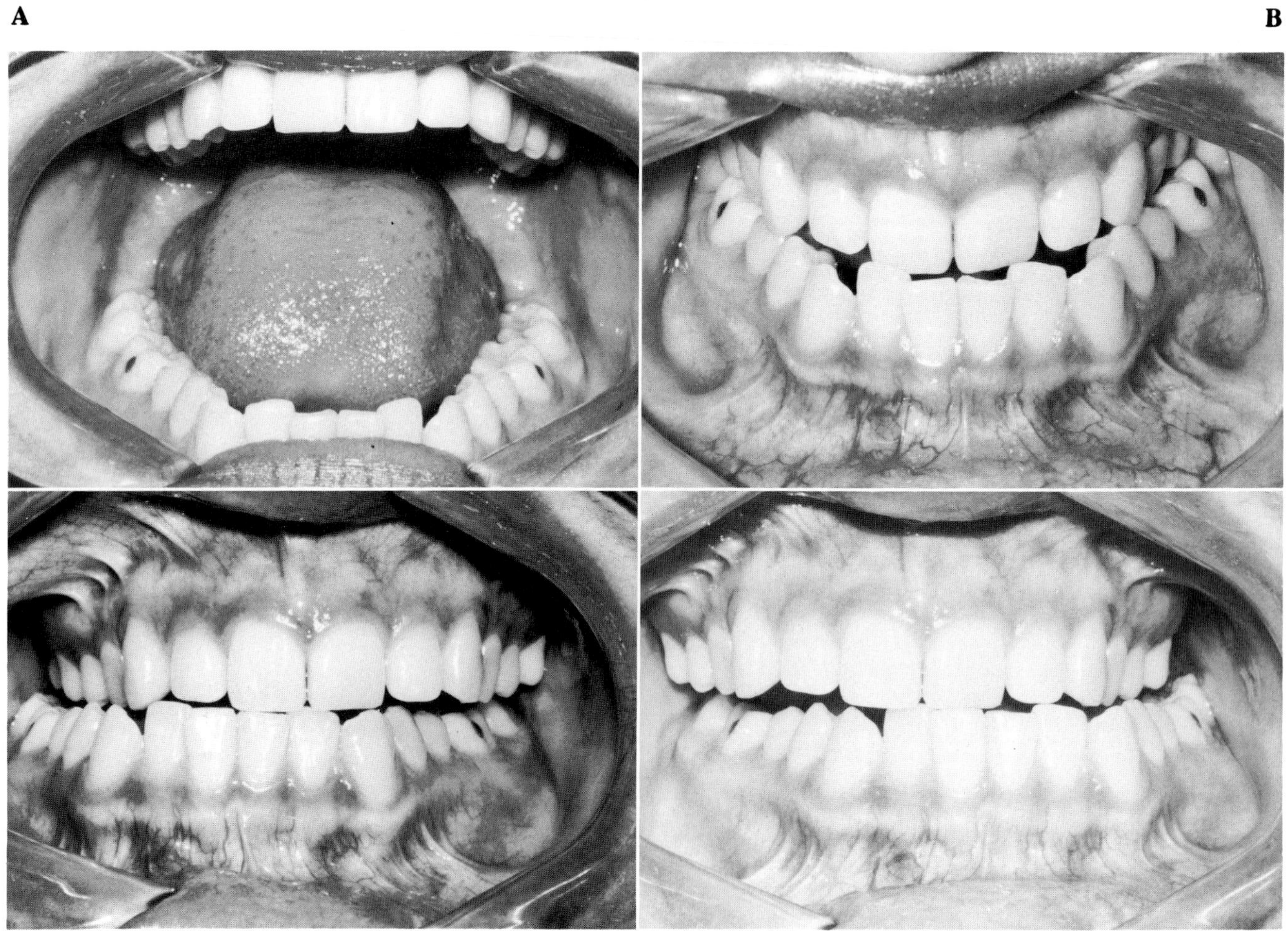

PLATE 3-5

Patients with disc derangements may have deviation of their movement patterns, a limited range of movement, or both. In the patient with clicking the jaw may deviate toward the side of the click, **A,** until the click occurs, and then return toward the midline, **B.**

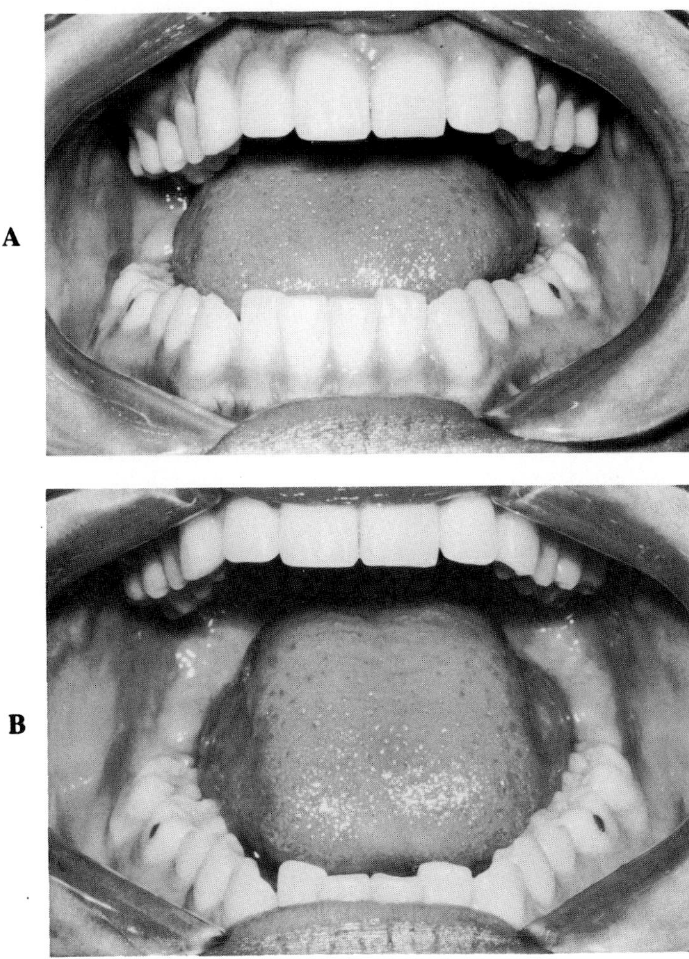

PLATE 3-6

Reciprocal clicking is the most common form of joint noise in patients with internal derangement. Reciprocal clicking refers to clicking during the closing (retrusive) movement preceded by a click during the opening movement. The position of the opening click is determined by measuring the vertical opening at the time the click occurs. As a general rule, the later the opening click, the greater the disc displacement. The position of the closing (retrusive) click is best determined by having the patient protrude the mandible maximally with the teeth in light contact, **A** and **B.** The patient then opens on a protruded pathway until the opening click occurs, **C** and **D.** The patient then closes along the protruded pathway with the teeth in light contact, **E** and **F.**

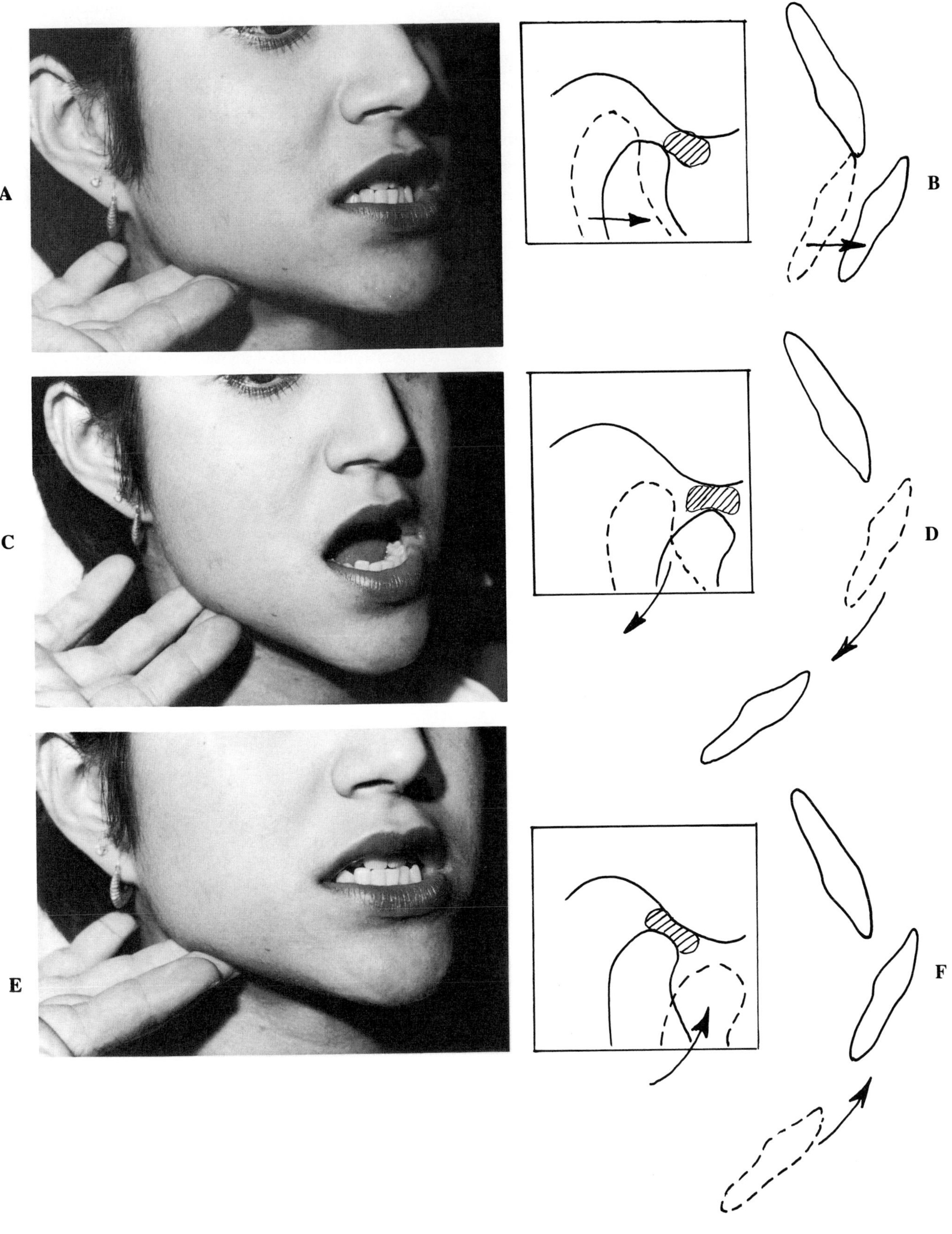
A
B
C
D
E
F

The mandible is slowly retruded toward the intercuspal position while the dentist lightly palpates the angles of the mandible, **G** and **H.** The position of the retrusive click is then noted, **I** and **J.** The click can be palpated at the mandibular angle, and the posterior mandibular teeth shift slightly upward as the click occurs. As a general rule, the closer the retrusive click is to centric occlusion (acquired occlusion) the better the prognosis is for nonsurgical treatment.

Not all reciprocal clicks represent disc displacement. Opening and closing clicks that occur in exactly the same position indicate deviations in form, usually an irregularity on the articular eminence.

Some patients will experience *locking* during examination, and others can intentionally produce locking. This should be observed and described as evidence of disc derangement.

Crepitus is defined as multiple scraping sounds and is generally considered to represent advanced disease. It frequently indicates a disruption of the disc or its attachment tissues.

It must be emphasized that although the presence of the described joint noises may technically indicate the presence of a disc derangement it should not automatically be assumed to be the cause of the patient's problem without other evidence.

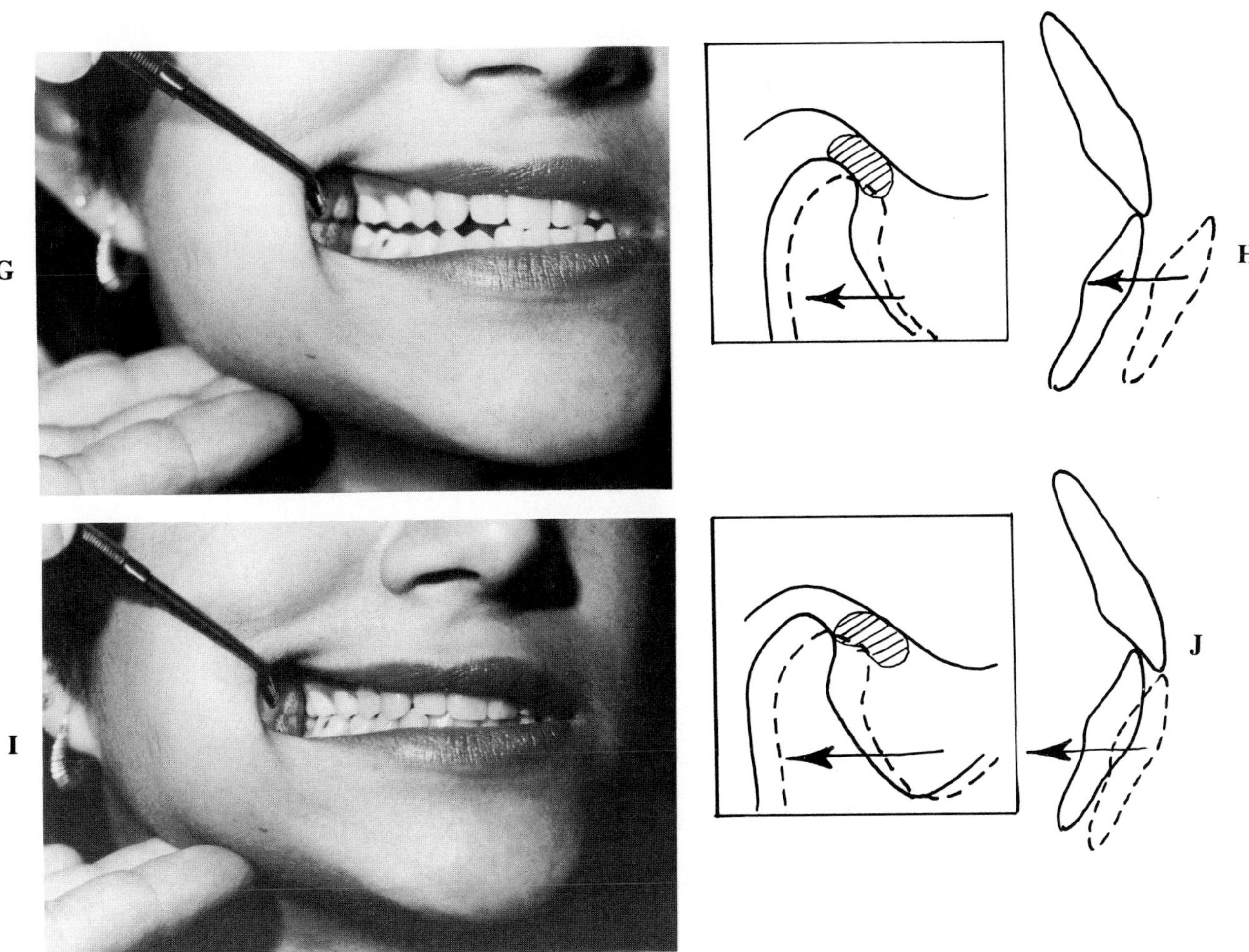
G
H
I
J

PLATE 3-7

Limited range of movement presents in three forms that usually occur together: limited opening with deviation, deviation on protrusion, and limited lateral movement. When the patient is in the closed-lock state, there is usually limited opening and deviation toward the affected side, **A.** The mandible will also deviate toward the affected side during protrusive movement. Lateral movement is decreased toward the opposite side, **B,** when compared to the unaffected side, **C.** There is generally some resilience to terminal stretch in both the maximal open and lateral positions, and increased joint pain is ellicited by terminal stretch. Increased joint pain may also occur during attempts to move the mandible posteriorly, that is, into centric relation. Loading the joint through upward pressure applied at the mandibular angle or by biting, usually on the opposite side, will also elicit increased joint pain in the affected side.

Patients with muscular disorders also may have limited opening and deviation to the affected side. Generally the deviation does not occur on protrusion nor are there limited lateral movements. Terminal stretch movements elicit pain along the temporalis insertion or pterygomasseteric sling and not within the joint.

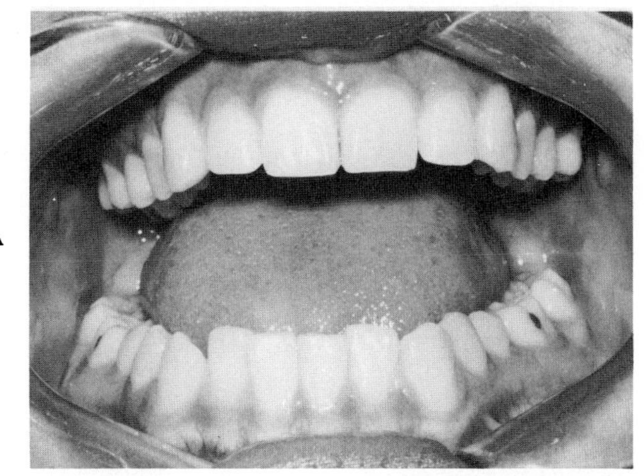

A

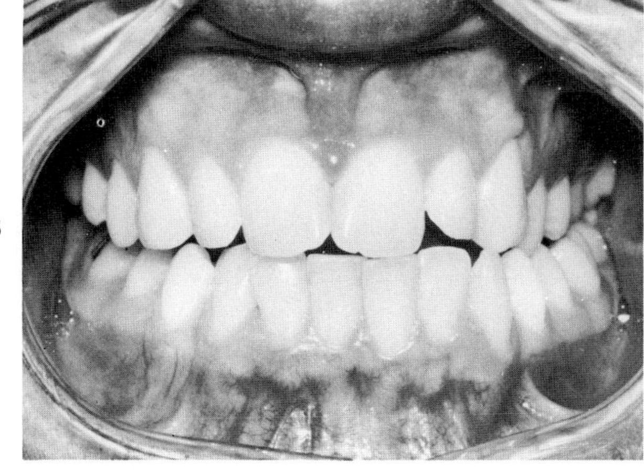

B

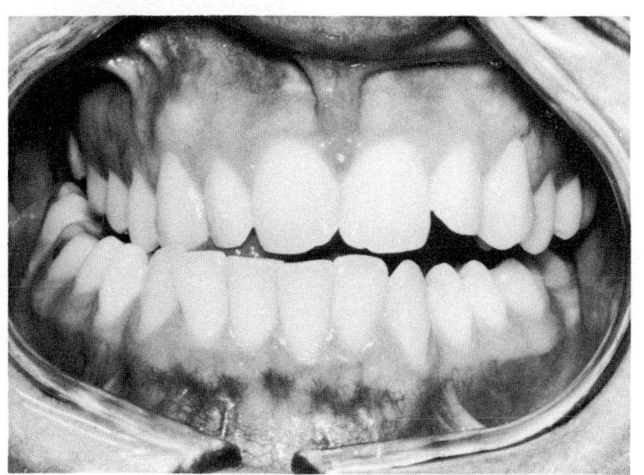

C

Muscular Examination

The masticatory muscles should be examined systematically. The head and neck should be inspected for soft tissue asymmetry or evidence of muscle hypertrophy. The patient should be observed for signs of jaw clenching or other habits. The muscles should be palpated for the presence of tenderness, fasciculations, spasms, and trigger points. Although subjective, an attempt should be made to grade the findings as, for example, mild, moderate, or severe. Moderate to severe muscle tenderness suggests a muscular disorder or at least a muscular component.

PLATE 3-8

A Palpation of the origin of the lateral pterygoid.
B Palpation of the insertion of the medial pterygoid intraorally.
C Palpation of the insertion of the medial pterygoid extraorally.
D Palpation of the insertion of the temporalis.

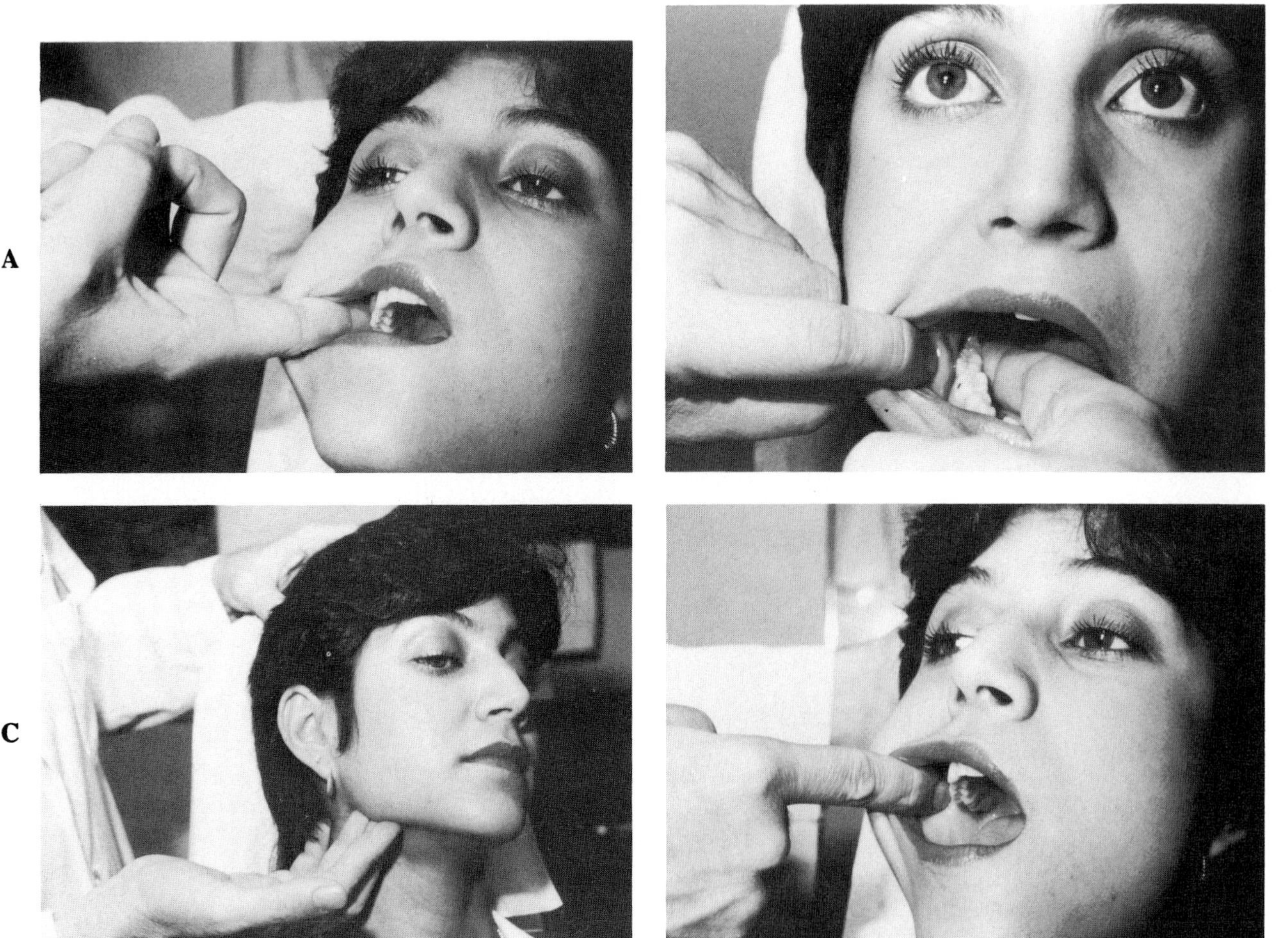

E Palpation of the posterior, middle, and anterior parts of the temporalis.
F Palpation of the masseter.
G Palpation of the sternocleidomastoid.

E

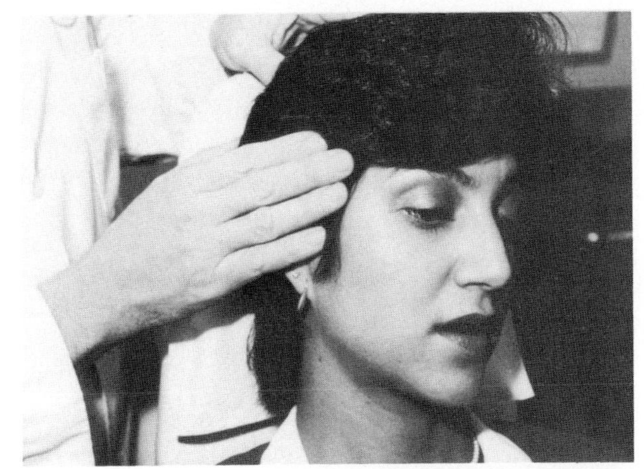

F

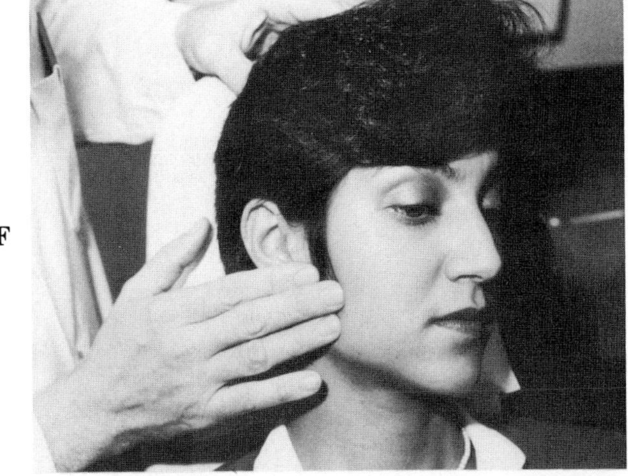

G

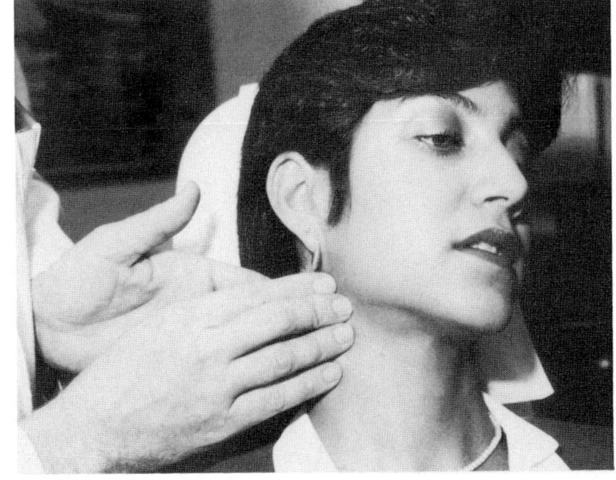

Dental Examination

The dental examination is important. Odontogenic sources of pain should be eliminated. The teeth should be examined for wear facets, soreness, and mobility, which may be evidence of bruxism. The number of teeth missing as well as the dental classification should be determined.

The significance of occlusal interferences is recognized as controversial; however, the occlusion should be evaluated. No occlusal findings are diagnostic of disc derangement; however, the occlusion may be important as an etiologic factor. Occlusal factors that have not been proven but are implicated include heavy incisal contacts (especially common in Class II Division 2 disorders), distal defective contacts, and missing posterior teeth.

PLATE 3-9

Maxillomandibular-skeletal relationship and dental, periodontal, and occlusal status should be thoroughly evaluated.

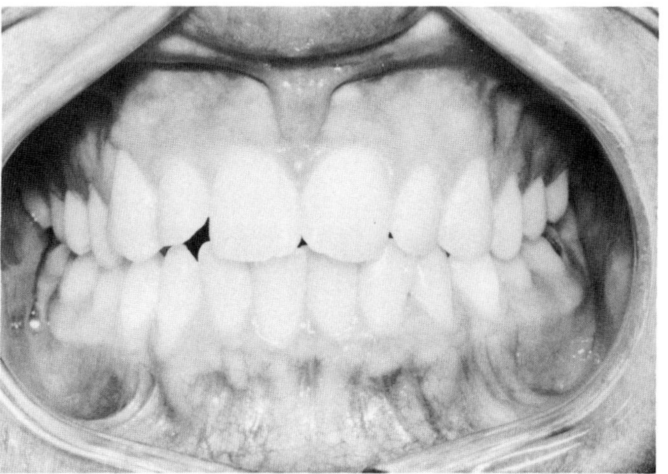

Cervical Examination

A cervical evaluation is important, especially in patients reporting neck and shoulder pains. This evaluation should include inspection of head and neck posture and search for evidence of muscle asymmetry or hypertrophy. The neck examination should include range of movement and palpation for muscle tenderness, fasciculations, spasm, or trigger areas. The presence of cervical joint noise should be noted.

CONVENTIONAL RADIOGRAPHY

The value of radiography of the TMJ in assessing osseous joint pathology is well recognized. It seems clear that patients suspected to have joint pathology should have some type of conventional radiograph to evaluate the joint structures. Various techniques—transcranial, lateral pharyngeal, panographic, etc.—exist. Each has its advantages and disadvantages. Presently no single technique can be recommended as superior.

Joint space analysis can be done only from transcranial or tomographic studies. The value of joint space analysis remains controversial; scientific evidence shows that a diagnosis of disc derangement cannot be made on the basis of joint space analysis alone.

TOMOGRAPHIC PROCEDURES

The benefits of tomographic radiographs are well recognized. Tomographic evaluation of the joint is recommended as a substitute for conventional radiography when available or as a more in-depth study of patients with osseous pathology demonstrated by conventional radiography.

SUMMARY: DIAGNOSTIC CATEGORIES AND THEIR CRITERIA

Anterior disc displacement with reduction

I. History
   A. Joint pain
   B. Clicking
II. Physical examination
   A. Joint tenderness
   B. Reciprocal clicking; clicks not occurring together
   C. Jaw deviated toward side of click until click occurs, then returns to midline
III. Routine radiographs (may show osteoarthrosis)

Anterior disc displacement with intermittent locking

I. Same as anterior disc displacement with reduction when clicking
II. Same as anterior disc displacement without reduction (closed-lock) when locked

Anterior disc displacement without reduction (closed-lock)

I. History
  A. Joint pain
  B. Limited opening
  C. Previous clicking with intermittent locking
  D. Sensation that something in the joint blocks opening
II. Physical examination
  A. Variable joint tenderness
  B. Limited opening and lateral movement toward opposite side
  C. Jaw deviates toward affected side
  D. Terminal stretch produces increased pain
III. Routine radiographs (may show osteoarthrosis)

Anterior disc displacement with perforation

I. History
  A. Joint pain
  B. Previous history of clicking, clicking with intermittent locking, and closed-lock
  C. Crepitus; grating, grinding noise
II. Physical examination
  A. Joint tenderness
  B. Crepitus
  C. Variable limited opening
III. Routing radiographs; generally show evidence of osteoarthrosis

chapter 4

Arthrography

Arthrography is defined as the injection of contrast material, radiolucent and/or radiopaque, into a synovial space followed by radiography of the joint. In the past few years arthrography of the TMJ has been employed routinely in many facilities throughout the country to visualize the joint soft tissues, specifically the disc and its attachments. The procedure is safe and effective in providing diagnostic information.

The following information may be obtained from an arthrogram:

1. Position of the disc relative to the condyle and articular eminence
   a. With mandible closed
   b. At various positions of mandibular movement
2. Morphology of the disc
3. Presence of tears (perforations) in the disc or its attachments
4. Presence of adhesions in the joint spaces
5. Presence of "loose bodies" in the joint spaces

INDICATIONS

The oral and maxillofacial surgeon needs a reasonably certain preoperative diagnosis before performing any operation to correct TMJ internal derangement. One purpose of TMJ arthrography is to confirm the diagnosis.

In some cases where the clinical diagnosis is certain there is controversy as to whether an arthrogram is needed before surgery. Certainly, an arthrogram is not required in those cases with evidence of osteoarthrosis on plain or tomographic radiographs. However, the surgeon may elect to obtain an arthrogram to have information about the soft tissues.

When the surgeon is not reasonably certain that the patient has internal derangement, an arthrogram is indicated. Additionally, the surgeon may desire specific information about disc position and morphology to plan the surgical procedure.

To some extent regional customs dictate the need for an arthrogram before surgery. An arthrogram may be used to document the diagnosis and the extent of derangement. Cases involved in litigation, bodily injury, or disability claims generally require extensive documentation, and obtaining a preoperative arthrogram in these situations seems prudent.

CONTRAINDICATIONS

Arthrography should be performed with caution in patients who have a history of reaction to iodinated contrast medium. Bleeding disorders and anticoagulation medication are relative contraindications. The surgeon and radiologist must weigh the value of the information that may be obtained against the risk to the patient. Computed tomography is an alternative procedure for these patients.

Arthrography should not be performed in the presence of localized skin infection because of the risk of introducing infection into the joint.

PATIENT PREPARATION

The purpose and procedure for the arthrogram are explained to the patient by the surgeon. We inform patients that they may have mild to moderate discomfort afterward and give them a prescription for a mild analgesic, for example, 30 mg of codeine. We also tell patients that the occlusion will feel different for approximately 12 to 24 hours after arthrography.

Patients are told about the possibility of facial muscle paralysis secondary to the local anesthetic and that this is temporary and will last about 2 hours. Patients who have a reducing disc are informed that occasionally the closed-lock condition occurs after the arthrogram and that this is also usually temporary.

We instruct patients to apply ice over the studied joint for 12 hours after the arthrogram and then to use moist heat until the discomfort and swelling from the procedure have resolved.

ARTHROGRAPHIC TECHNIQUE

PLATE 4-1

The patient is placed on the fluoroscopic table in a lateral recumbent position with the head tilted on the table top. This allows the joint to project over the skull above the facial bones. The side of the face to be examined is uppermost. Having the patient open and close the mouth several times while under fluoroscopic observation allows rapid identification of the condyle, fossa, and eminence. The skin over the joint area is prepped with iodine and isolated using either sterile towels or a sterile plastic drape.

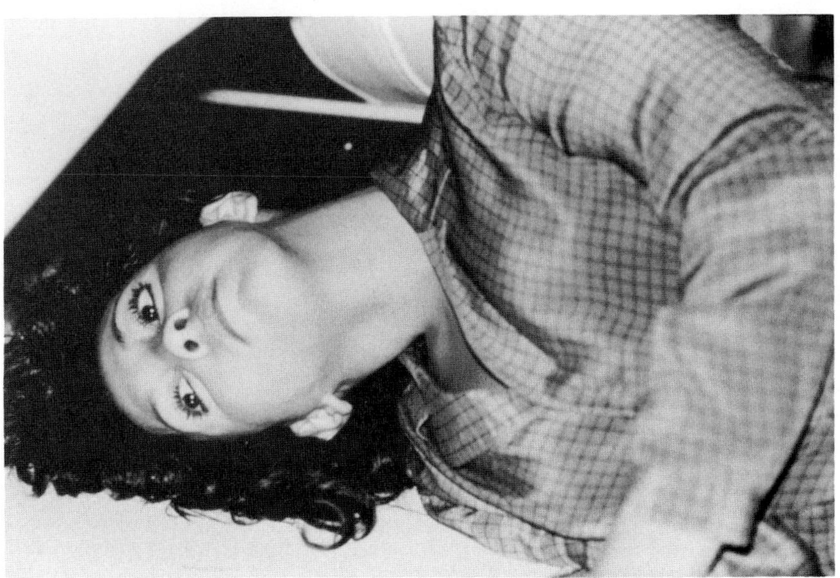

PLATE 4-2

A Under fluoroscopic guidance, the posterosuperior aspect of the mandibular condyle is identified. Local anesthetic is infiltrated into the region. A ¾ or 1¼ 23-gauge scalp vein needle and attached tubing are filled with contrast material; care is taken to eliminate air bubbles. We put 3 ml of diatrizoate meglumine (Reno-M-60) or iothalamate meglumine (Conray) and 0.03 ml of 1 : 1,000 epinephrine into a 5 ml syringe.

B Oriented perpendicular to the skin, the needle is introduced into a predetermined region of the condyle with the mandible in the closed position. After the needle is advanced, fluoroscopic observation ensures correct positioning. When the condyle is touched, the patient is instructed to open the mouth slightly, and the needle is guided behind the posterior slope of the condyle.

A

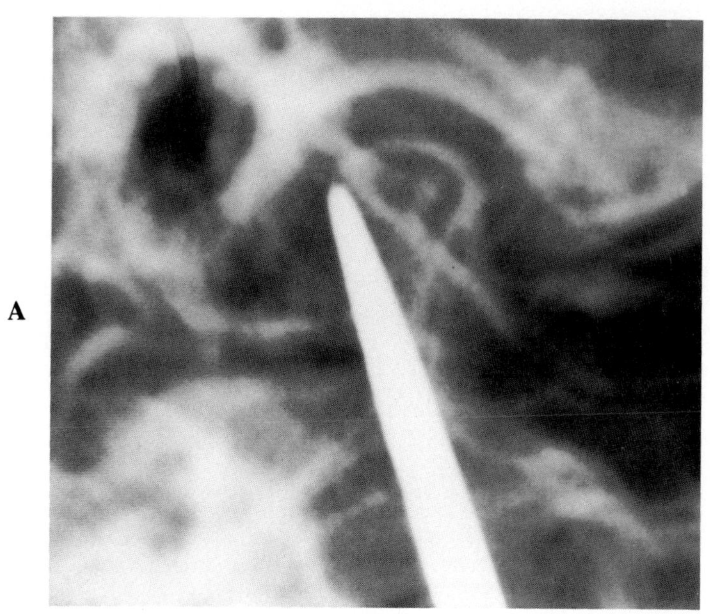

B

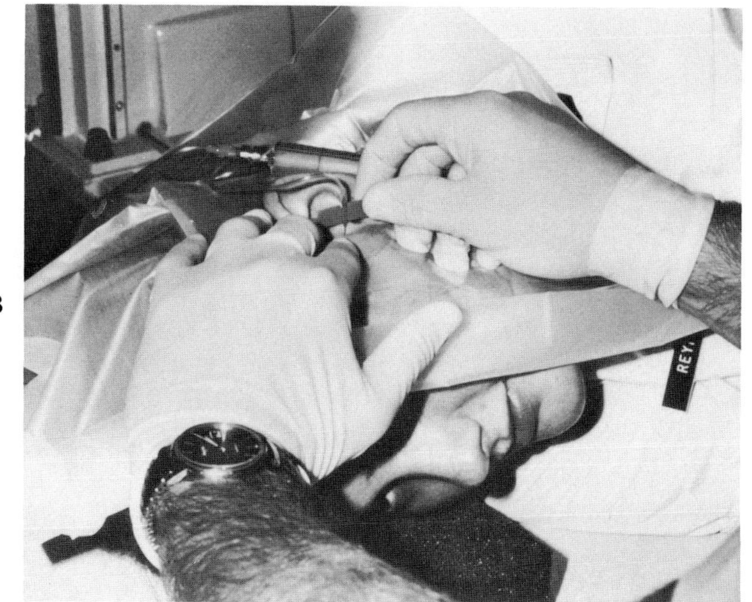

C and **D** On fluoroscopic observation the needle must be *perfectly contiguous* with the posterior margin. If *space exists* between the needle and the posterior margin, the needle *will not be in* the lower joint space and should be repositioned until it is correctly located.

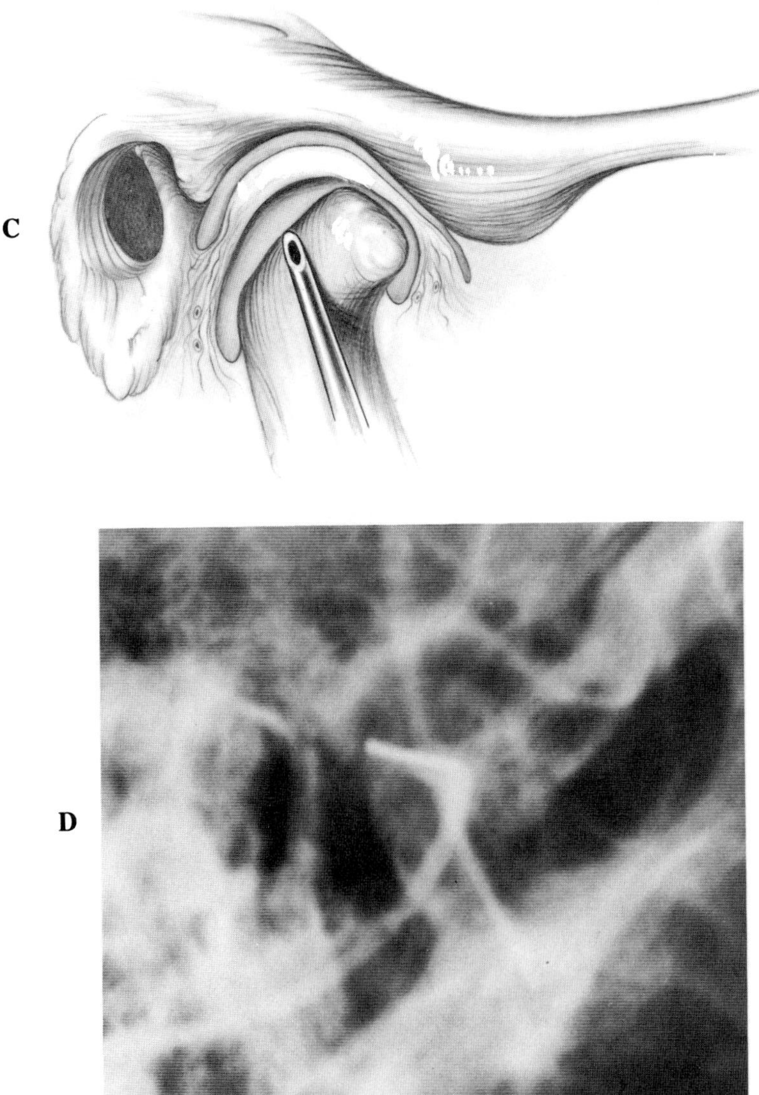

E and **F** When needle placement is correct, the patient is instructed to open and close the mouth slowly. On fluoroscopic observation the needle tip should move with the condyle. It should remain contiguous with the posterior margin during the first part of movement. A slight separation of the needle and the posterior margin may occur about midopening of the mouth.

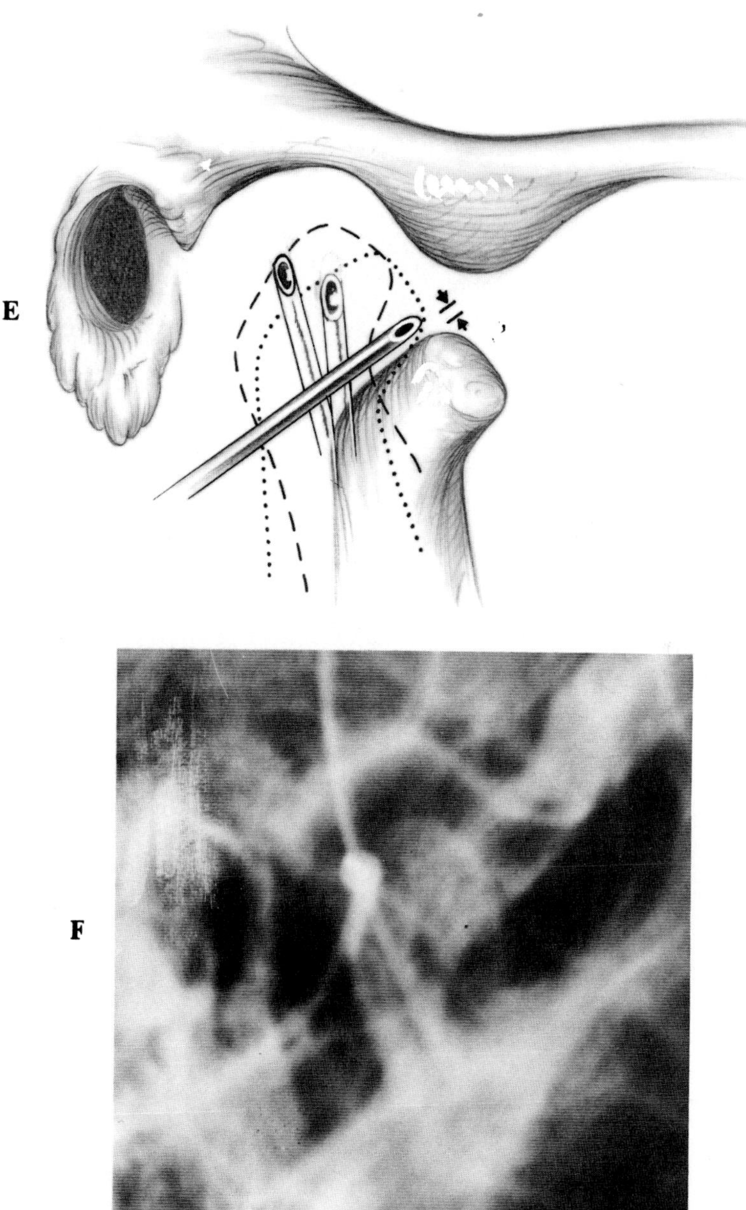

G and **H** A test injection of contrast material, approximately 0.1 to 0.2 ml, is injected. The contrast material should flow freely anterior to the condyle when the needle is properly placed in the lower joint space. A total of about 0.5 ml of contrast material completes the injection.

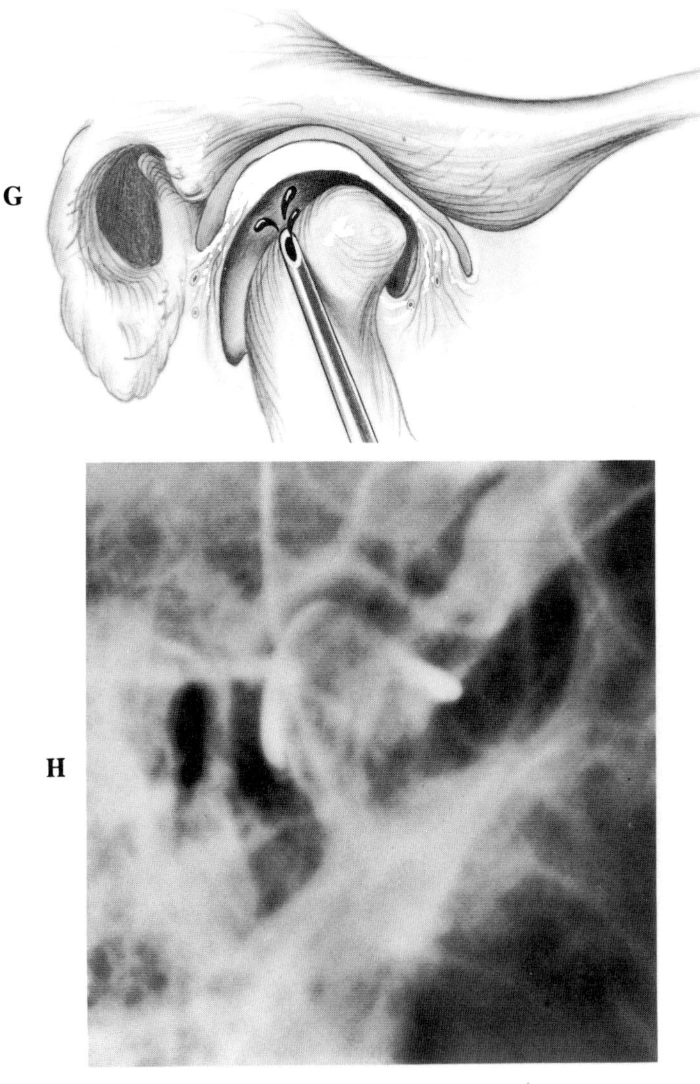

I and **J** If the needle is not correctly placed in the lower joint space, contrast material may collect around the tip of the needle as the material is injected. One should immediately stop the injection and reposition the needle. *Failure to recognize this is one of the most common mistakes* while performing arthrography.

I

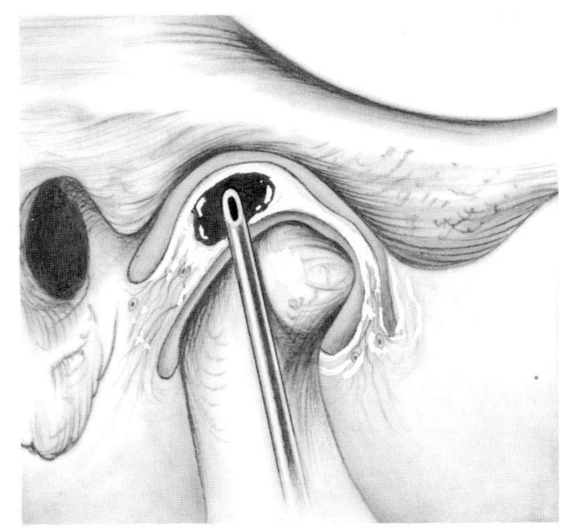

J

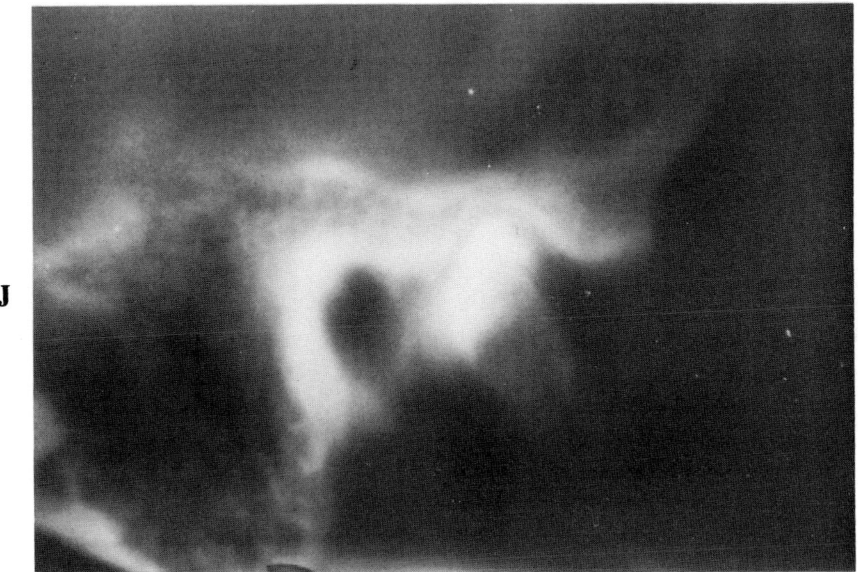

K and **L** After successful injection of the lower joint space the joint is fluoroscopically observed during movement. If the *diagnosis is certain,* the needle is withdrawn and fluoroscopic-videotape images are recorded during opening and closing movements of the mandible. Spot lateral radiographs under fluoroscopic guidance are obtained, completing the study.

Plate 4-2

K

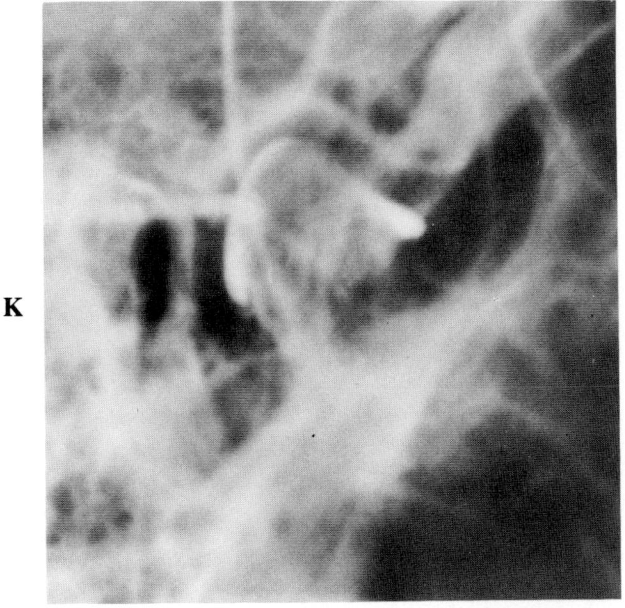

L

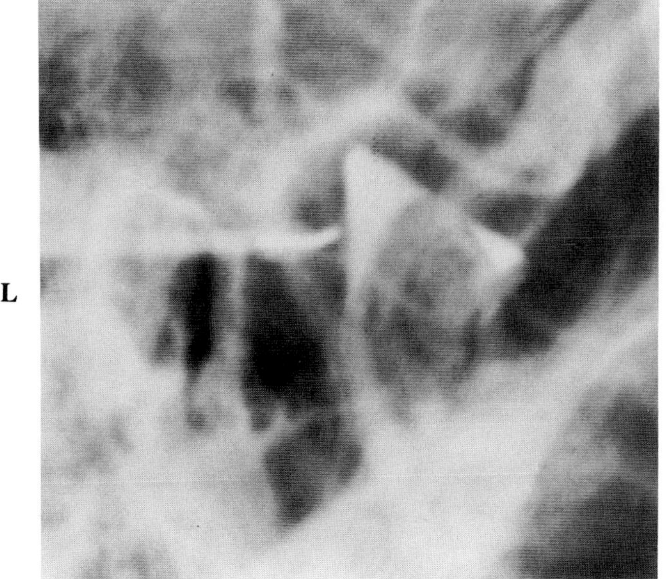

PLATE 4-3

A and **B** If the *diagnosis is uncertain* from the lower joint space, the upper joint space should be injected before the needle is removed from the lower joint space. The needle is directed against the posterior slope of the articular eminence. As bone contact is obtained, the position is checked fluoroscopically. If the position is correct, the needle should be advanced into the upper joint space. A test injection of contrast material of approximately 0.1 to 0.2 ml is given, and the contrast material should flow freely into the upper joint space.

After successful injection of the upper joint space the joint is observed fluoroscopically. Additional contrast material may need to be injected into the lower space. If the *diagnosis is certain,* the needles are withdrawn, and fluoroscopic-videotape images are recorded during opening and closing movements of the mandible. Spot lateral radiographs under fluoroscopic guidance are obtained, completing the study.

A

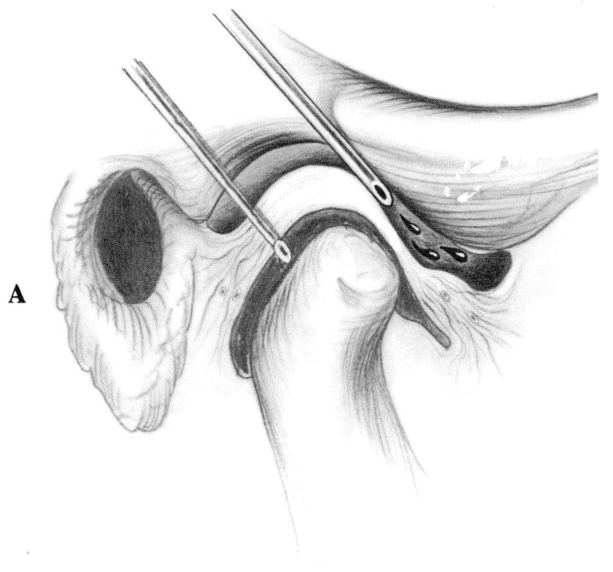

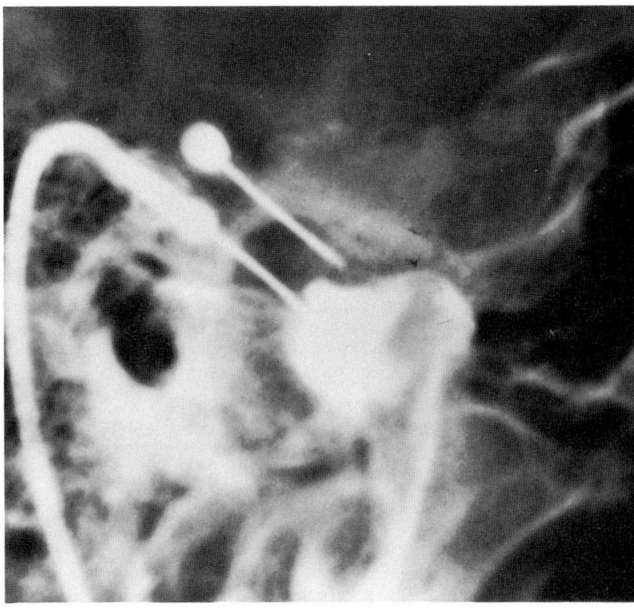

B

C and **D** If the *diagnosis is uncertain* or if additional information is needed, tomograms are obtained. A bite block is used to keep the mandible open and steady while doing the open-mouth tomograms.

NOTE: Some clinicians prefer to routinely inject both joint spaces before tomography. Unquestionably this provides more information, but the need for the additional information is controversial. Presently the controversy remains unresolved, and the decision to inject only the lower space or both spaces routinely depends on the clinician's preference.

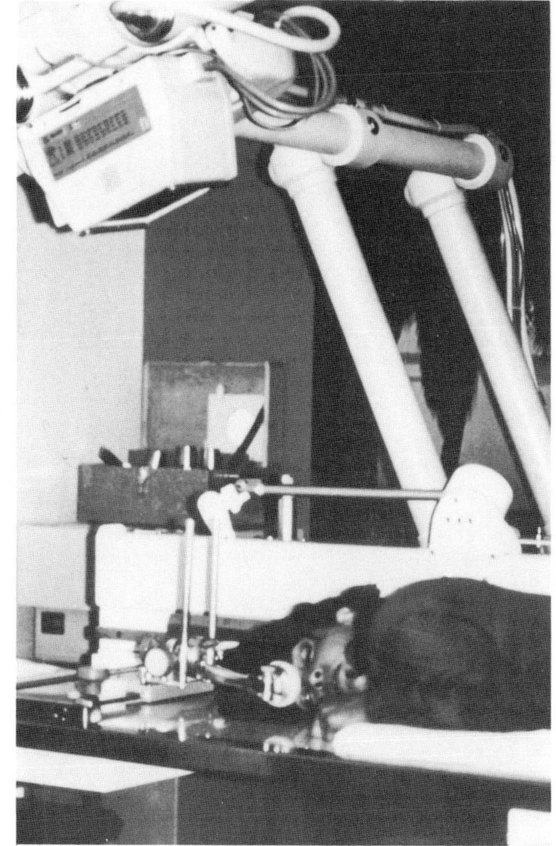

C

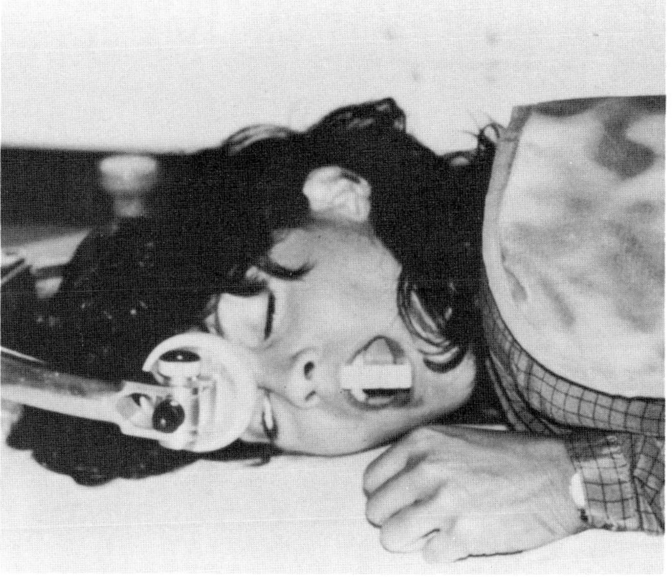

D

INTERPRETATION

Normal Lower Joint Space (Tomogram)

PLATE 4-4

A and **B** The normal lower joint in the closed mouth position is contiguous with the articular surface of the mandibular condyle and extends only slightly anterior to the condyle. Anteriorly the lower joint space forms a small, teardrop configuration directed obliquely downward.

A

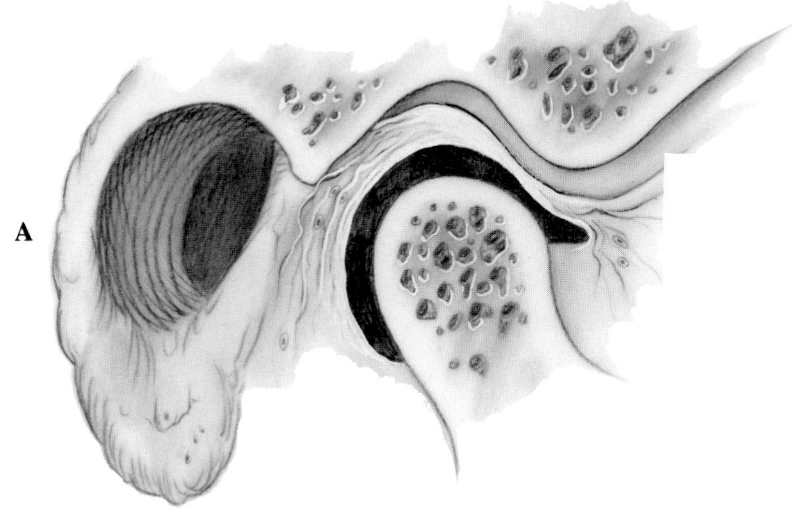

B

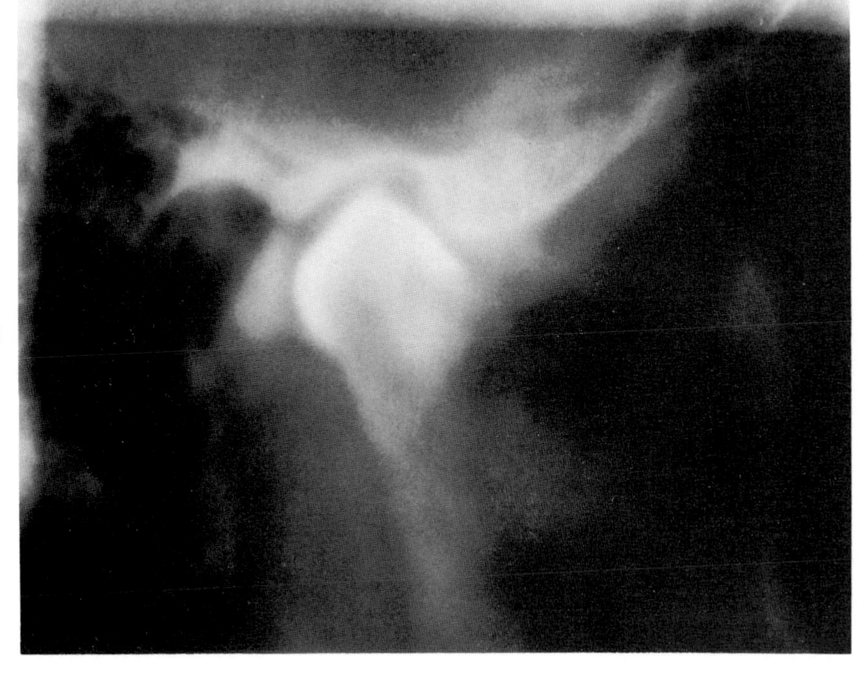

C and **D** As the mandible opens, the condyle rotates into the intermediate zone of the articular disc. Contrast material flows posteriorly as the joint space opens behind the condyle. In the midopen position, contrast material is seen anteriorly and posteriorly to the condyle. The superior margin of the lower joint space is concave both anteriorly and posteriorly to the condyle. These concave superior margins reflect the anterior and posterior bands of the disc.

Contrast material remaining anterior to the condyle in the midopen position is *frequently misdiagnosed* as anterior displacement without reduction. Injection of the upper joint space decreases the possibility of this misdiagnosis.

C

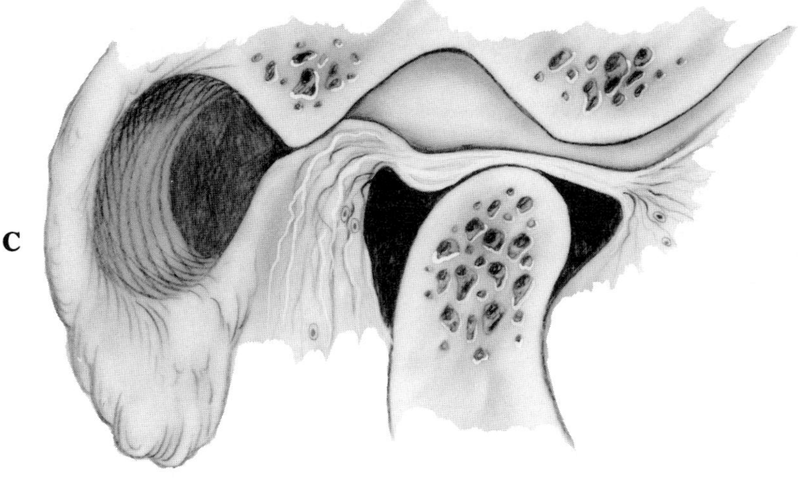

D

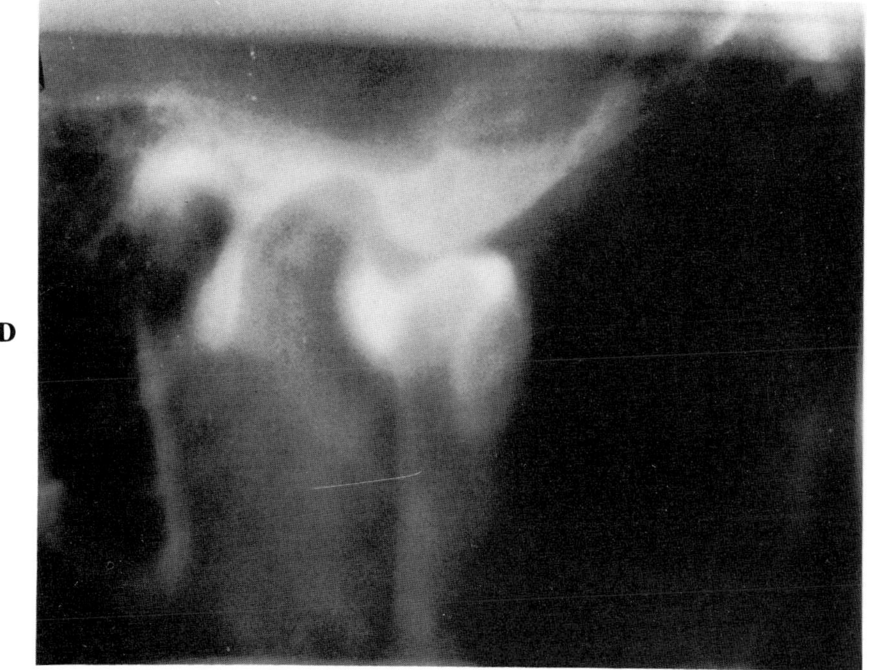

E and **F** In the maximum open position more contrast material flows posteriorly, and only a thin curvilinear rim of contrast material remains along the anterosuperior margin of the condyle. The joint space behind the condyle is smoothly concave along the superior margin.

E

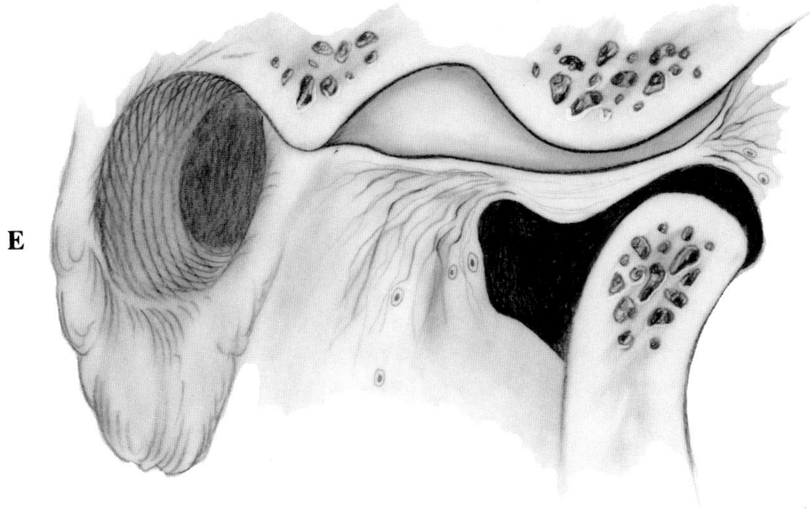

F

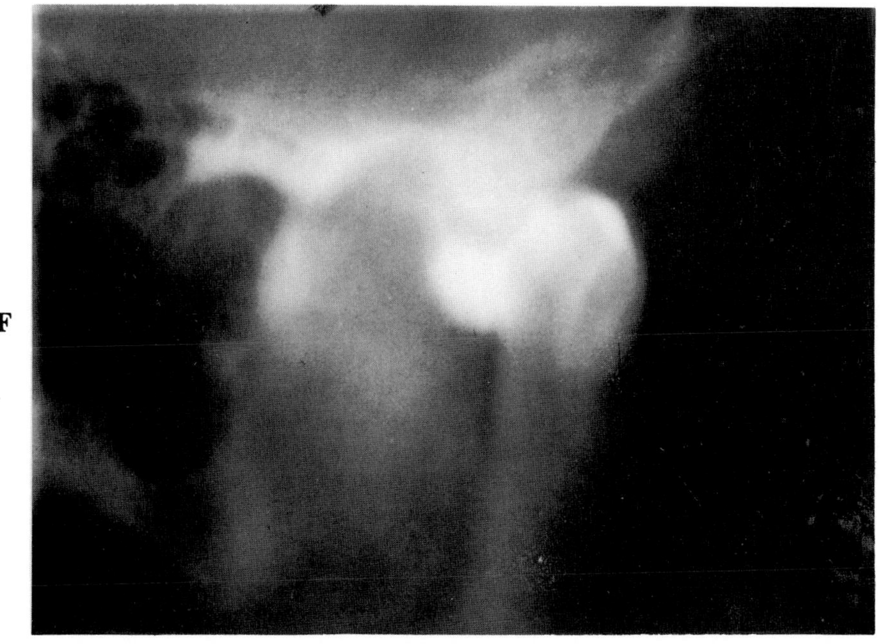

Normal Upper and Lower Joint Spaces (Tomogram)

With both joint spaces injected the disc can be indirectly visualized as the radiolucent area between the contrast-filled joint spaces.

PLATE 4-5

A and **B** In the closed-mouth position the upper joint space is contiguous with the glenoid fossa and articular eminence. The upper joint space always extends farther anteriorly than the lower joint space. The lower joint space is contiguous with the articular surface of the mandibular condyle and extends only slightly anterior to the condyle. The posterior band of the disc is above the anterosuperior surface of the condyle, and the intermediate zone and anterior band lie along the posterior slope of the articular eminence.

A

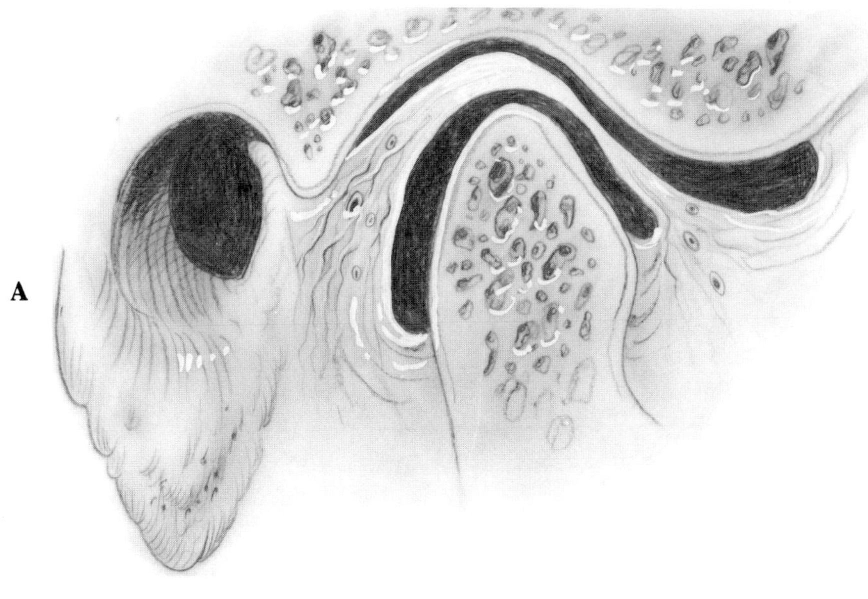

B

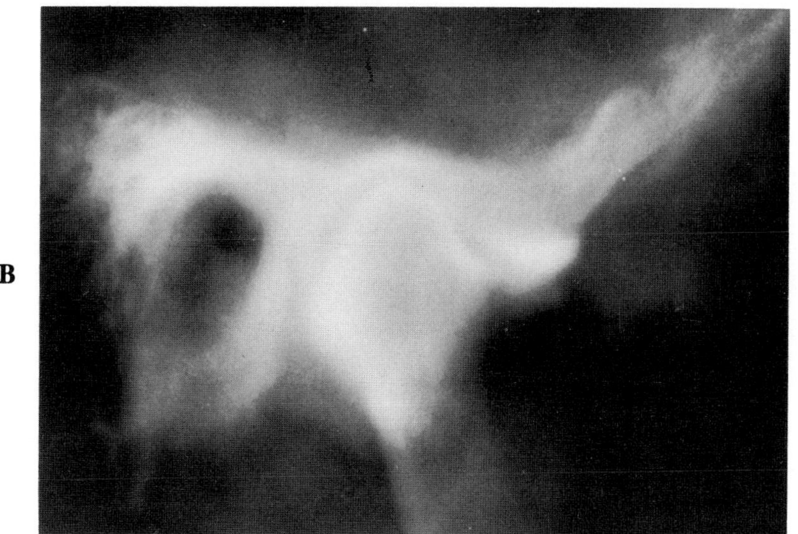

C and **D** As the mandible opens, the condyle rotates into the intermediate zone of the articular disc. Contrast material flows posteriorly as the joint spaces open behind the condyle and in the articular fossa. Contrast material in the upper joint space completely fills the articular fossa. The inferior margin of the upper joint space is smooth and essentially flat. The superior margin of the lower joint space is concave both anteriorly and posteriorly to the condyle. These concave margins delineate the anterior and posterior bands of the disc. The thin area between these bands is the intermediate zone.

C

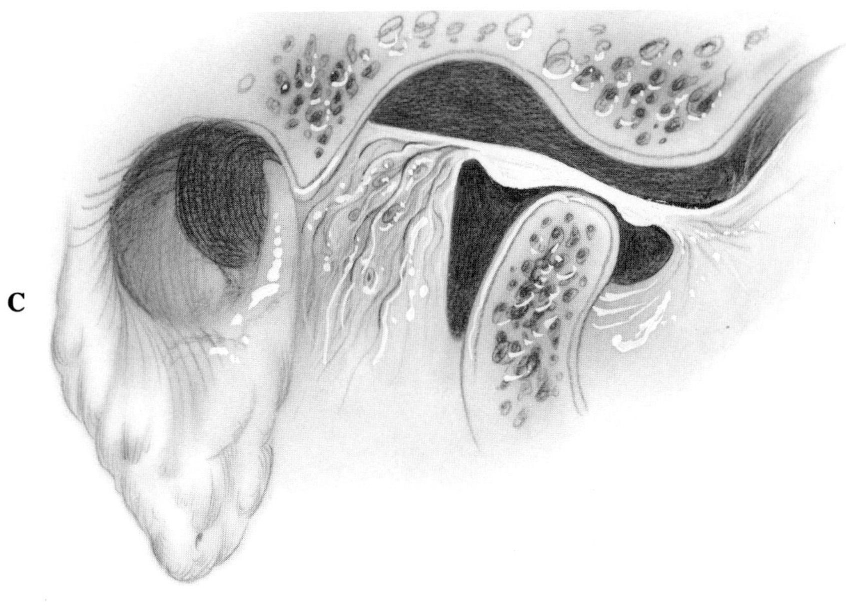

D

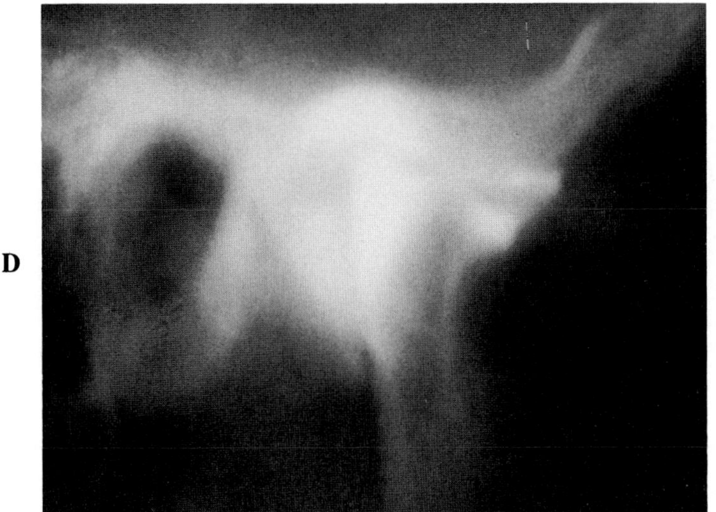

E and **F** In the maximum open position more contrast material flows posteriorly. The disc is positioned slightly posterior in its relationship to the condyle. The anterosuperior surface of the condyle is below the anterior band, and the posterior band and intermediate zone of the disc are positioned above and posterior to the posterosuperior aspect of the condyle.

E

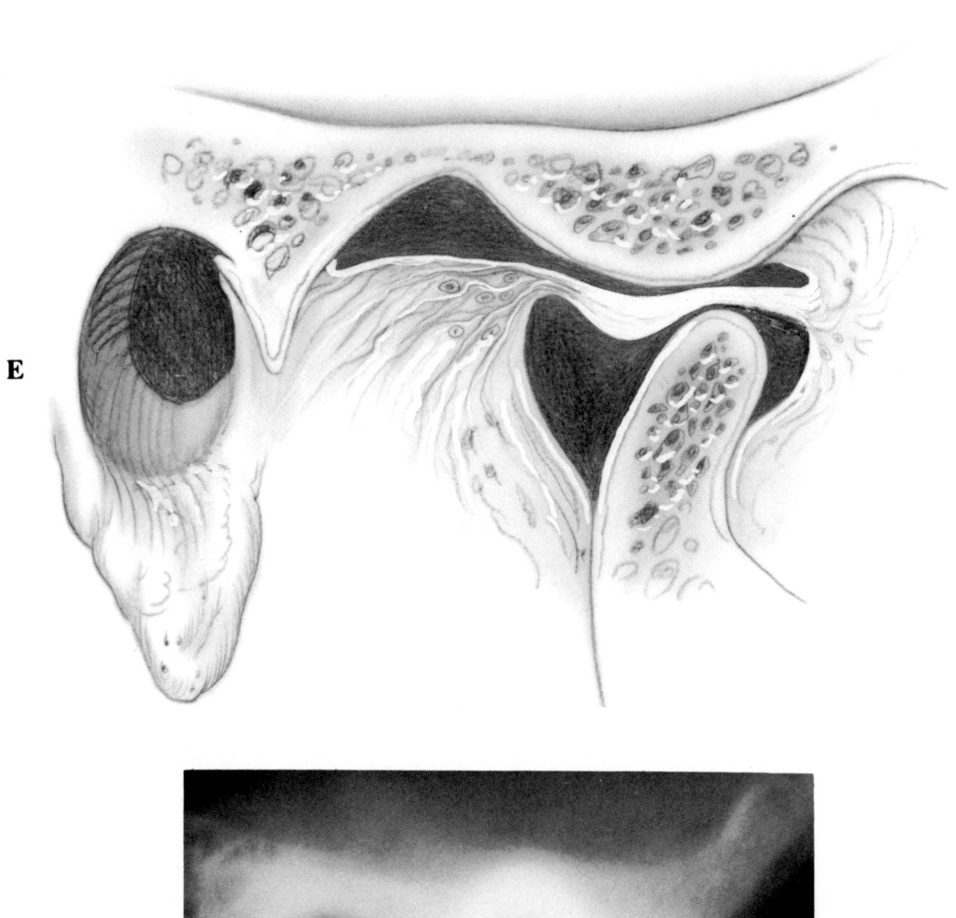

F

Disc Displacement with Reduction—Lower Joint Space (Plain Film)

PLATE 4-6

A and **B** In the closed-mouth position the lower joint extends farther anteriorly than normal. Compare with Plate 4-5, **A** and **B.** The posterior band of the disc is in front of the condyle.

A

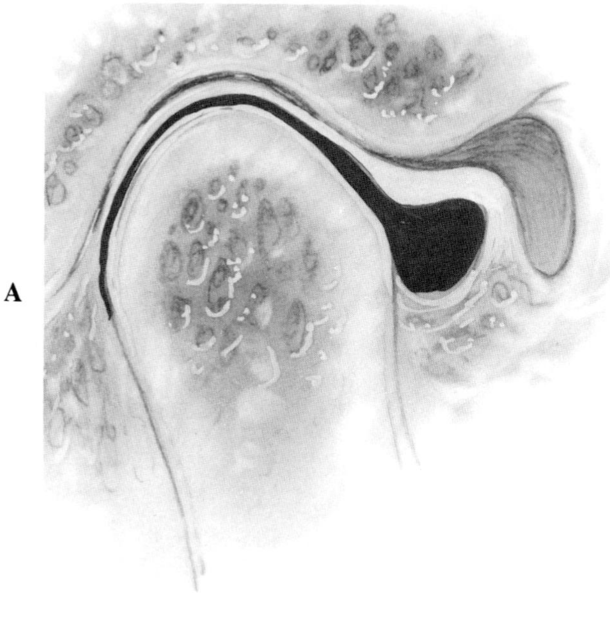

B

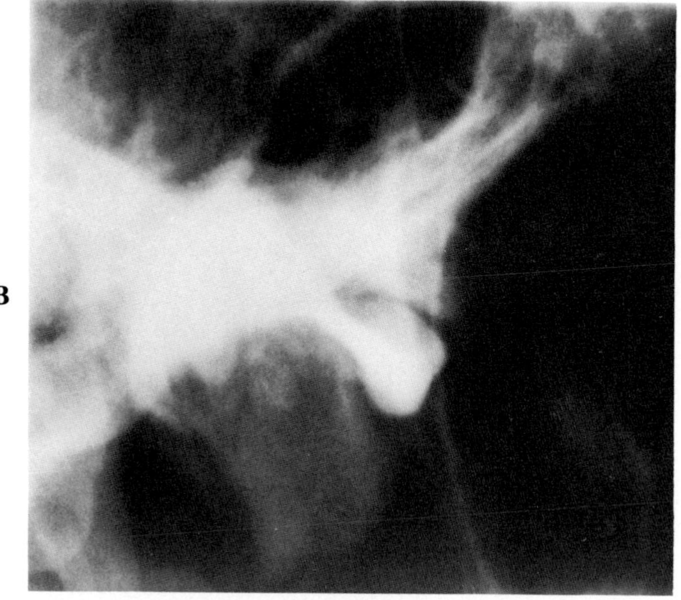

C and **D** As the mandible opens, the condyle pushes against the posterior band of the disc. The lower joint space changes shape as the disc folds upward through the intermediate zone. The posterior band of the disc is indicated by the concave superior margin of the lower joint space in front of the condyle.

E and **F** After the opening click occurs the arthrogram appears normal.

C

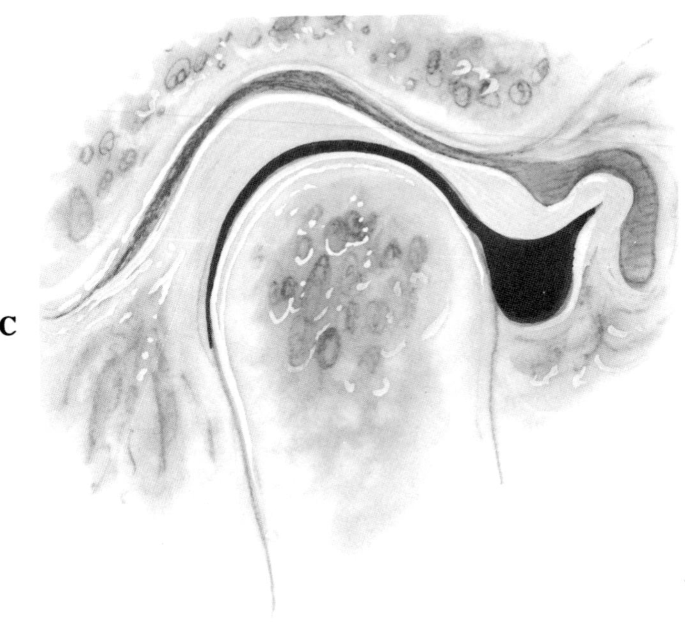

D

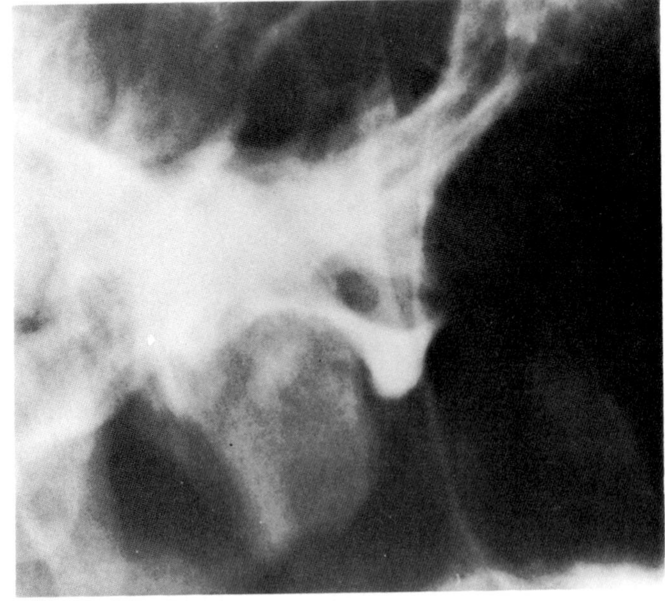

E

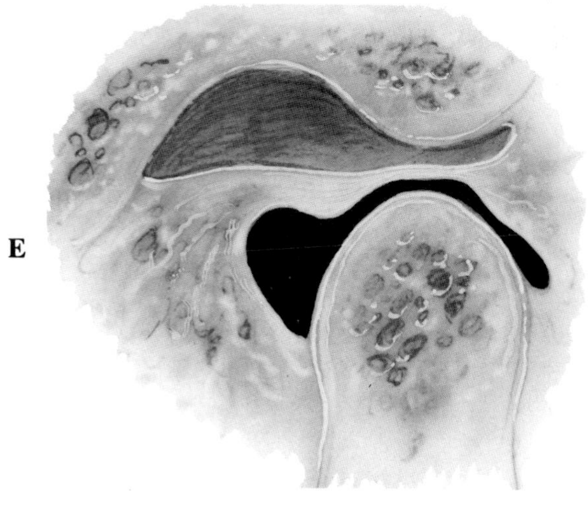

F

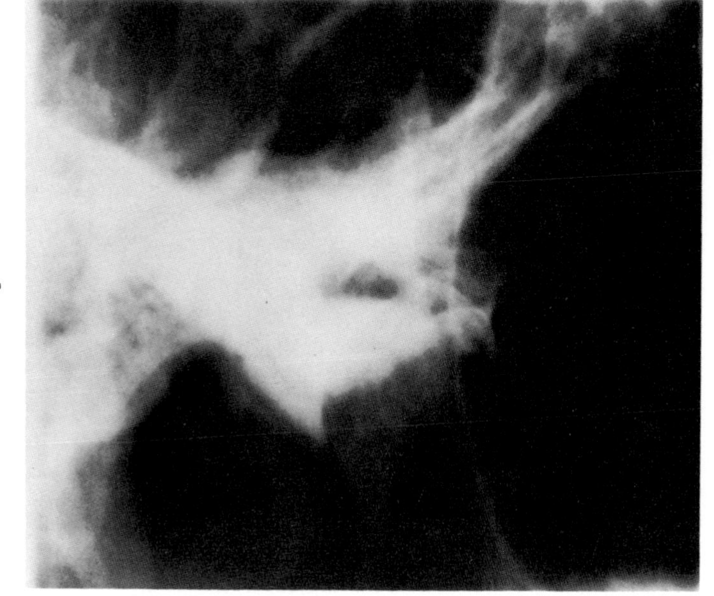

Disc Displacement with Reduction—Both Joint Spaces (Plain Lateral Film)

PLATE 4-7

A and **B** In the closed-mouth position the lower joint space extends as far forward as the upper joint space. The anterior part of the upper joint space is very large and not contiguous with the articular eminence. Compare with Plate 4-6, **A** and **B.** The disc is anterior to the condyle.

A

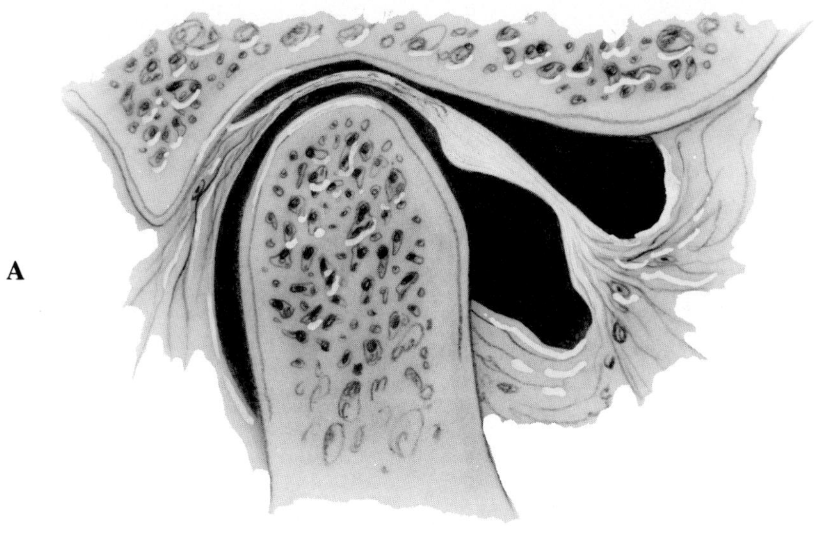

B

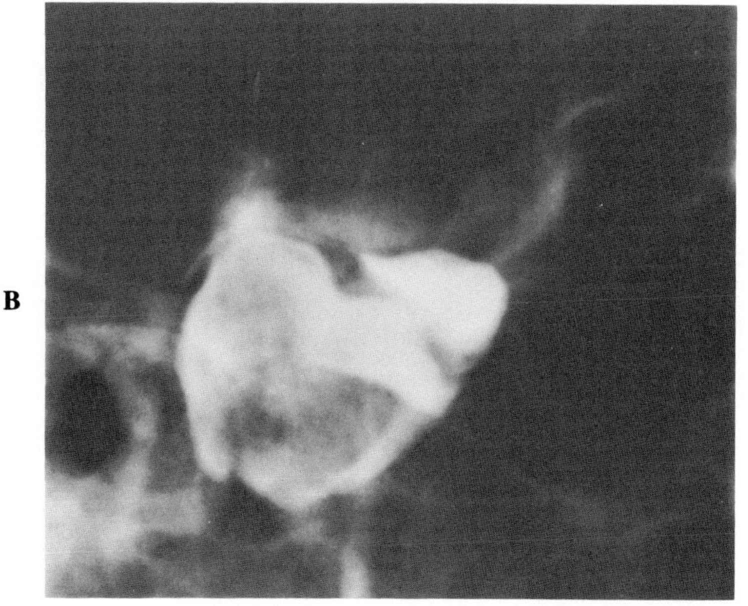

C and **D** As the mandible opens, the condyle pushes against the posterior band of the disc. The lower joint space becomes triangular as the disc folds upward through the intermediate zone. The inferior margin of the upper joint space delineates the superior surface of the disc.

E and **F** After the click occurs the arthrogram appears normal.

C

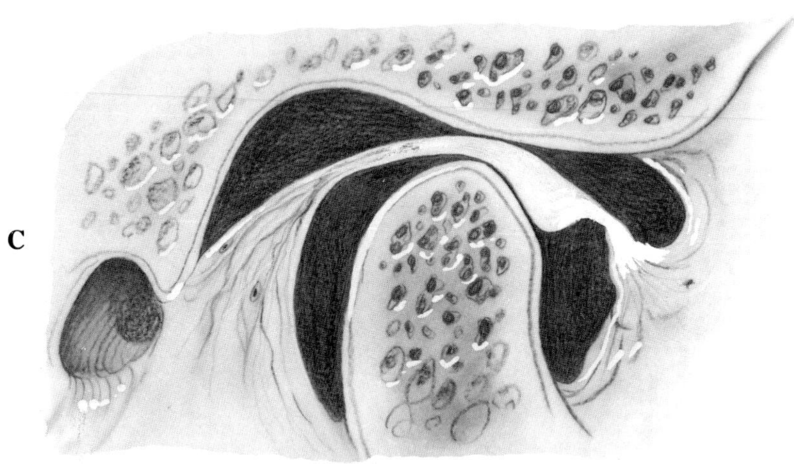

D

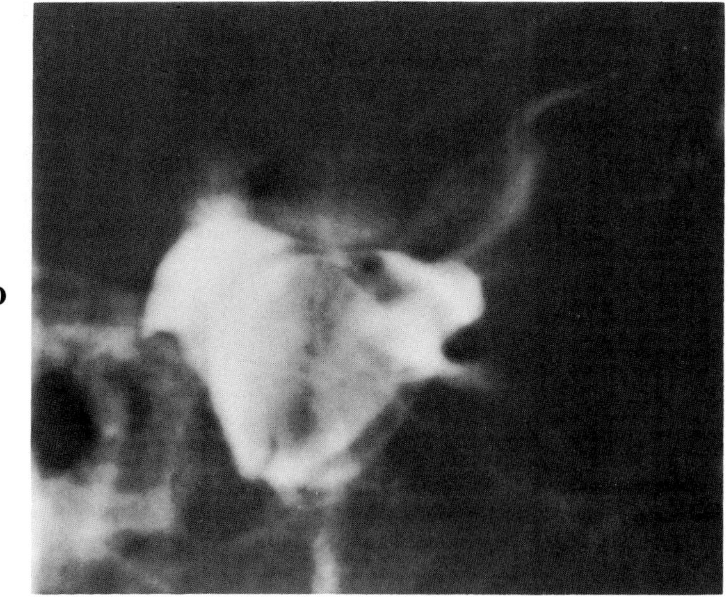

E

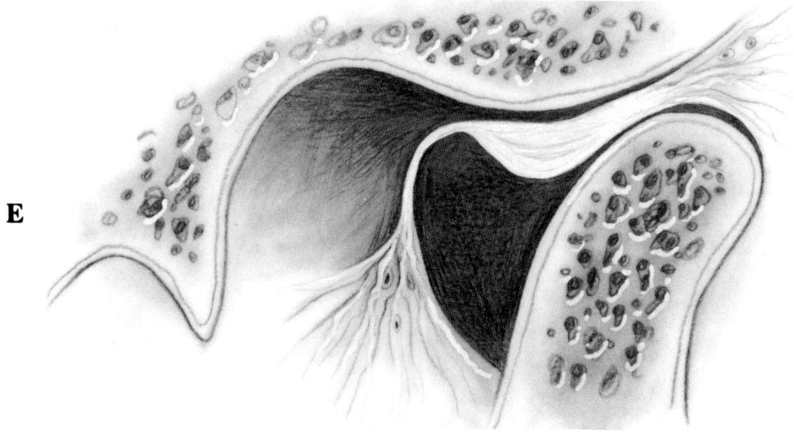

F

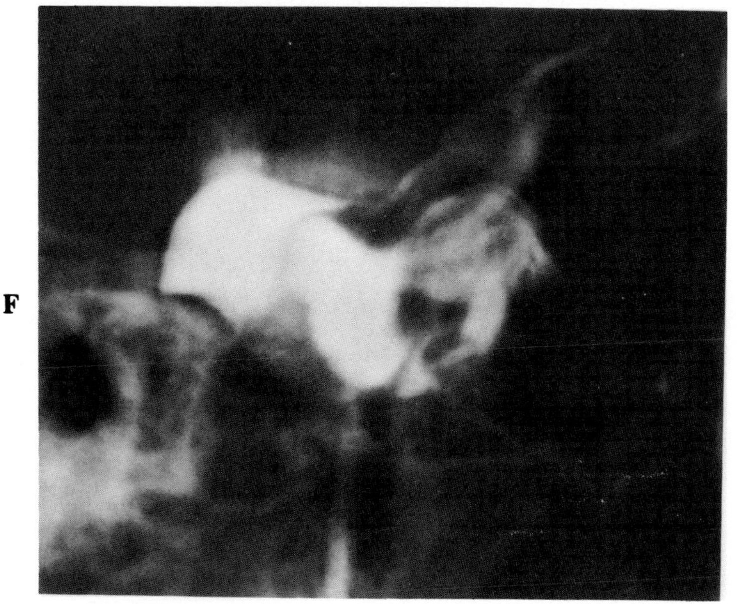

Disc Displacement with Reduction—Both Joint Spaces (Tomogram)

PLATE 4-8

A and **B** In the closed-mouth position the lower joint space extends farther anteriorly than normal. The upper joint space appears normal. The posterior band of the disc is anterior to the condyle.

A

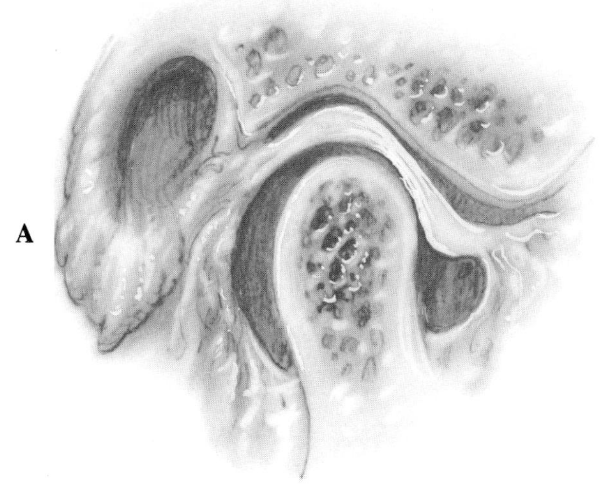

B

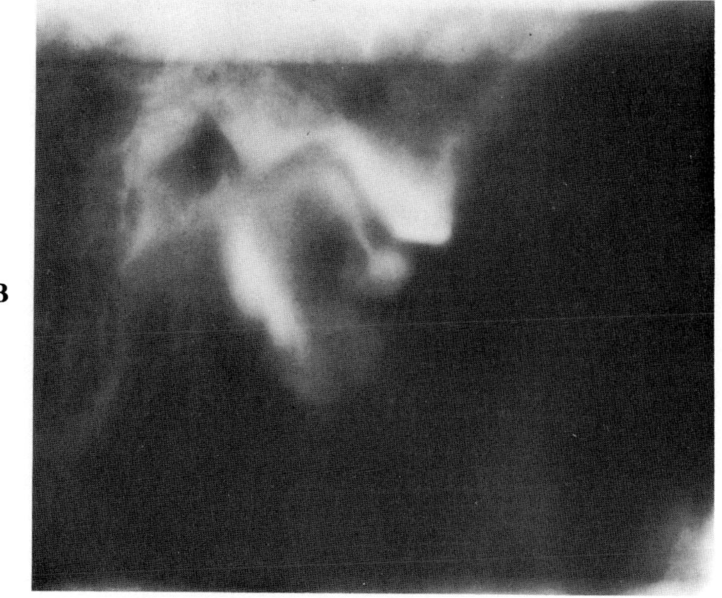

C and **D** As the mandible opens, the condyle pushes against the posterior band of the disc. The lower joint space becomes thinner as the disc folds downward through the intermediate zone. The anterior part of the upper joint space becomes triangular, with the apex pointing downward. Compare with Plate 4-8, **C** and **D.**

E and **F** After the click occurs the arthrogram appears normal.

C

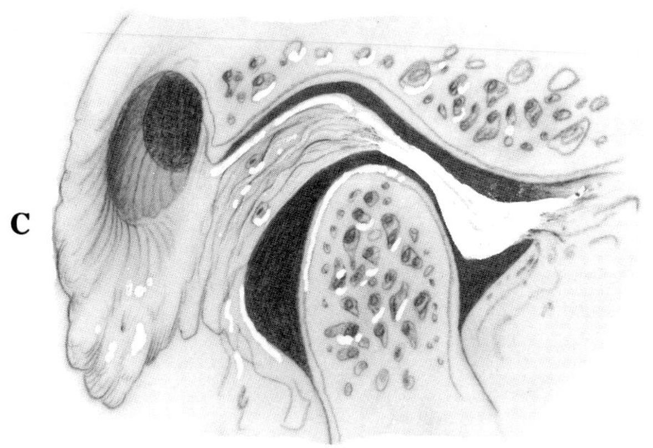

D

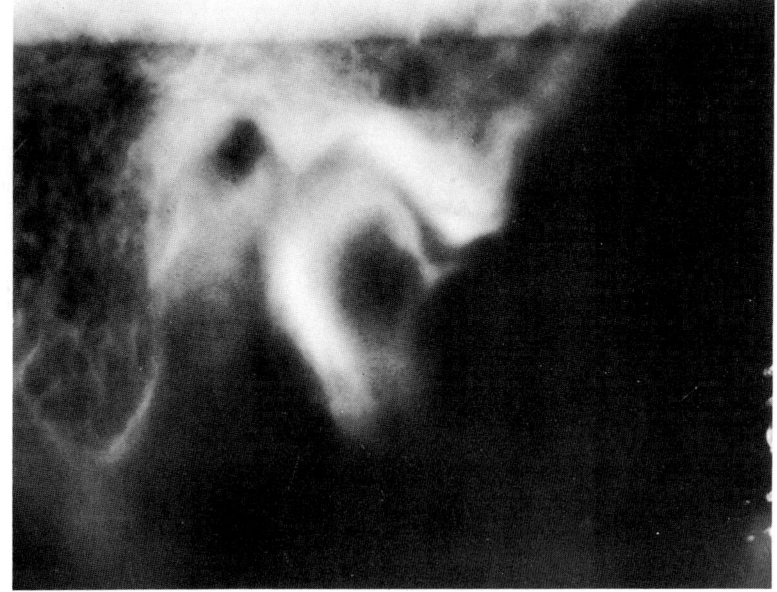

E

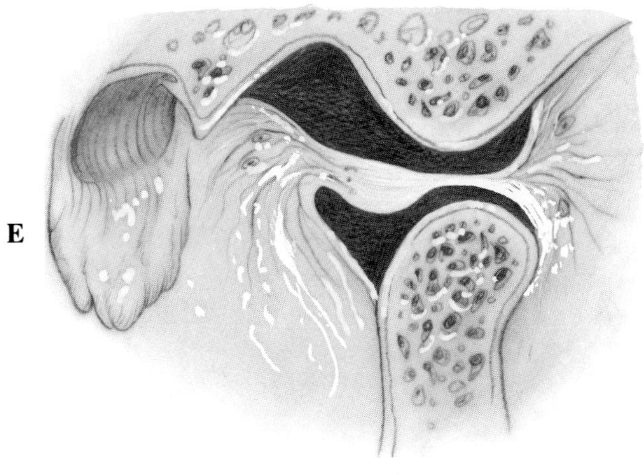

F

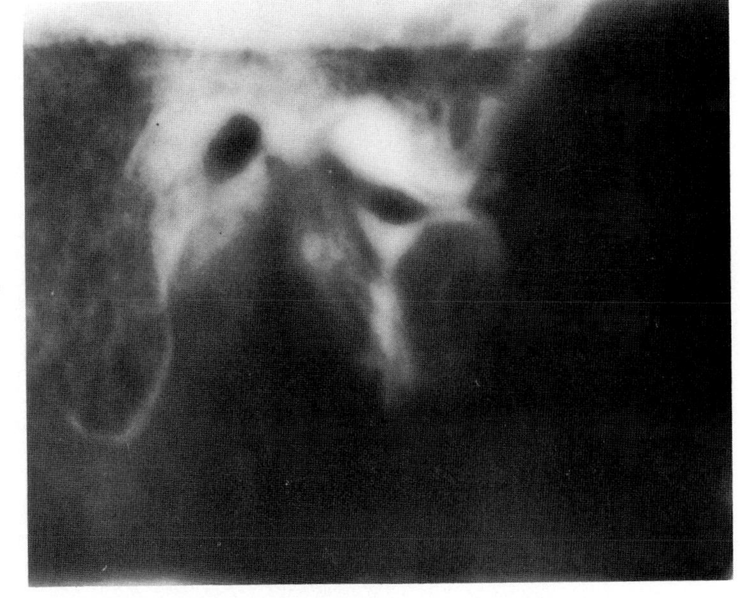

Disc Displacement without Reduction—Lower Joint Space (Plain Film)

PLATE 4-9

A and **B** The lower joint space extends farther anteriorly than normal. The posterior band of the disc, indicated by the concave superior margin of the lower joint space, is anterior to the condyle.

A

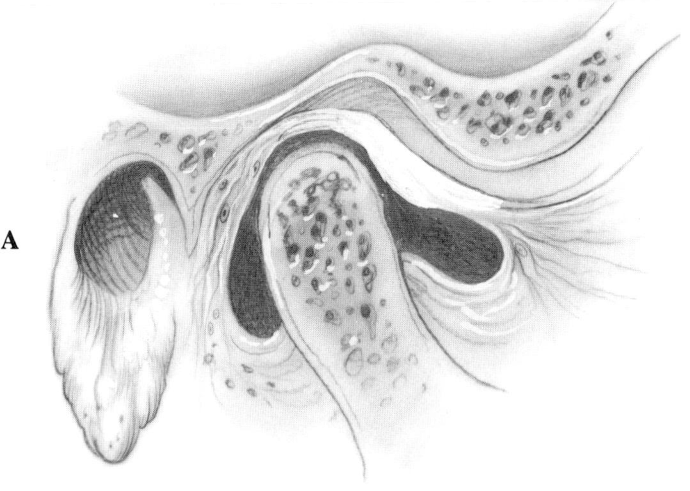

B

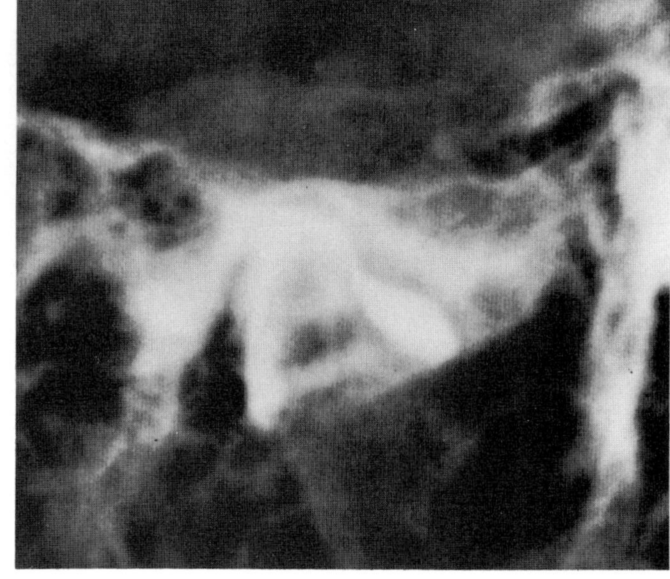

C and **D** As the mandible opens, the condyle pushes against the posterior band of the disc. The lower joint space changes shape as the disc folds upward through the intermediate area. During maximum opening the disc does not reduce to a normal position. Note that the condyle does not translate very far.

C

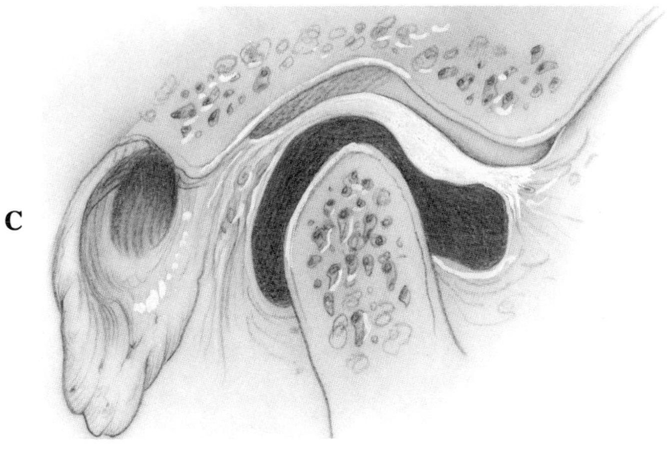

D

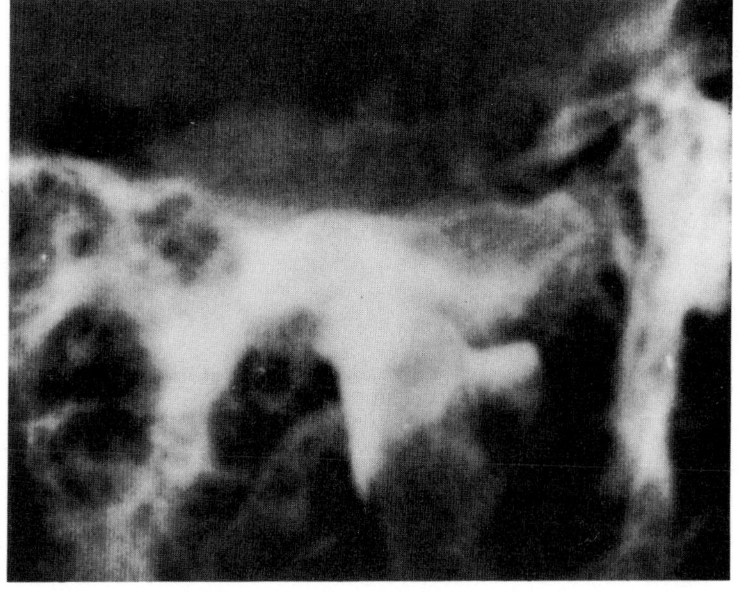

Disc Displacement without Reduction—Lower Joint Space (Tomogram)

PLATE 4-10

A The lower joint space extends farther anteriorly than normal. The concave superior margin of the lower joint space in front of the condyle indicates the position of the posterior band of the disc. The convex area is the intermediate zone, and the most anterior concave margin is the anterior band.

B As the condyle translates, the disc is pushed anteriorly and folds upward through the intermediate zone.

C The disc does not reduce even though the condyle has translated to the height of the articular eminence.

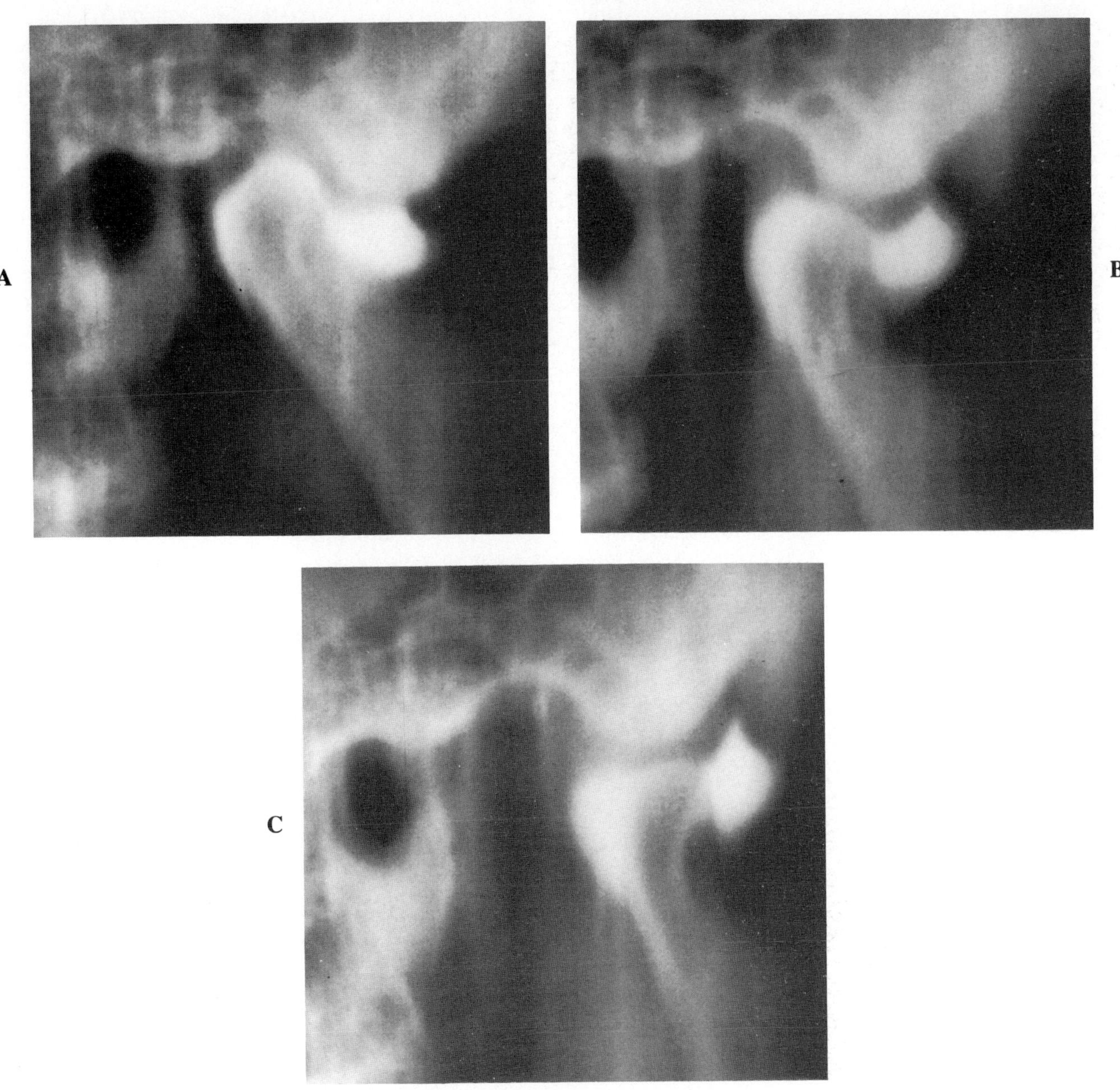
A
B
C

Disc Displacement without Reduction—Upper and Lower Joint Spaces (Tomogram)—cont'd

PLATE 4-11

A and **B** The lower joint space extends quite far anteriorly. The upper joint space appears normal. The disc is anterior to the condyle.

A

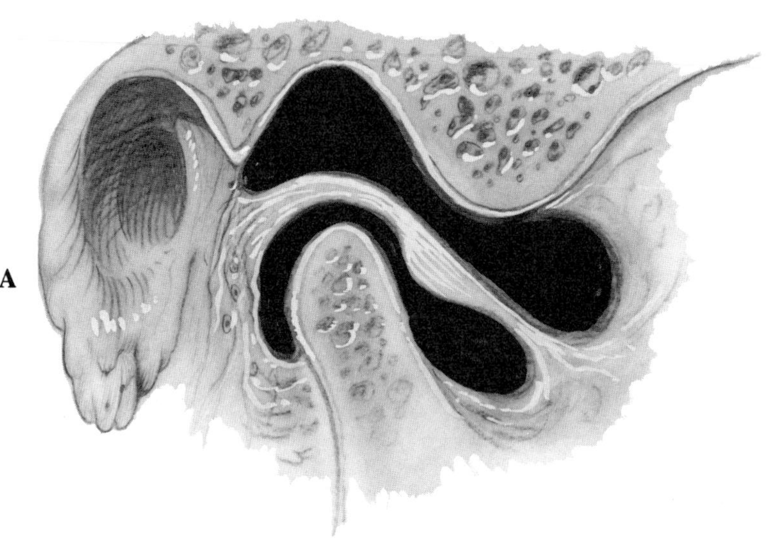

B

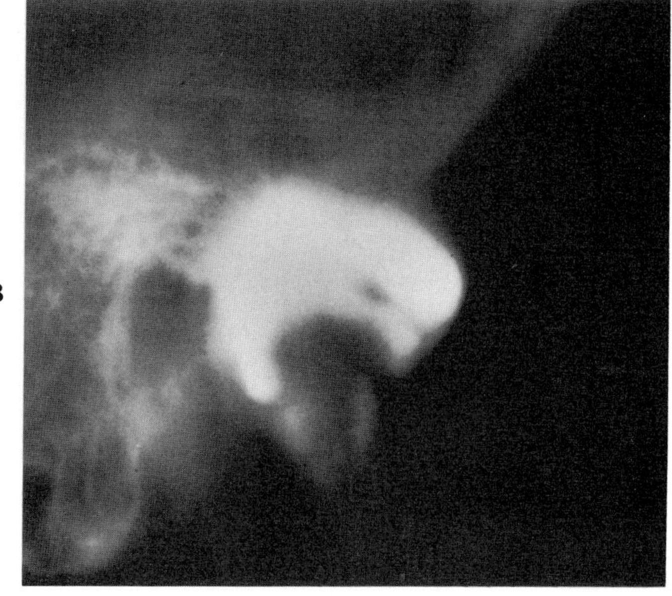

C and **D** As the mandible opens, the condyle pushes against the posterior band of the disc. The disc folds upward through the intermediate zone and does not reduce to a normal position.

C

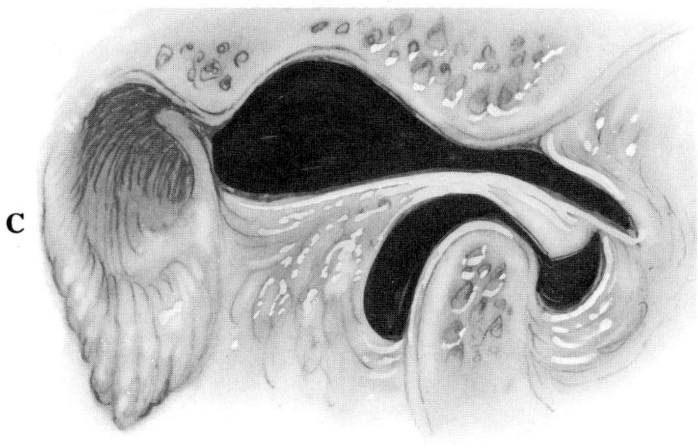

D

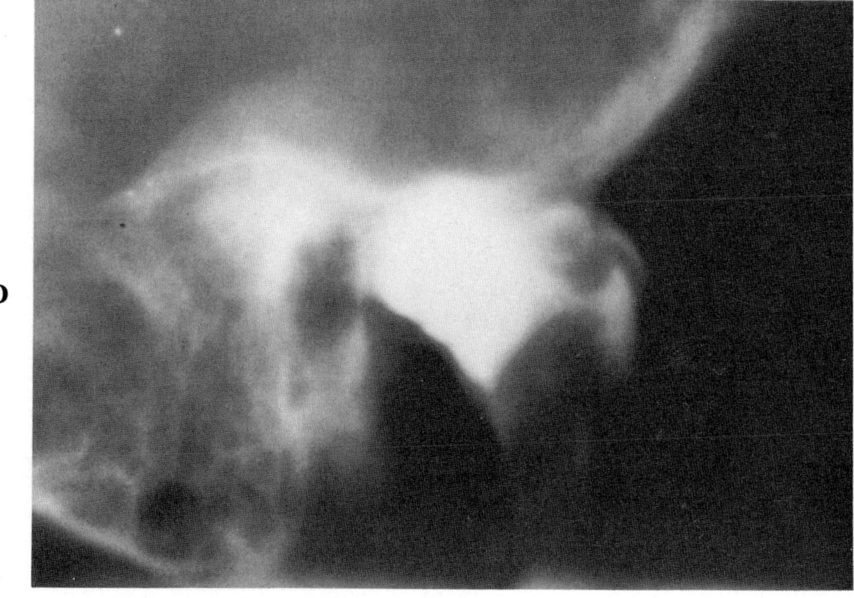

Disc Displacement without Reduction—Upper and Lower Joint Spaces (Tomogram)—cont'd

PLATE 4-12

A and **B** The lower joint space extends very far anteriorly and is larger than normal. The upper joint space is not contiguous with the articular eminence. The very thick disc is anterior to the condyle. The intermediate zone and anterior band extend beyond the height of the articular eminence.

A

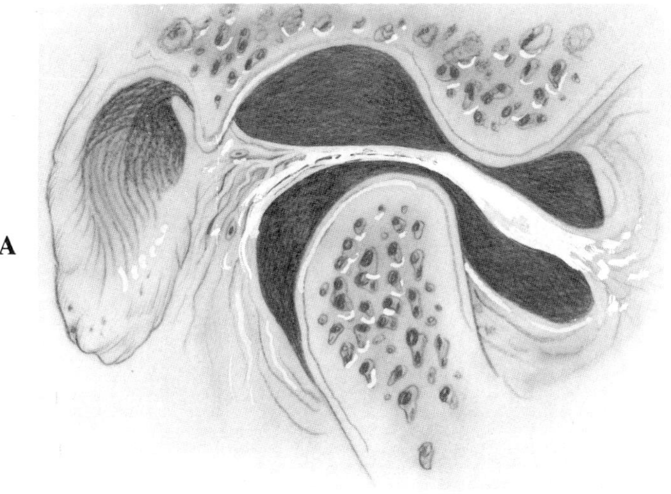

B

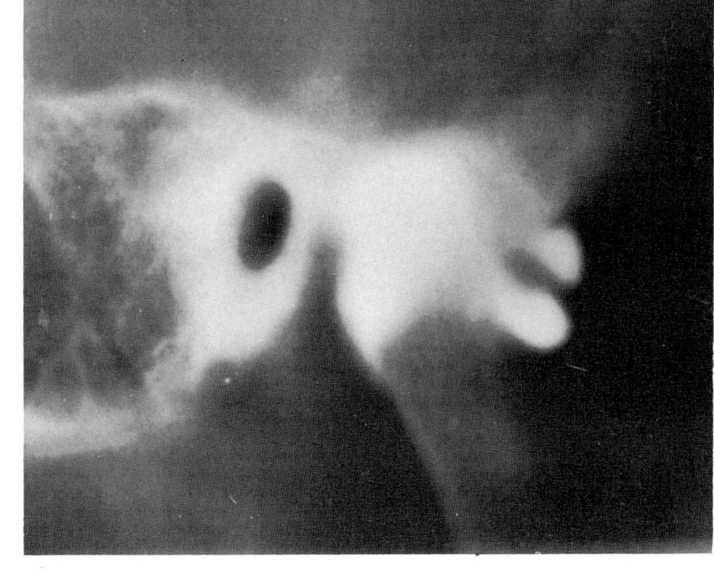

C and **D** During opening of the mandible the disc is pushed anteriorly and folds upward through the intermediate zone. Note the thin margin of contrast material in the upper joint space that delineates the superior surface of the disc. The condyle translates very well.

C

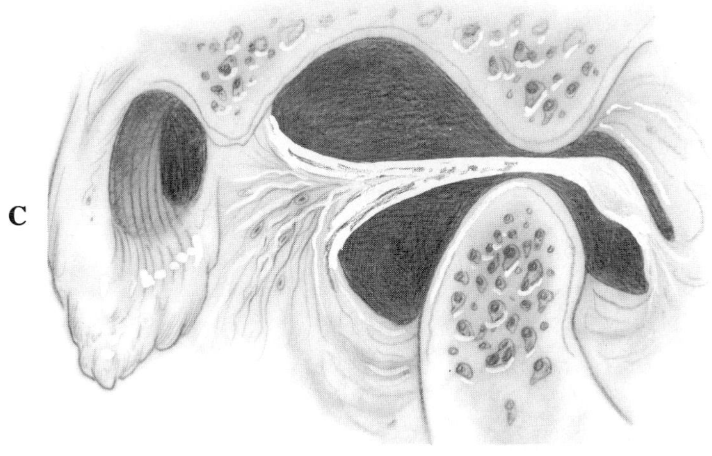

D

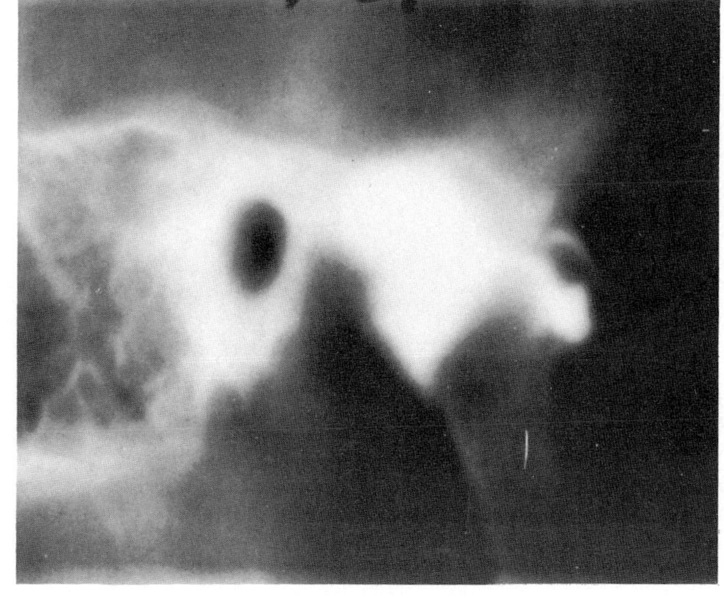

Disc Displacement without Reduction—Perforation (Plain Film)

PLATE 4-13

A Perforation of the disc or its attachments is indicated by the simultaneous filling of both joint spaces when only one space has been injected. This arthrogram shows that both the upper and lower spaces have been injected. Note the needle in the lower joint space. The disc is also displaced anteriorly. Only a small amount of disc remains.

B The disc does not reduce on opening.

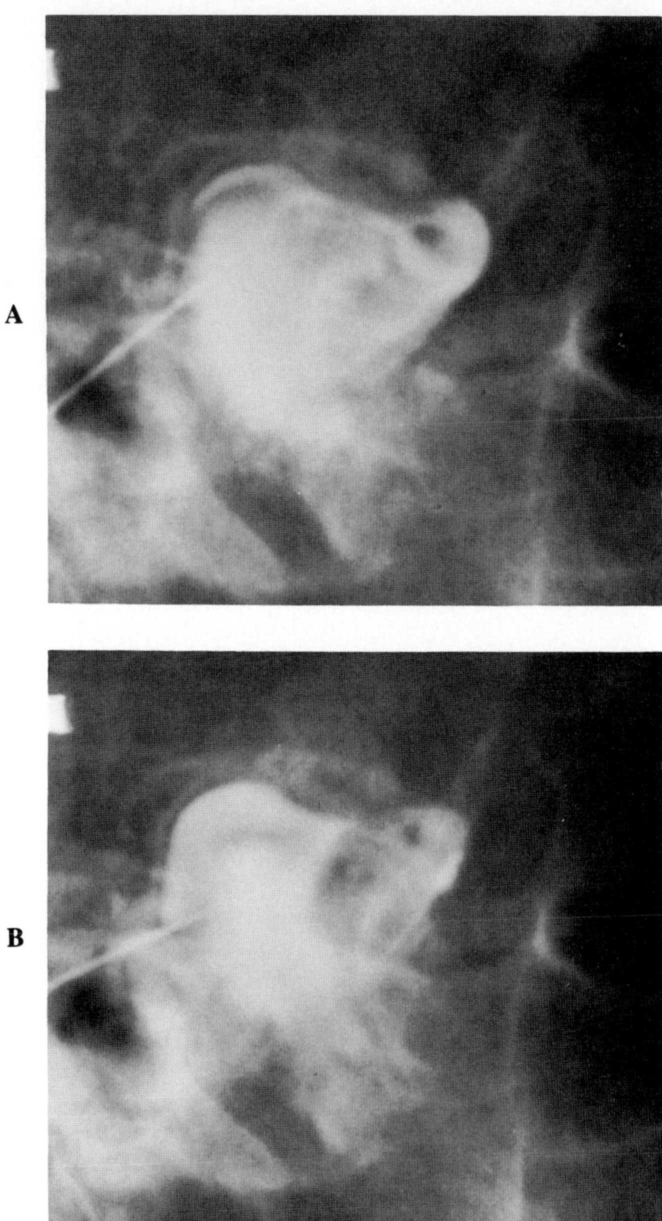
A
B

Disc Displacement without Reduction—Perforation and "Loose Body" (Tomogram)

PLATE 4-14

A and **B** During this arthrogram both joint spaces fill simultaneously when the lower joint space is injected. This indicates a perforation of the disc or its attachments. The disc is also anteriorly displaced, as demonstrated by the anterior extension of the lower joint space.

A

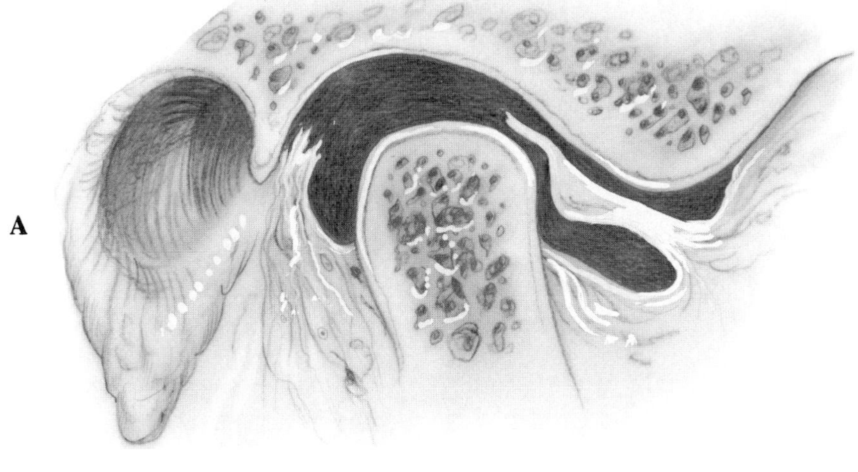

B

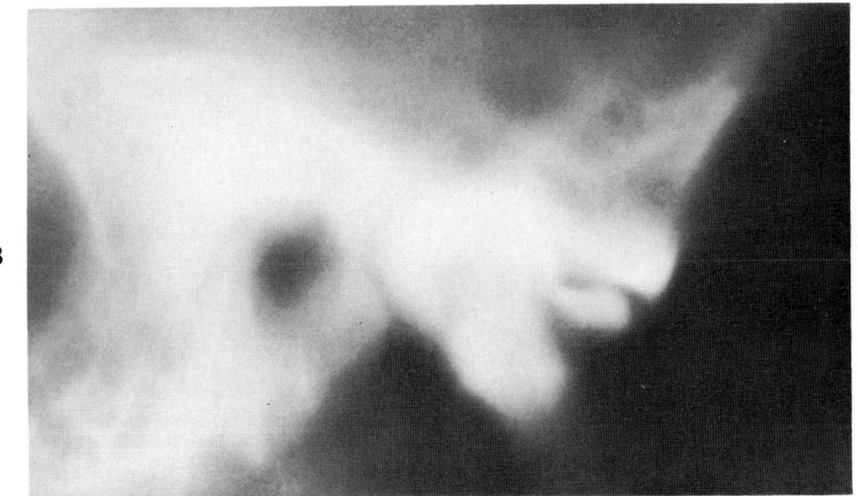

C and **D** During opening of the mandible the condyle pushes the disc forward and the disc folds upward through the intermediate area. Note the thin margin of contrast material delineating the superior surface of the disc. Also note the radiolucent round object in the lower joint space. This is a loose body, as may be seen in synovial chrondrometaplasia. It may also represent an air bubble accidently injected into the lower joint space.

C

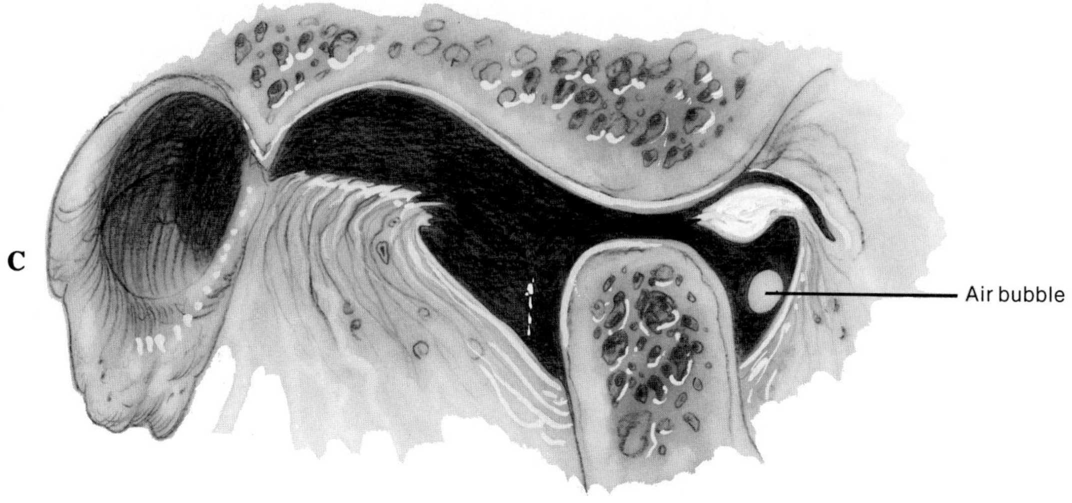

D

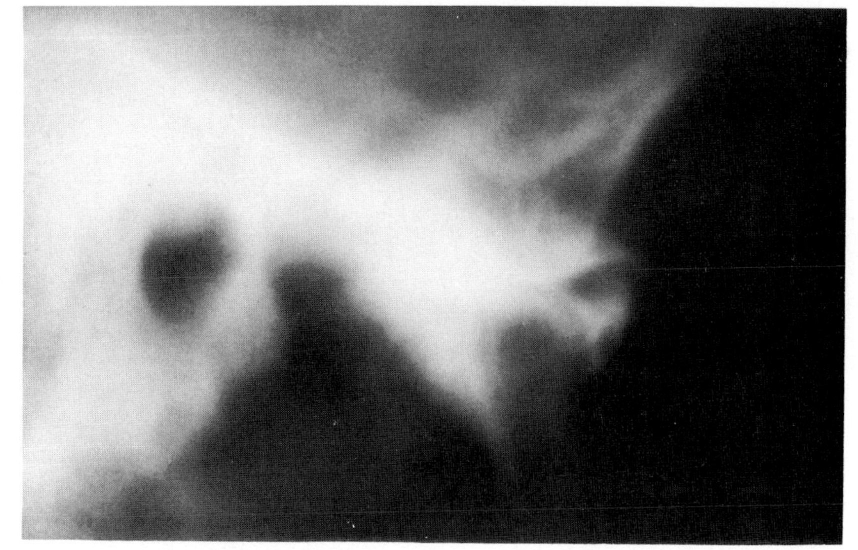

Disc Displacement and Adhesions in the Upper Joint Space

PLATE 4-15

A and **B** This very thick disc is displaced anteriorly. The upper joint space is not smooth and uniformly dense with contrast material. There are two filling defects in the upper joint space, which indicate fibrous adhesions.

A

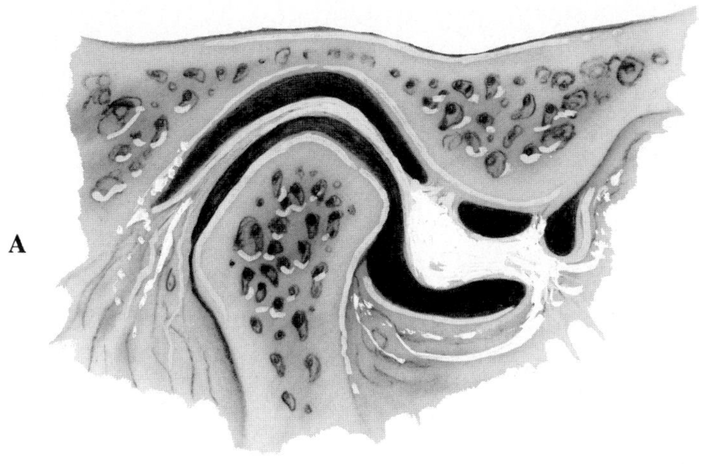

B

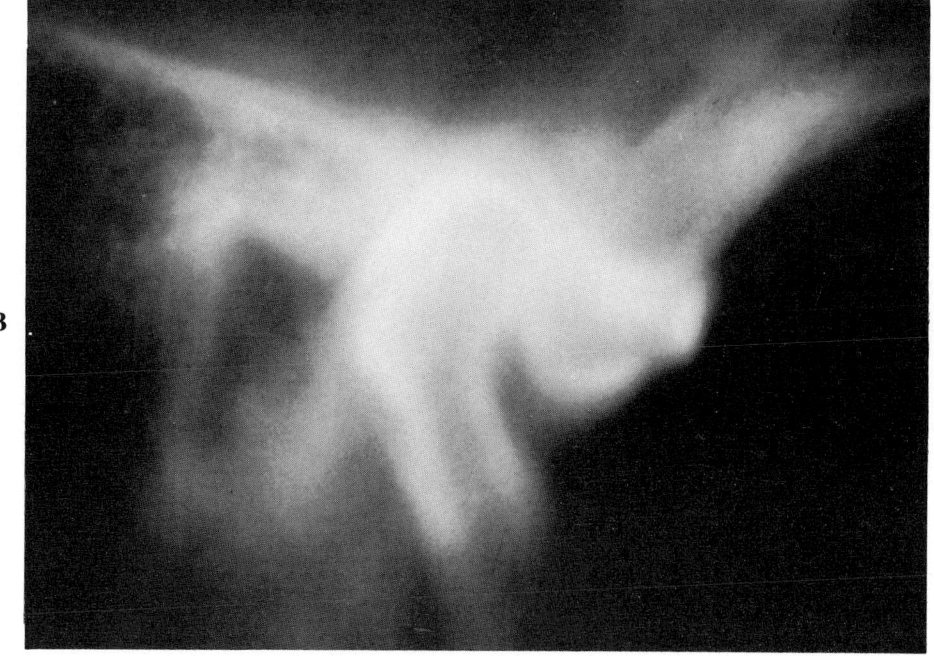

Arthrographic Findings Compared to Surgical Findings

In our experience of having compared arthrographic and surgical findings in several hundred cases arthrography has proven to be a reliable method for determining position, morphology, and integrity of the disc. Plates 4-16 to 4-20 illustrate some comparisons of arthrographic and surgical findings.

PLATE 4-16

A This arthrogram shows that the disc is anteriorly displaced in front of the condyle.

B The upper joint space has been opened. The disc is displaced anteriorly, as shown by the arthrogram.

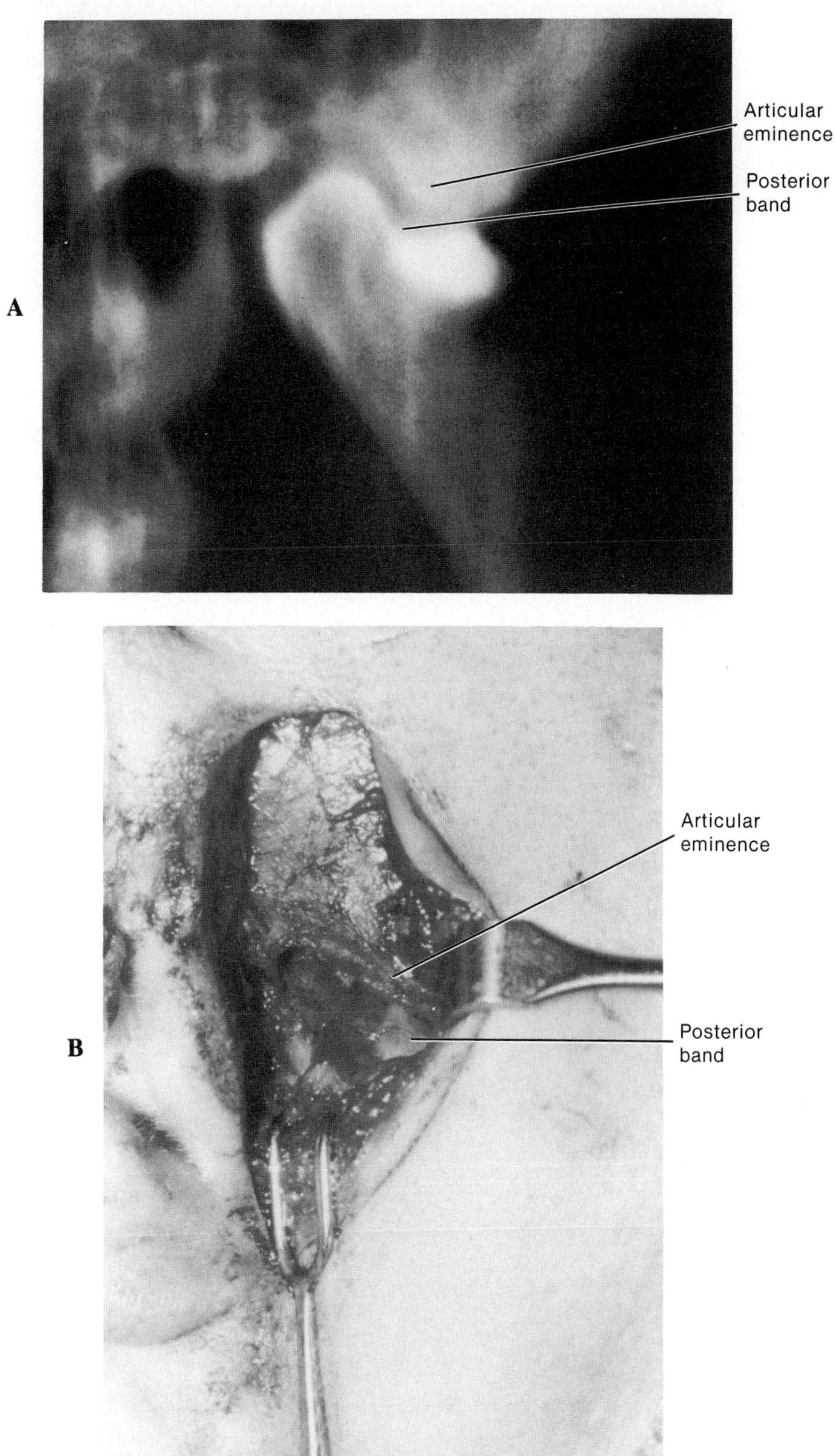
A
Articular eminence
Posterior band
B
Articular eminence
Posterior band

PLATE 4-17

A This arthrogram shows the disc folded downward through the intermediate zone as the condyle pushes against the posterior band.

B The upper joint space has been opened. The disc folds downward through the intermediate zone as the condyle is moved anteriorly. Compare the triangular area of the upper joint space with the same area in **A.**

A

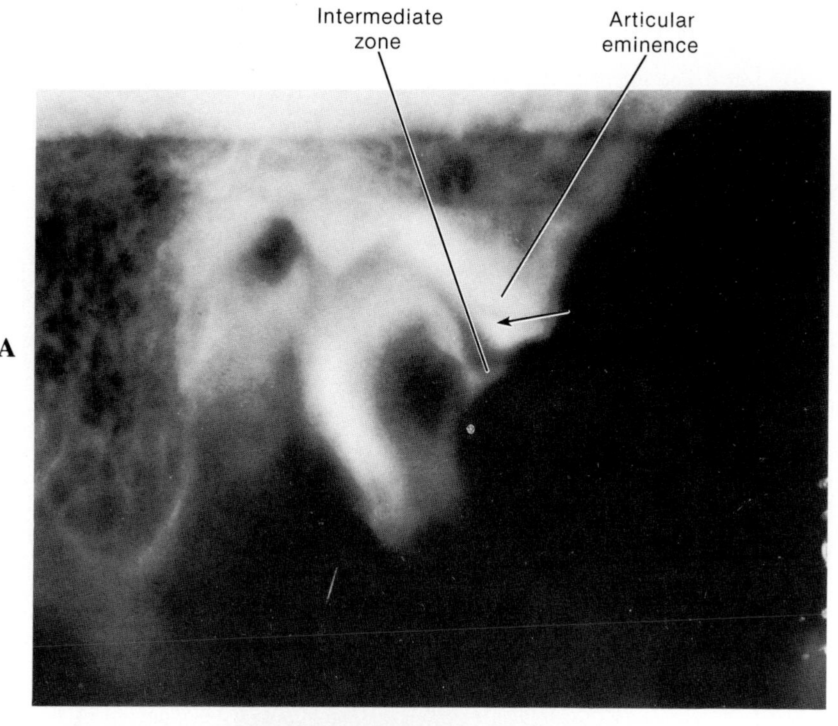
Intermediate zone
Articular eminence

B

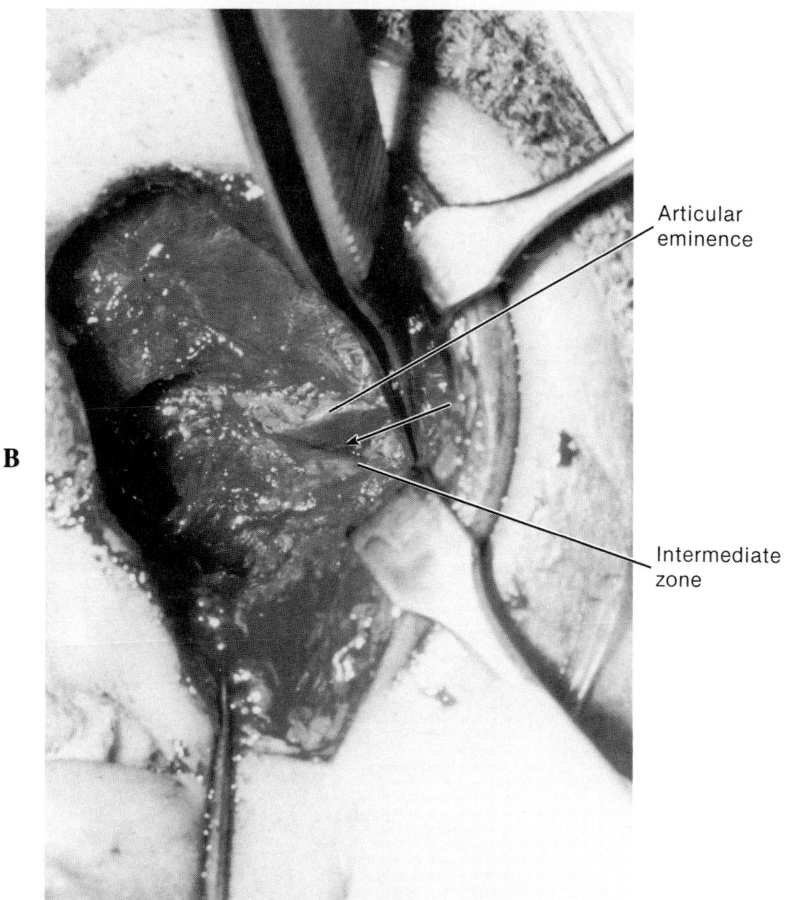
Articular eminence
Intermediate zone

PLATE 4-18

A This arthrogram shows anterior displacement of the disc.

B The upper joint space has been opened. The disc is anteriorly displaced.

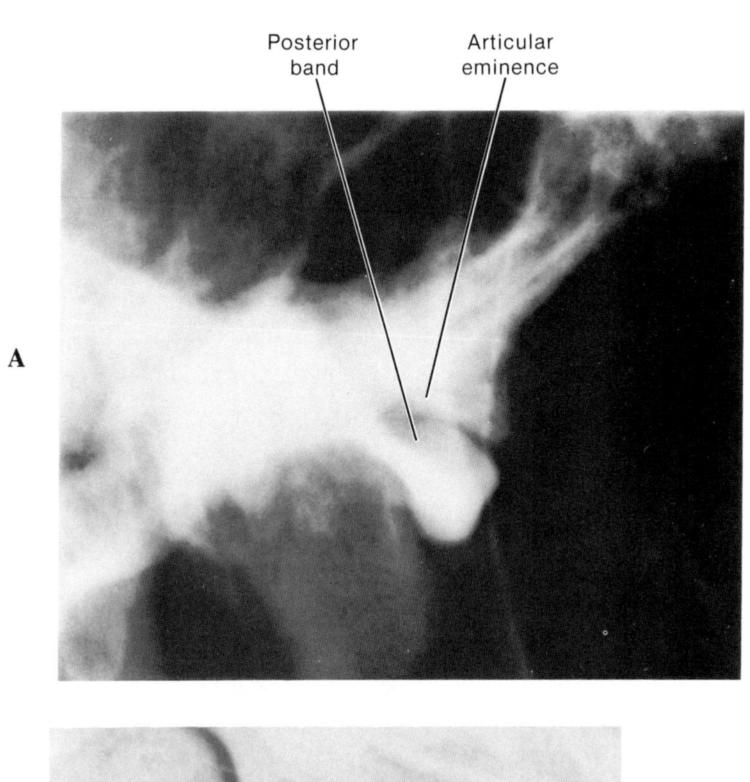

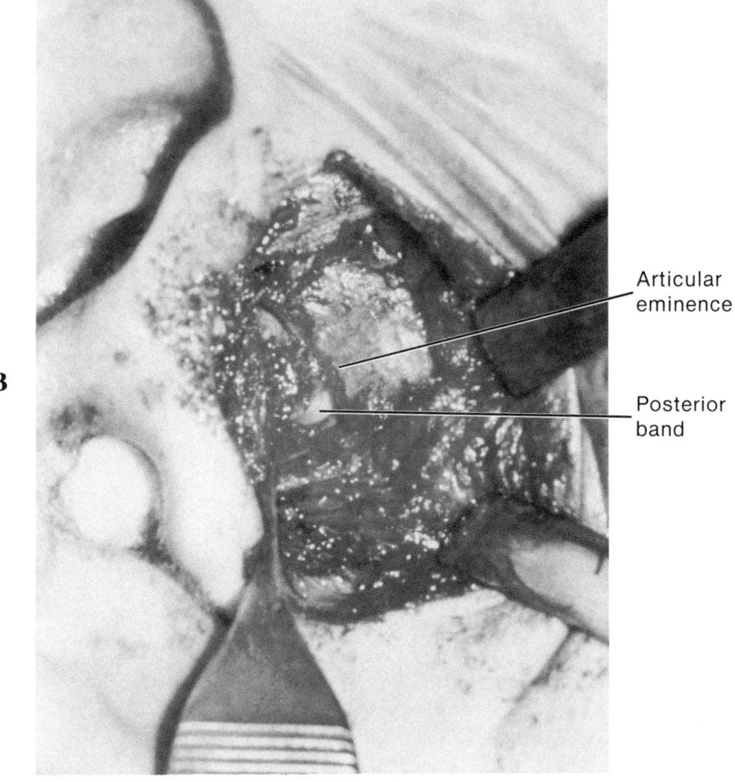

C This open-mouth arthrogram shows reduction of the disc to a normal position.
D The condyle has been moved anteriorly and the disc is reduced to a normal relationship with the condyle.

C

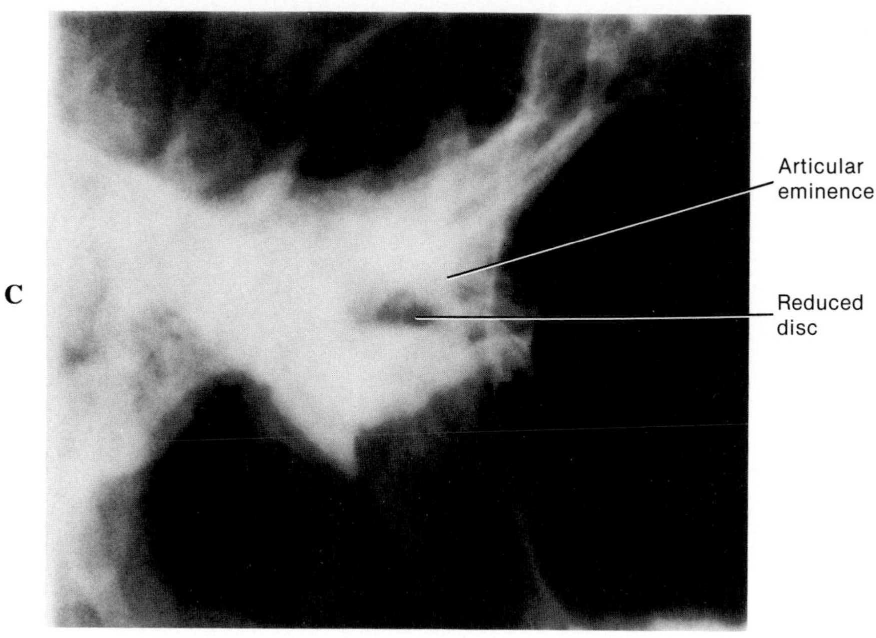

D

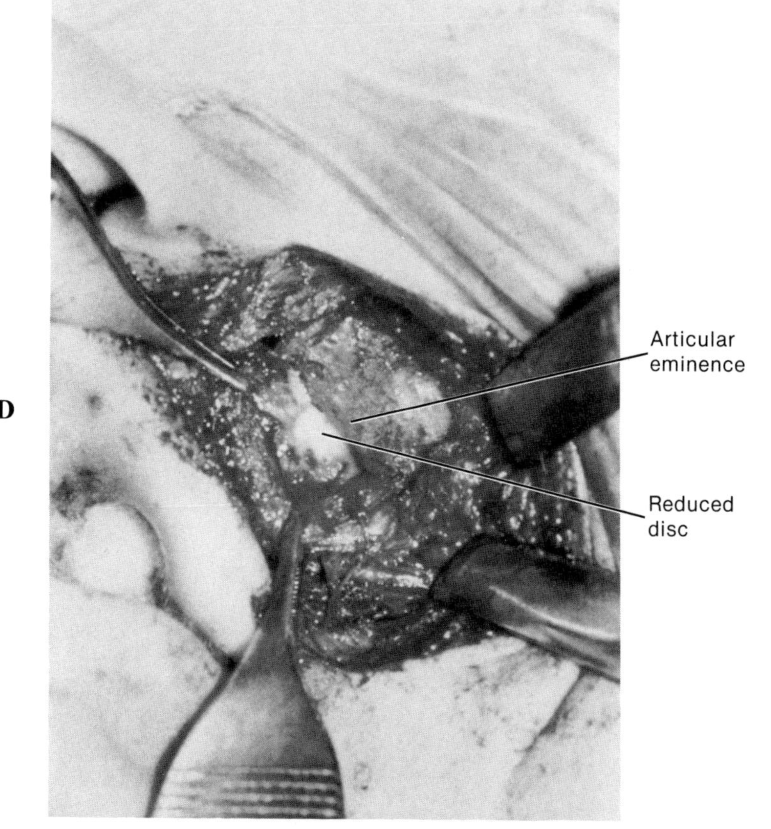

PLATE 4-19

A This arthrogram demonstrates anterior displacement of the disc. The posterior band is thick and has a convex inferior surface. The intermediate zone is quite narrow.

B The disc has a thick posterior band and a convex inferior surface. The intermediate zone is very narrow.

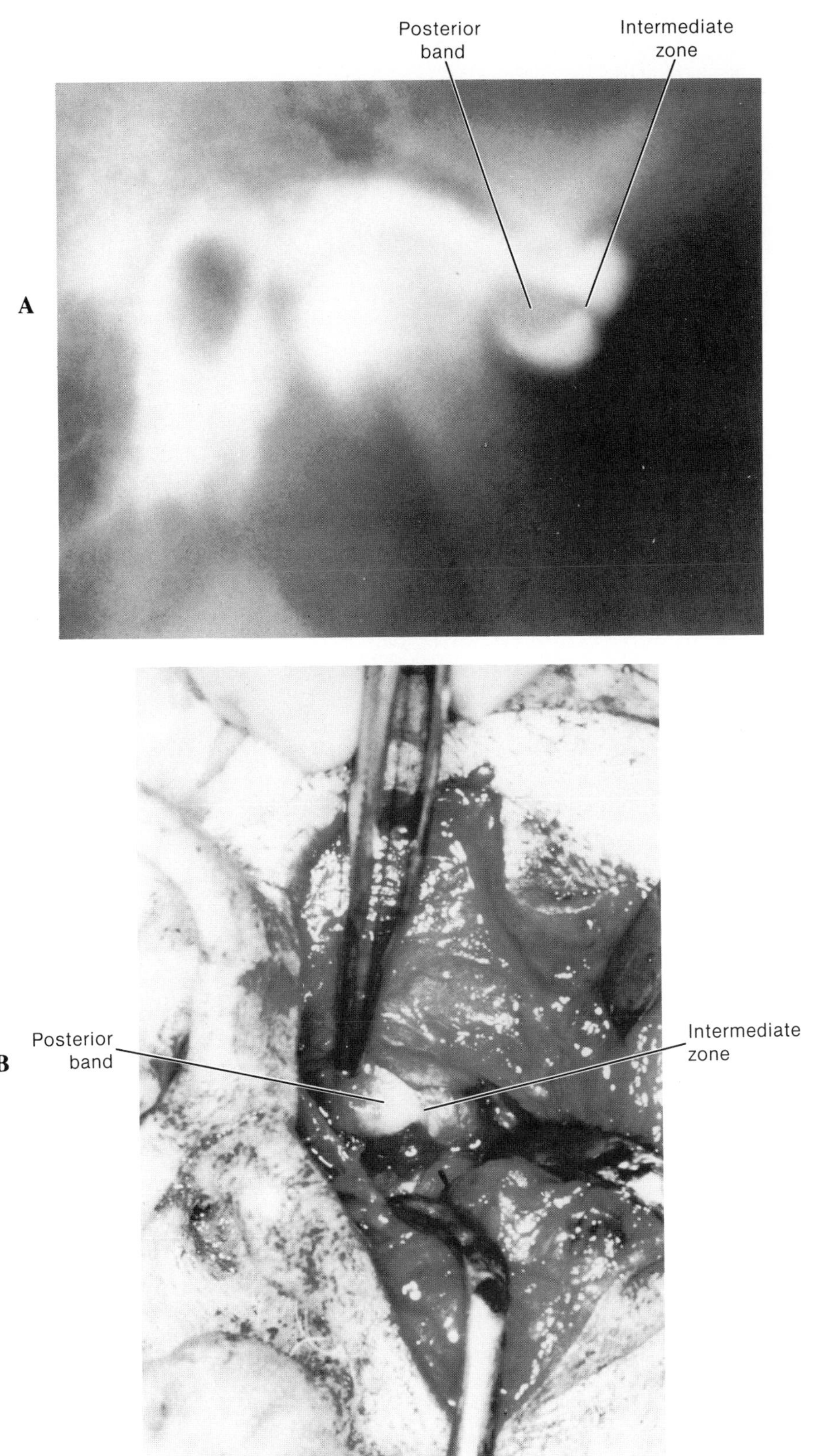
Posterior band
Intermediate zone
A
Posterior band
B
Intermediate zone

PLATE 4-20

A This arthrogram demonstrates a perforation of the disc or its attachments.

B The perforation is large and located at the junction of the posterior band and posterior attachment tissue.

A

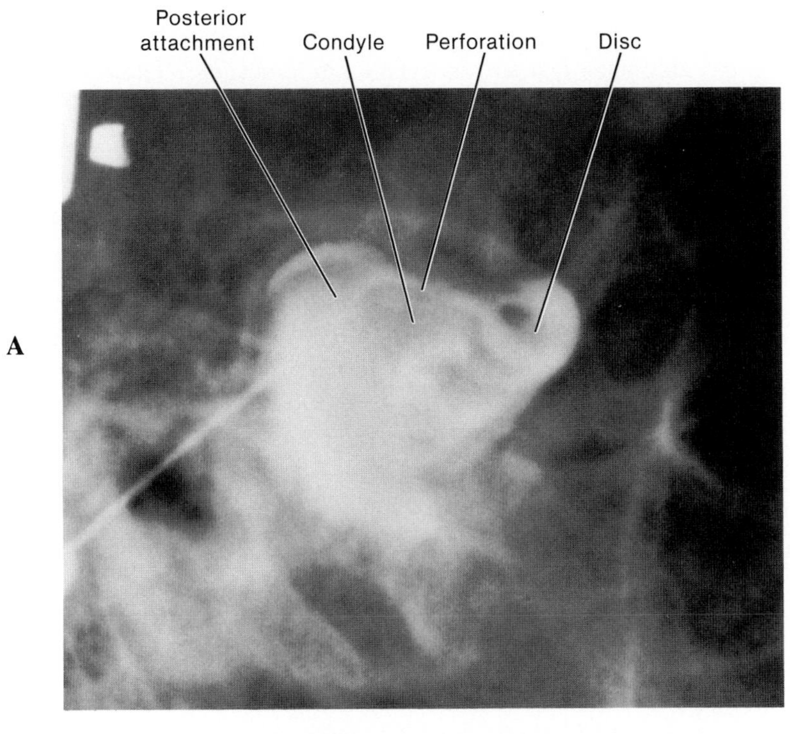
Posterior attachment
Condyle
Perforation
Disc

B

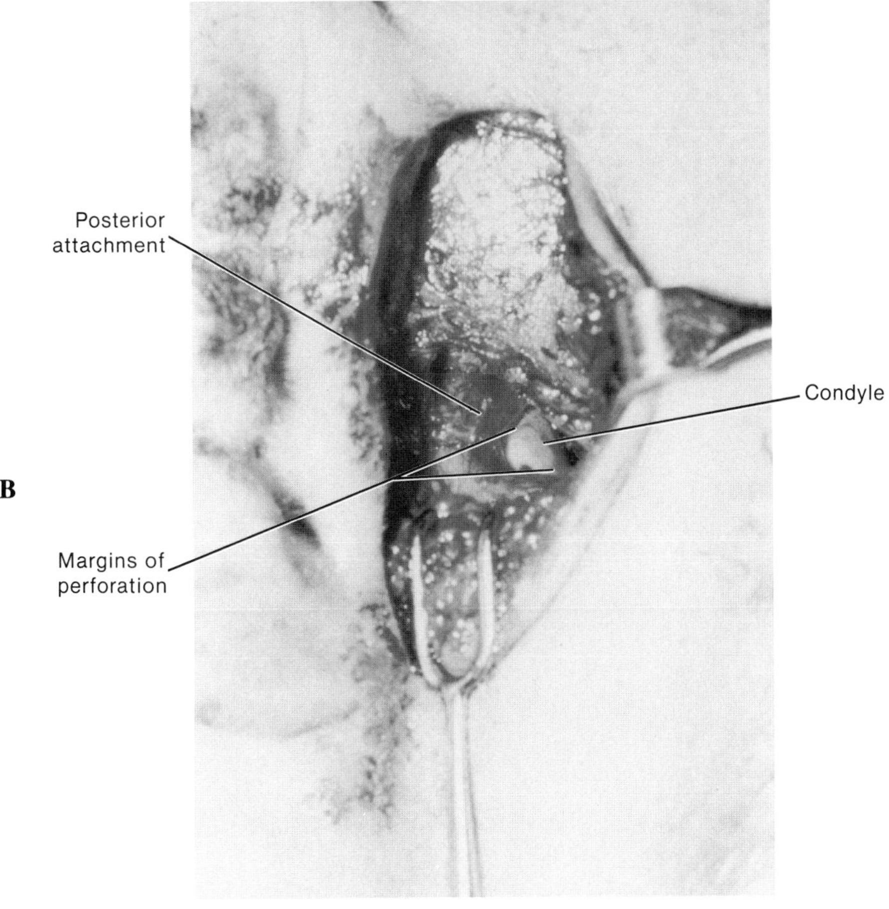
Posterior attachment
Condyle
Margins of perforation

COMPLICATIONS

Arthrography has proven to be a safe procedure. The few complications reported are as follows:

1. *Facial muscle paralysis secondary to the local anesthetic*. This is temporary and resolves as the anesthetic wears off. The patient should be cautioned to protect the involved eye until the paralysis has resolved. Reassurance of the patient that the paralysis is temporary is important.
2. *Hematoma over the joint area*. If a hematoma occurs, it is managed with immediate pressure followed by the application of ice packs over the area. The next day moist heat is used over the area. The hematoma usually resolves in 3 to 4 days.
3. *Closed-lock*. Occasionally a patient who has a reducing disc will develop closed-lock after the arthrogram. This is more likely to occur in patients who have intermittent closed-lock. The patient should be reassured that the problem usually resolves in a few days.
4. *Infection*. There have been no documented cases of infection following an arthrogram.
5. *Broken catheter tip*. When a catheter is placed into the joint space, there is the possibility for the tip to break off. We are aware of three cases. The needle should not be moved in and out of the catheter because of the possibility of cutting the catheter tip with the needle. During movement of the condyle the catheter may become folded and break during removal. If the catheter tip breaks, it should be surgically removed.

chapter 5

Surgery

The surgical treatment of TMJ internal derangement consists of two basic procedures: disc repositioning and disc removal. Several variations of these two procedures may be performed. We do not believe that surgeons should limit themselves to either disc repositioning only or discectomy (meniscectomy) only, but feel that there are specific indications for each procedure.

As a result of accumulated experience with a number of techniques and with the development of new diagnostic procedures, appropriate indications for these surgical procedures have evolved. When the procedures are used in the appropriate setting, a high rate of success can be expected.

The purpose of this chapter is to describe the indications and surgical techniques for disc repositioning procedures and meniscectomy (discectomy) with placement of an alloplastic fossa implant (Silastic or Proplast/Teflon).

INDICATIONS

The decision to perform TMJ surgery is predicated on *documentation of TMJ disc derangement* and its role as a *major source of the patient's pain and/or dysfunction*. The pain and/or dysfunction should be of such magnitude as to *constitute a disability* to the patient. Surgical treatment is *not recommended for preventive measures* at this time.

Experience has shown that *most patients benefit from appropriate nonsurgical therapies*. The probability of successful nonsurgical therapy depends on the degree of pathology. Preliminary evidence suggests that there is a high probability of success with nonsurgical therapy in patients with early derangements, and a lower probability of success in patients with advanced derangements.

Patients should be informed of the potential risks and benefits of both nonsurgical and surgical treatments and should be involved in the decision as to the type of treatment. This may include nonsurgical or surgical treatments alone or in combination.

Some patients with diagnosed internal derangement may also have psychologic disorders and/or muscle disorders such as myofascial pain and dysfunction. When these problems exist, they must be evaluated and their management included in the overall treatment plan.

PATIENT PREPARATION

Patient preparation for surgery is mandatory if successful results are to be obtained consistently. Experience has shown that well-informed patients do better during all stages of the treatment. The risks and benefits of the proposed treatment, the procedure, the hospital experience, the postsurgical management, and the expected results are discussed with the patient and preferably with a spouse, other relative, or friend at least 1 week before surgery. The patient is encouraged to ask questions and is given the opportunity to seek another opinion. This same information is reviewed by the surgeon with the patient the day before the surgical procedure is to be performed. A specific TMJ surgical consent form may be helpful in organizing these points and documenting them before surgery. An example is included for evaluation and possible use.

RICHARD S. RUTKOWSKI, D.D.S., INC.
BRUCE SANDERS, D.D.S., INC.
JOHN W. GIVEN, D.D.S., INC.
Oral and Maxillofacial Surgeons

Diplomates of the American Board of
Oral and Maxillofacial Surgery

CONSENT FOR TEMPOROMANDIBULAR JOINT (T.M.J.) SURGERY

NAME ______________________________

PROCEDURE ______________________________

____

I. Dr. Rutkowski/Sanders/Given have explained to me about the pathology (disease)that exists in my right and/or left temporomandibular joints (lower jaw joints). I understand that my condition of limited or compromised function and/or pain may be secondary to a number of possible processes including, but not limited to traumatic injury, malocclusion, articular disc displacement (cartilage dislocation), degenerative joint disease, inflammation, infection, arthritis, developmental or congenital defect or tumor (neoplastic process). I understand that the surgery to be performed is an exploratory procedure and the treatment rendered at that time will be based on the finding's during surgery. Surgical treatment may include, meniscus repair, meniscectomy (removal of cartilage), placement of an implant, eminectomy, or condylectomy.

II. Complications of such surgery can include but are not limited to facial nerve paralysis with inability to close eyelid on the affected side, and inability to wrinkle the forehead, post operative infection, resultant malocclusion (incorrect bite) and limited opening, lack of improvement or worsening of pain and jaw dysfunction;further degenerative changes with the T.M.J.. I understand that this surgery is performed through an incision on the side of my face, in front of my ear and there will be a post operative scar.

III. I understand that future treatments required may include physical therapy, splint therapy, restorative dentistry, orthodontics, orthognathic surgery (jaw repositioning), and further reconstructive T.M.J. surgery which include implant removal.

IV. I understand that there is no guarantee given for the correction of my subjective symptoms and/or objective physical findings.

I have read this consent and have been offered a full explanation of its contents. I understand the document and hereby give my informed consent for surgery.

______________________________ ______________________________

Witness Date Patient (or legal guardian) Date

SURGICAL TECHNIQUES

Disc Repositioning, Recontouring, and Repair with or without Arthroplasty

PLATE 5-1

A The preauricular region is prepped and draped so that the ear and lateral canthus of the eye are exposed. The hair in the temporal region can be shaved, although recently we have not found this necessary. A sterile plastic drape is used to keep the hair out of the surgical field. Cotton soaked in mineral oil is placed into the external auditory canal.

B The incision is outlined at the junction of the facial skin with the helix of the ear. The incision line is injected with 2% lidocaine and 1 : 100,000 epinephrine to decrease the superficial bleeding. NOTE: The inferior extent of the outlined incision should be placed in the natural skinfold and not as drawn here.

C A large towel clamp is placed at the mandibular angle to allow movement of the condyle and inferior retraction of the condyle during the procedure. The towel clamp is placed posteriorly to the facial artery and vein and below the mandibular canal.

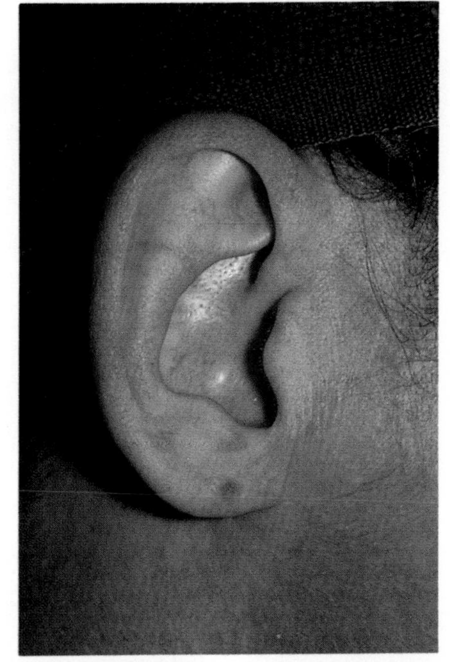

A

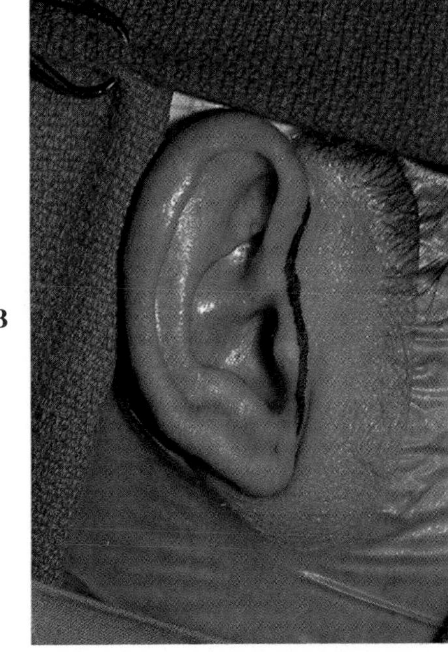

B

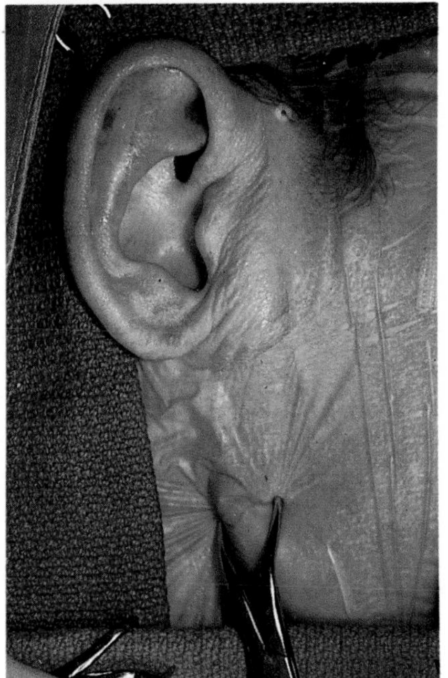

C

PLATE 5-2

A and **B** The incision is made and extended through skin and subcutaneous tissues to the depth of the temporalis fascia. It is important that all bleeding be controlled as the dissection proceeds. This is best done with electrocautery.

C The superior part of the flap is extended anteriorly by blunt dissection with a periosteal elevator. The flap is developed inferiorly adjacent to the external auditory cartilage. It should be remembered that the external auditory cartilage runs anteromedially and the inferior dissection is parallel to the cartilage.

Usually a vein crosses the lateral aspect of the articular fossa. This vein is a visual landmark for identifying the correct depth of the capsule. The vein should be dissected out, clamped, divided, and ligated or cauterized.

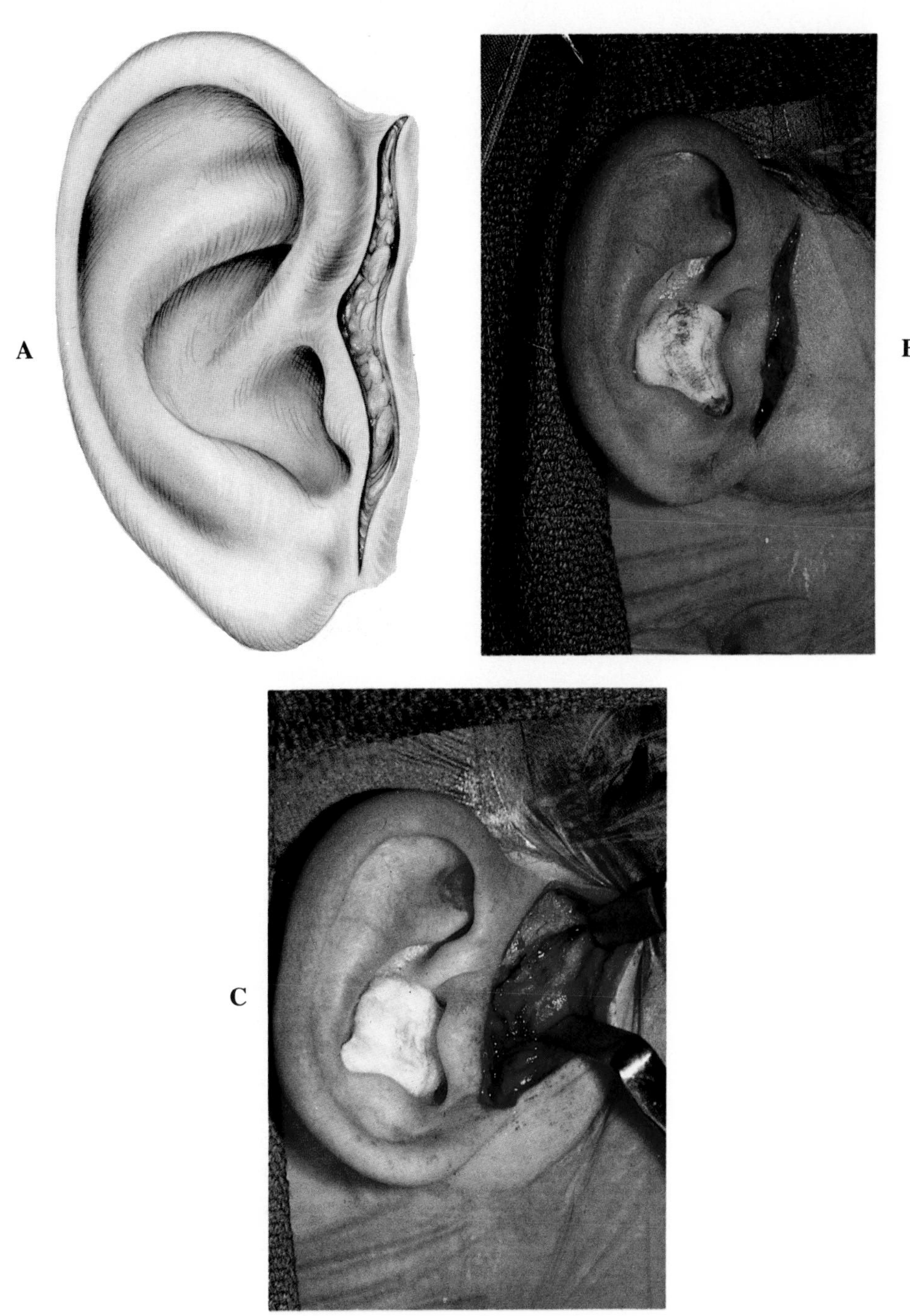
A
B
C

D and **E** An oblique incision, parallel to the temporal branches of the facial nerve, is made through the superficial layer of temporal fascia. The incision extends to bone over the lateral part of the fossa. Its inferior aspect should be no farther than 8 mm in front of the tragus of the ear. The lateral aspect of the fossa is exposed by blunt dissection with a periosteal elevator.

D

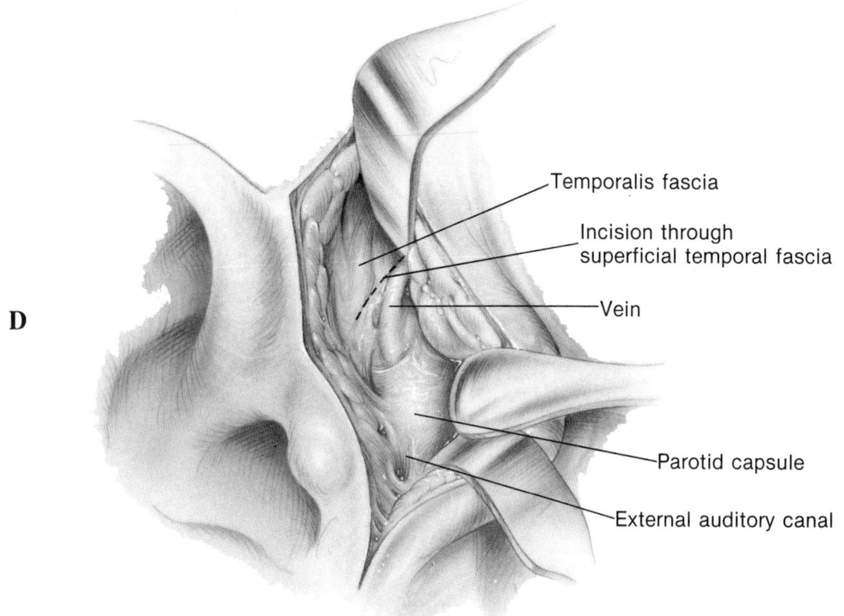

E

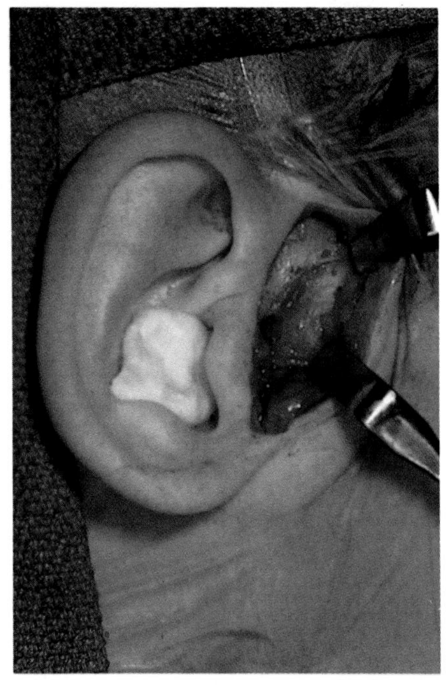

F and **G** Inferiorly a pocket is developed between the parotid and the TMJ capsules using blunt scissors. The superficial tissue is then released posteriorly by sharp dissection with the scissors.

F

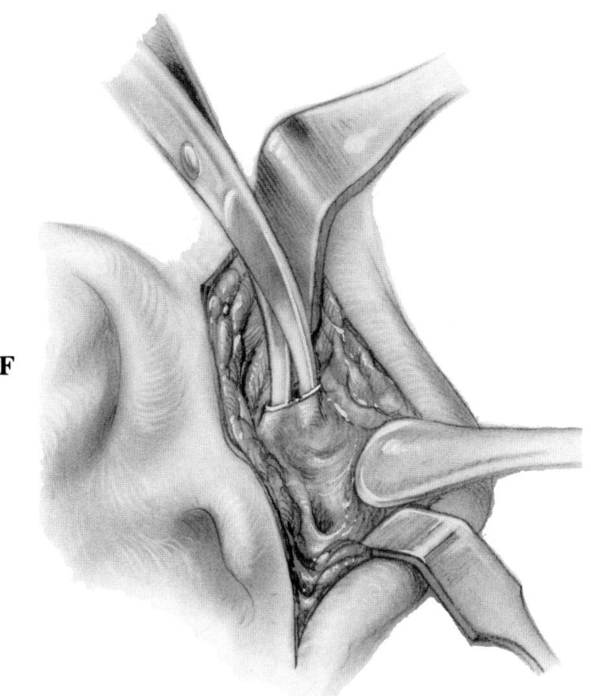

G

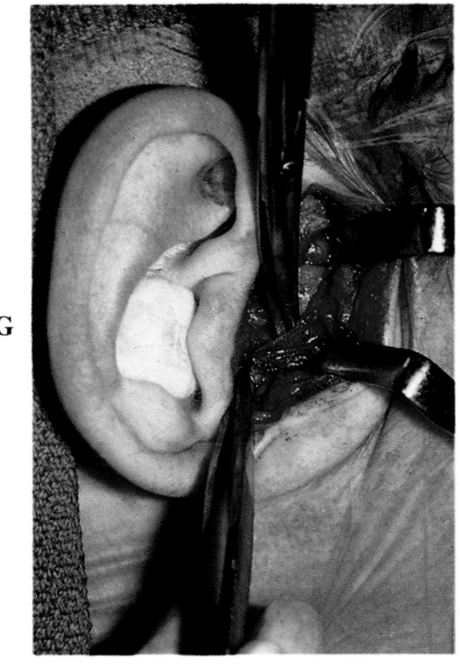

H and **I** The TMJ capsule is now exposed with blunt dissection using a periosteal elevator. The capsular exposure should extend at least to the height of the articular eminence.

NOTE: This dissection is a conservative modification of the Al-Kayat and Bramley approach. It allows the dissection down to the capsule to stay beneath the branches of the facial nerve, thereby protecting the nerve.

H

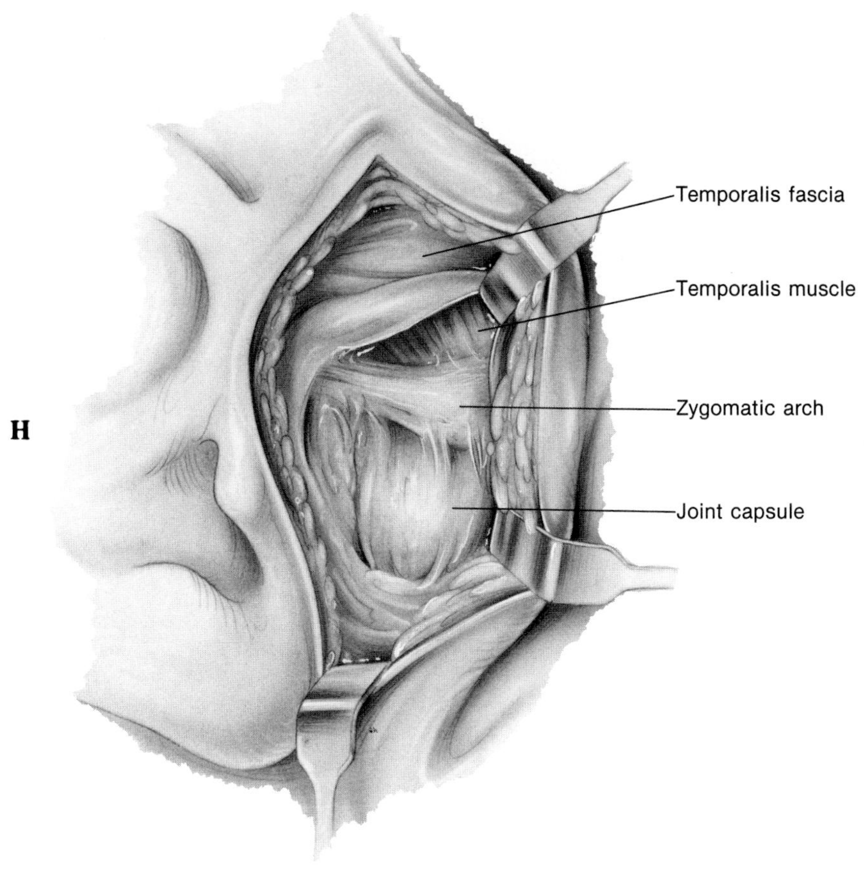
Temporalis fascia
Temporalis muscle
Zygomatic arch
Joint capsule

I

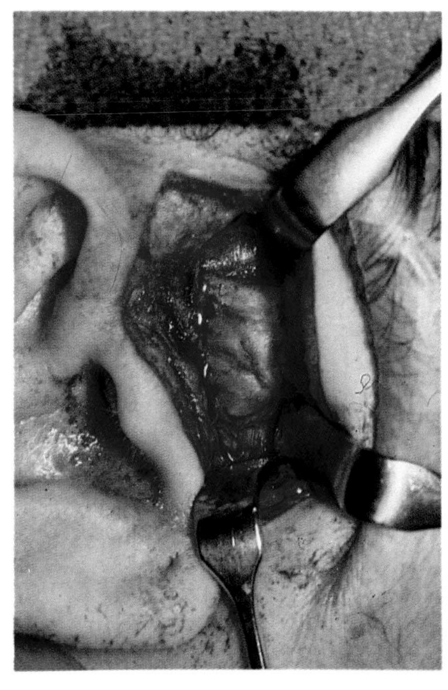

PLATE 5-3

A and **B** With the condyle distracted inferiorly, pointed scissors enter the upper joint space anteriorly along the posterior slope of the eminence. The opening is extended anteroposteriorly by cutting along the lateral aspect of the eminence and fossa. The inset shows the position of the incision in the frontal plane. The incision is continued inferiorly along the posterior aspect of the capsule until the capsule blends with the posterior attachment of the disc.

C The capsule is reflected laterally, opening the upper joint space. The disc and its attachments can now be visualized and inspected as to position, movement, and integrity.

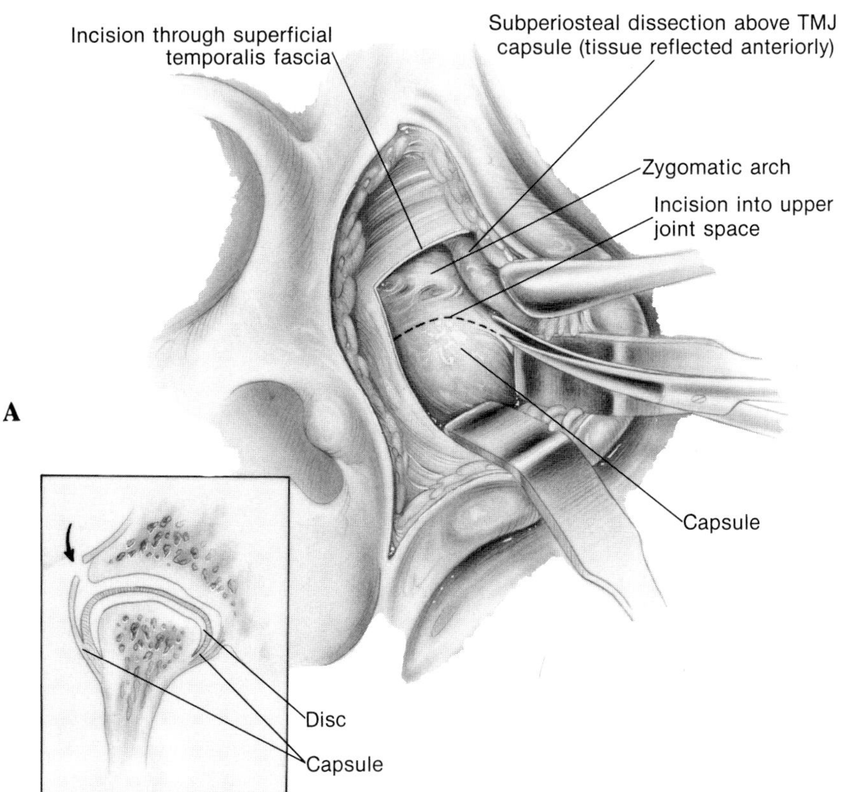

The decision to reposition, recontour, and/or repair a disc is based on the following findings:

1. The disc can be repositioned to a normal anatomic relationship with the condyle and fossa and is not under tension in this position.
2. The disc is essentially normal as to shape and thickness. Abnormal thickenings can be recontoured if the overall disc thickness is sufficient, at least 2 mm.
3. The disc appearance is essentially normal, that is, white, firm, and glistening, and not erythematous or soft.
4. Perforations are small and have at least one aspect adjacent to vascularized tissue. Large perforations can be repaired only if they are in the posterior attachment tissues.

B

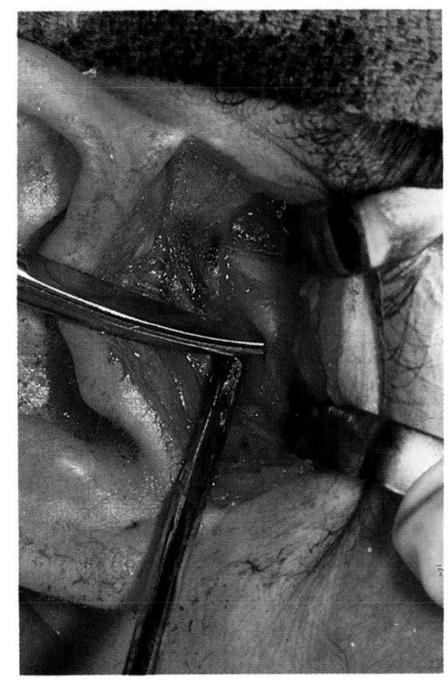

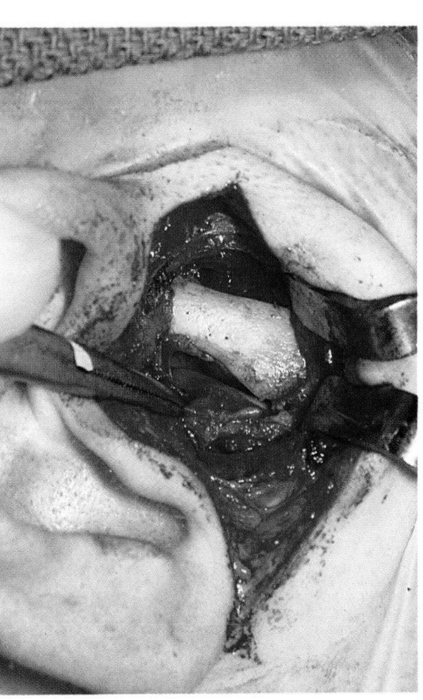

C

PLATE 5-4

A The position of the disc relative to the condyle and fossa is examined at rest and during movement. The disc is displaced anteriorly and the condyle is articulating against the posterior attachment tissues.

B The disc can be reduced in many cases by moving the condyle anteriorly while holding the posterolateral edge of the disc with tissue forceps. This disc is now reduced, demonstrating that it can be repositioned correctly. The disc is essentially normal in appearance, and there are no perforations.

A 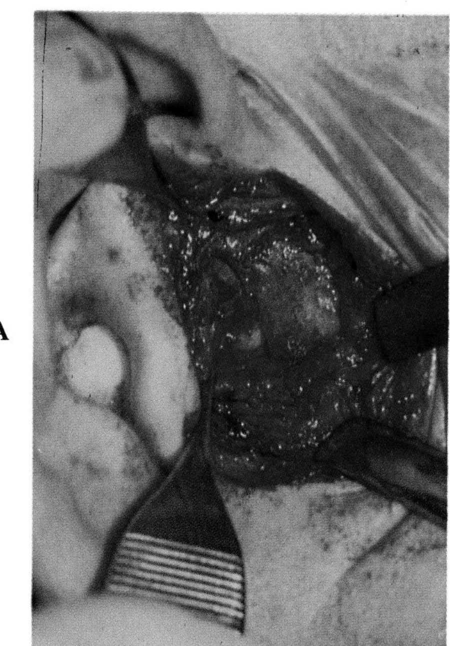

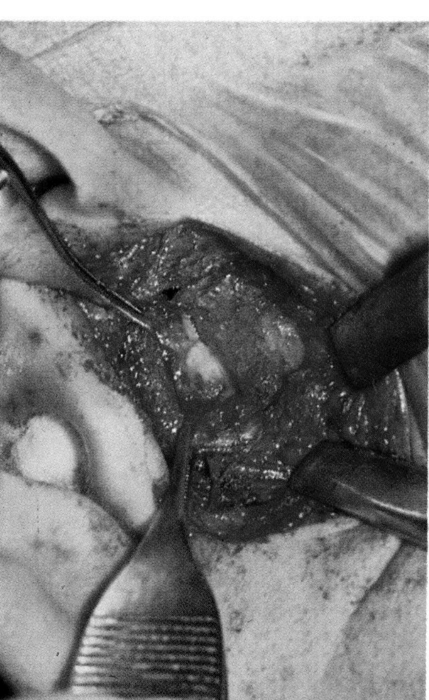 B

C and **D** In this case only posterior attachment tissue can be seen. The disc is displaced quite far anteriorly and there are no perforations. The disc does not reduce during movement of the condyle.

E and **F** If the surgeon grasps the posterolateral aspect of the disc, it can be repositioned to a normal relationship with the condyle and eminence. The disc's appearance is essentially normal, and this disc therefore does not need to be removed.

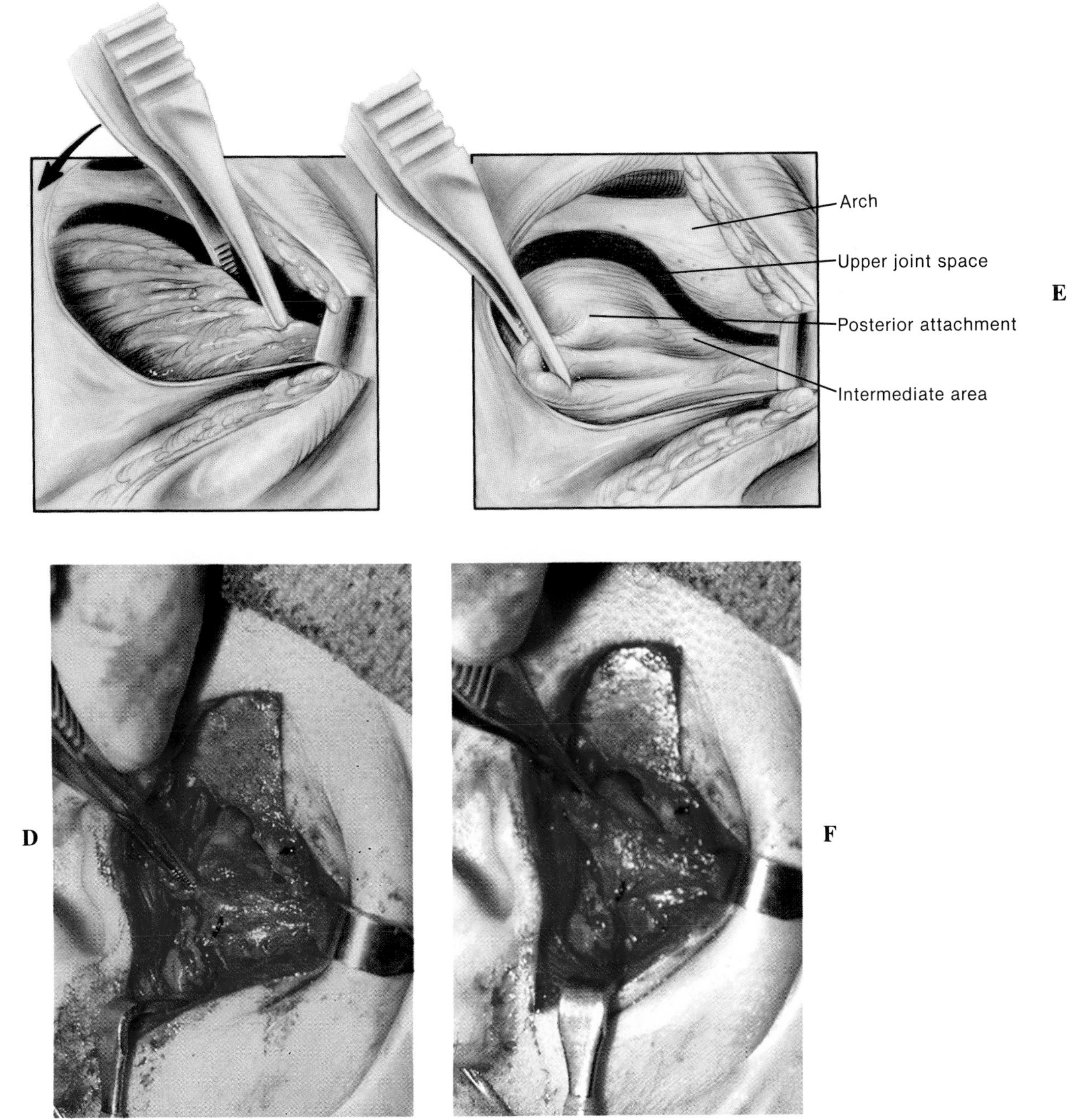

PLATE 5-5

A In some cases the lateral aspect (tubercle) of the articular eminence is quite prominent and obstructs visualization and access into the upper joint space.

B and **C** In these cases the lateral aspect of the eminence is removed using a unibeveled chisen and osteotome. Only the lateral aspect is removed, not the entire eminence. The inset shows a frontal view of the bone being removed.

D Removal of the lateral aspect of the eminence increases visualization and access to the articular structures. Rough bone surfaces are smoothed using a bone file.

A

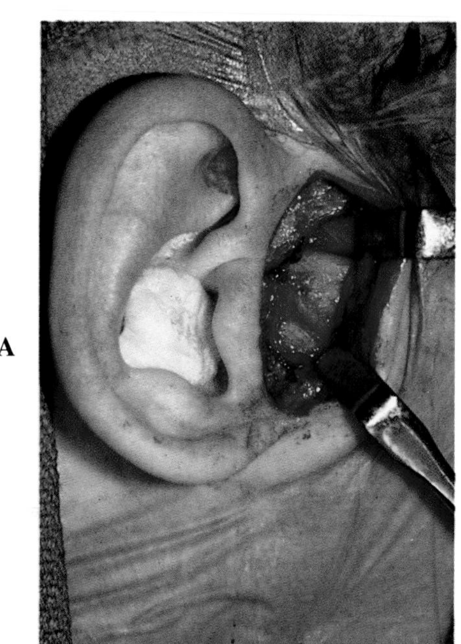

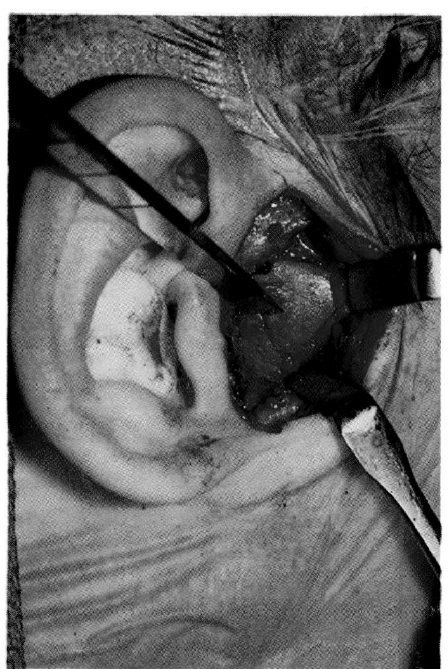

C

D

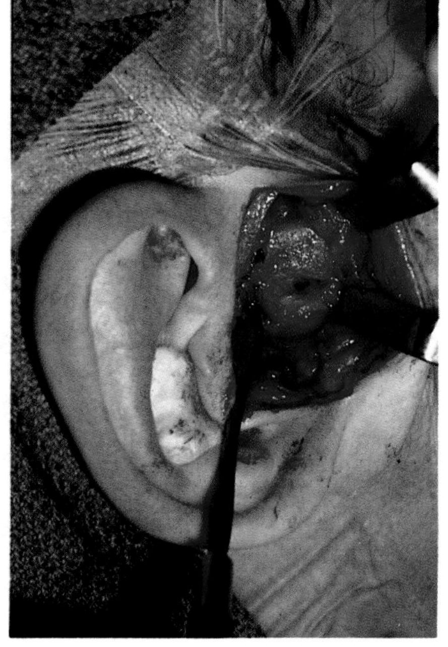

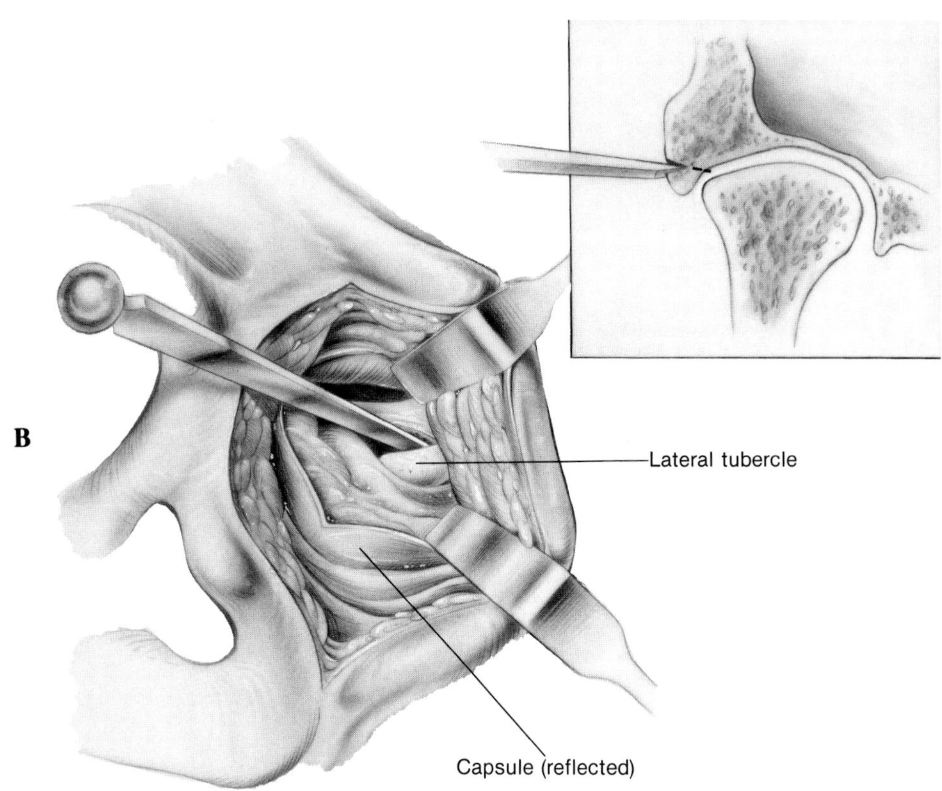
B
Lateral tubercle
Capsule (reflected)

PLATE 5-6

A and **B** The lower joint space is opened by making an incision in the disc along its lateral attachment to the condyle within the lateral recess of the upper joint space. The inset shows a frontal view of its position. The incision is extended posteriorly into the posterior attachment tissues.

C and **D** The lower joint space is opened. Brisk hemorrhage may occur from the cut posterior attachment tissue.

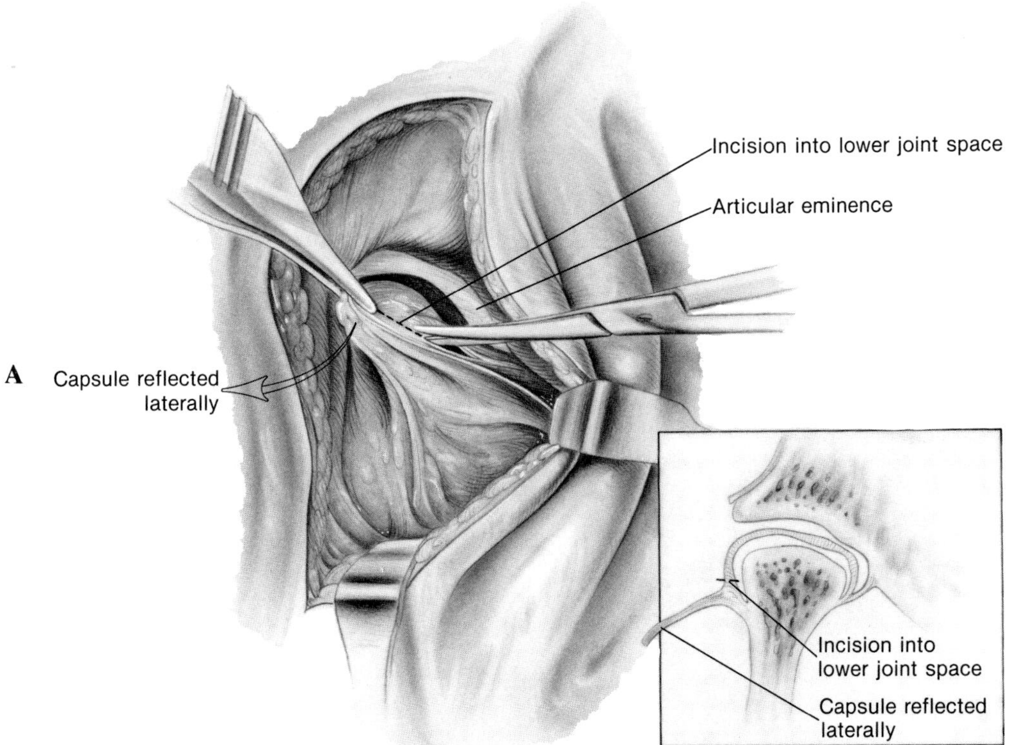

B

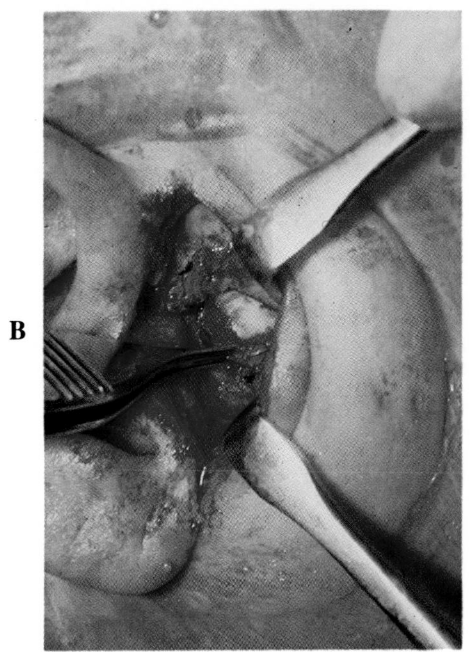

D

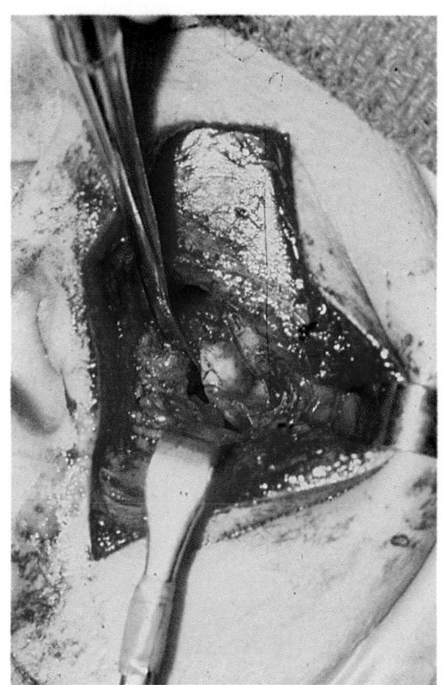

C

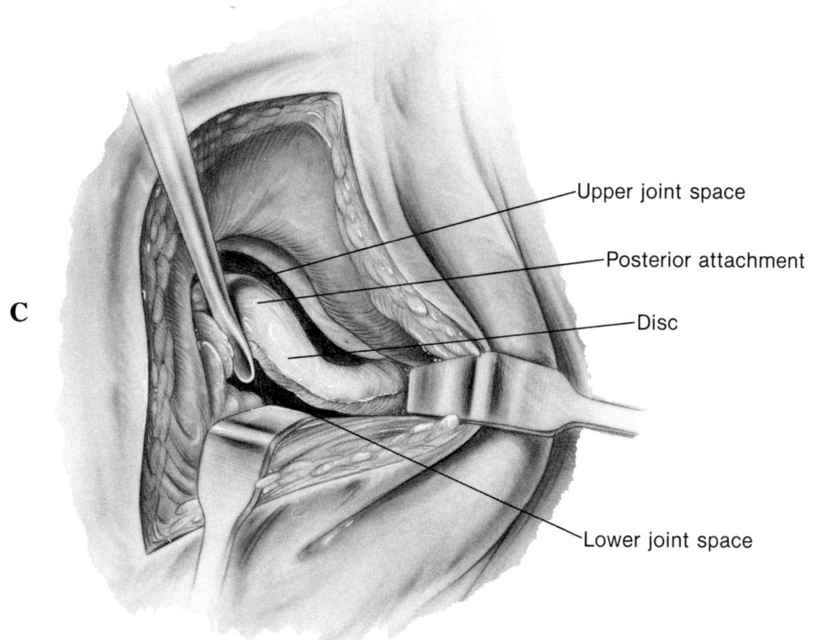
Upper joint space
Posterior attachment
Disc
Lower joint space

E and **F** A small DeBakey vascular clamp is placed as far posteriorly as possible across the posterior attachment tissues to control the hemorrhage.

Before the lower joint space is opened, the amount of tissue to be removed from the posterior attachment to correctly reposition the disc should have been determined. The determining factors are the distance and the direction the disc must be moved to position it in a normal relationship with the condyle and eminence. Each case is individually planned to correct the specific derangement present.

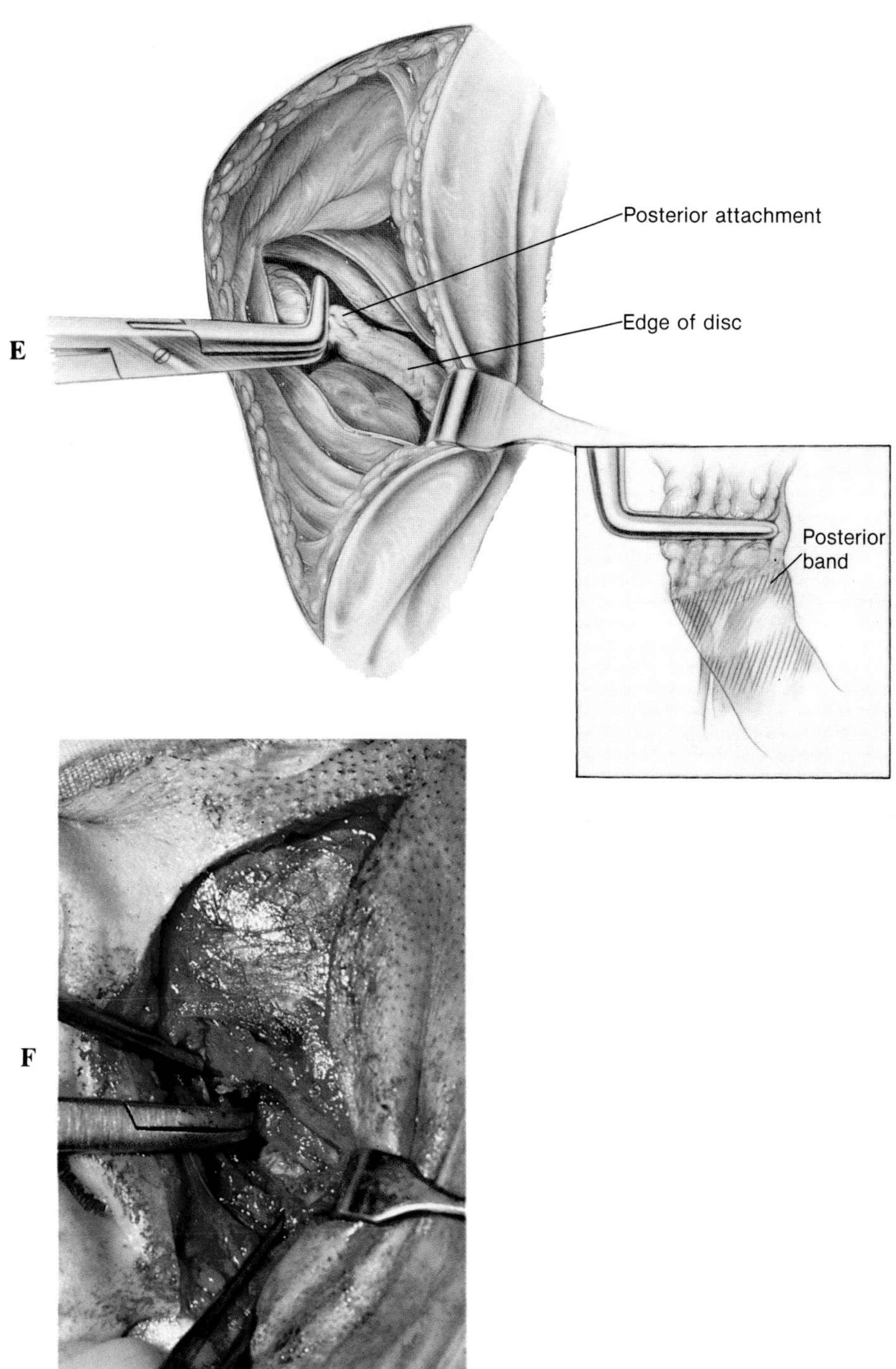
Posterior attachment
Edge of disc
E
Posterior band
F

PLATE 5-7

A and **B** This case illustrates a partial disc displacement in which the lateral aspect of the disc is displaced anteriorly. The medial attachment is normal. One can visualize that a wedge should be removed to allow the lateral edge of the disc to rotate posteriorly around the medial attachment.

C and **D** The appropriate wedge of tissue is removed using scissors. An edge of tissue should be left remaining anterior to the DeBakey clamp. If necessary, the anterior incision can extend into the disc. This removed tissue should be sent for histologic examination.

A

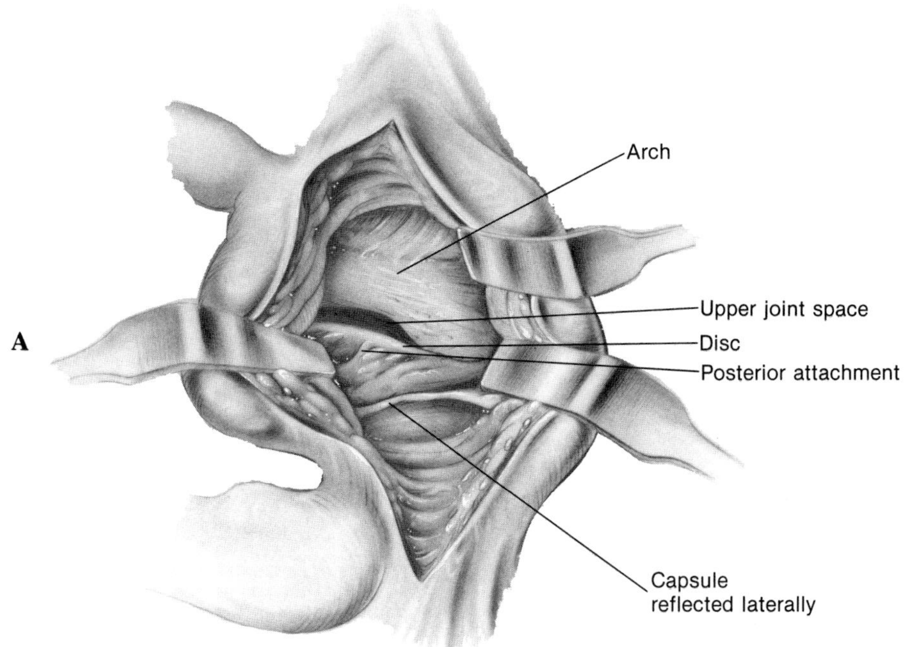

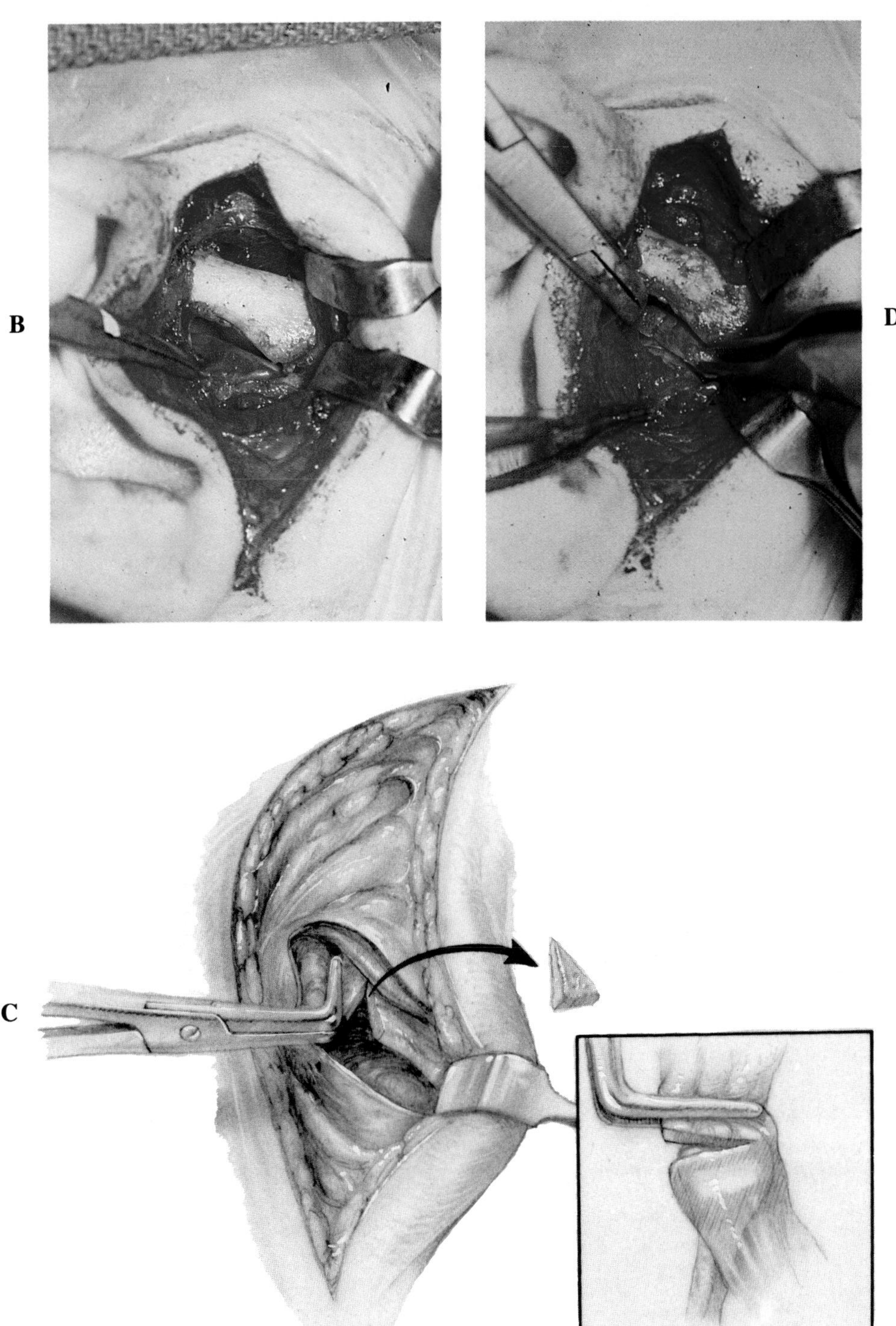
B
D
C

E This case illustrates complete anterior disc displacement.

F The wedge of tissue to be removed is wider than in the previous case, and the incision must extend farther medially to reposition the disc correctly. The inset shows this from above.

E

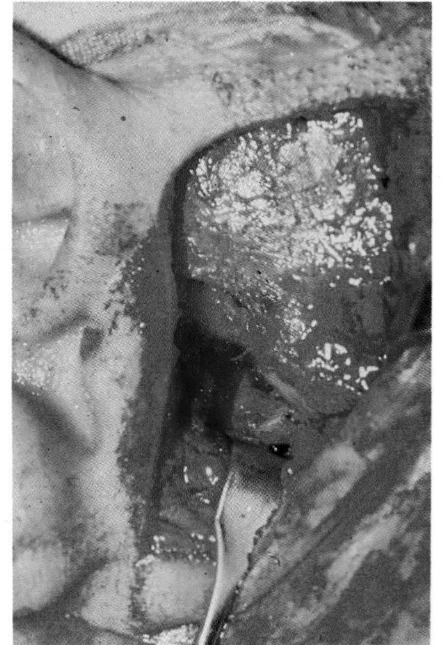

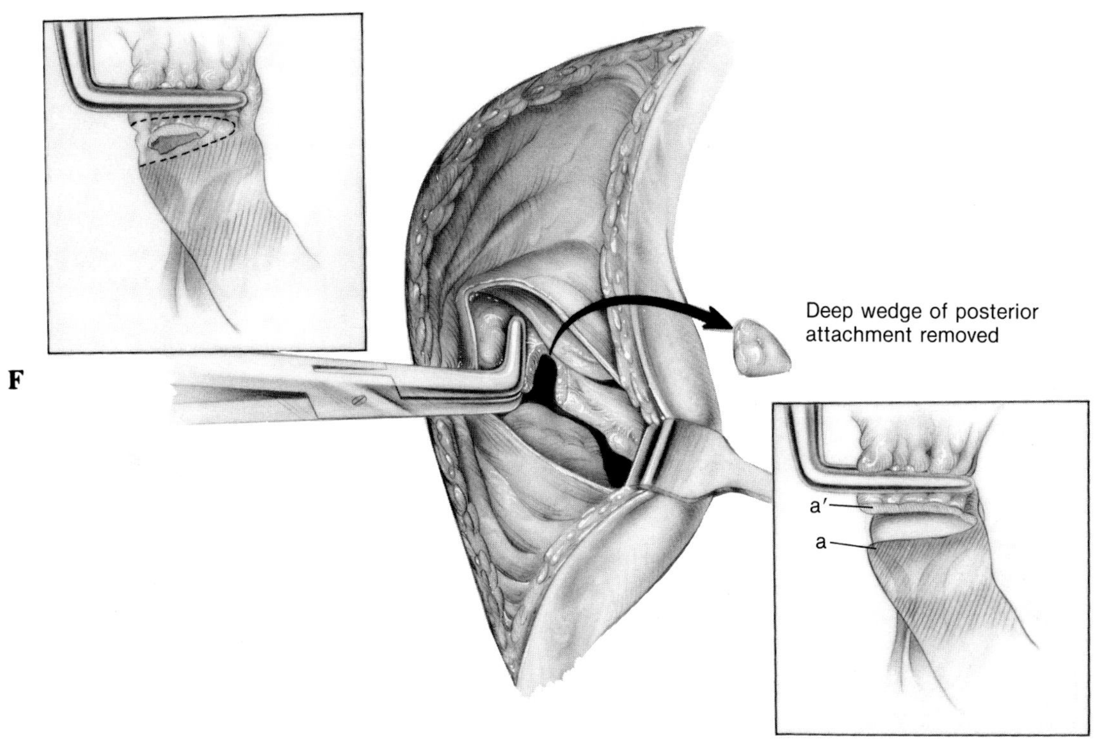
F
Deep wedge of posterior attachment removed
a′
a

G The appropriate wedge of tissue has been removed, leaving an edge of tissue in front of the condyle.

H This case illustrates a perforation at the junction of the posterior band and the posterior attachment. The disc can be repositioned in a normal relationship.

I The perforation is included within the wedge of tissue removed to reposition the disc.

The disc contour is examined, and should show the disc to be essentially biconcave in appearance. On the average the posterior band is 3 mm thick, the intermediate zone 1 mm thick, and the anterior band 2 mm thick. Abnormal thickenings or ridges can be reduced using either a #11 or a Beaver blade. The objective of disc recontouring is to establish a more normal contour and allow normal condyle-disc function.

G

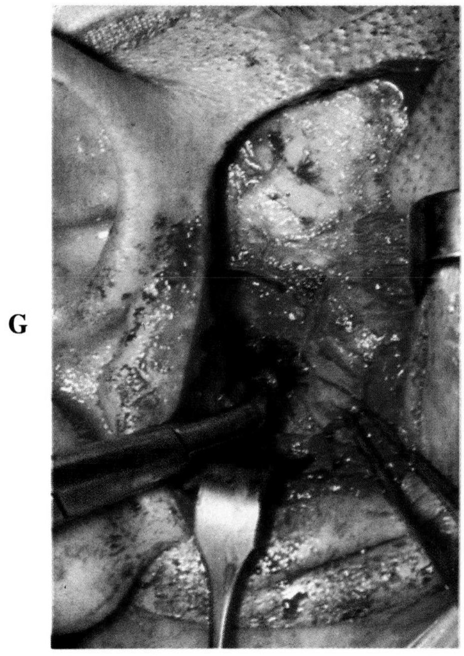

H

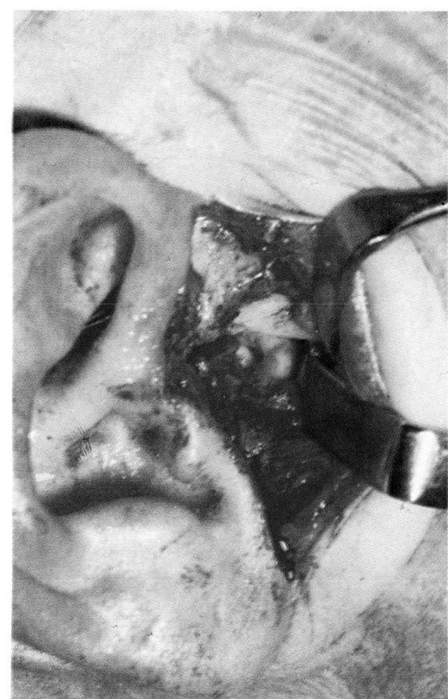

I

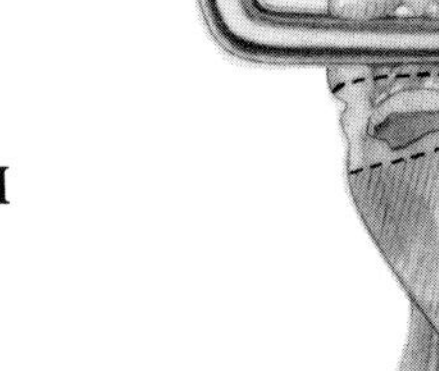

PLATE 5-8

A There is a thick ridge on the inferior surface of the disc, which would interfere with normal condyle-disc function.

B and **C** Using a knife the surgeon removes the ridge of tissue from the inferior surface of the disc to allow normal function. After removal of this ridge, the posterior band should be at least 2 mm thick.

D The condyle and articular eminence are inspected for evidence of osteoarthrosis, which is typified by areas of erosion with breaks in the articular connective tissue. Osteophytes may be present. Areas of osteoarthrosis are smoothed using a reciprocating bone file. Only minimal reduction is performed and only in areas of erosion or osteophyte formation.

The disc is repositioned and the incision in the posterior attachment tissues is closed using interrupted vertical figure-of-eight sutures. The suture material is 4-0 Mersilene on an S-2 spatula needle. Sutures are placed about 2 mm apart with the knots buried. If the tissue is thin, simple interrupted sutures are used. Castroviejo needle holders are used to place the sutures.

A

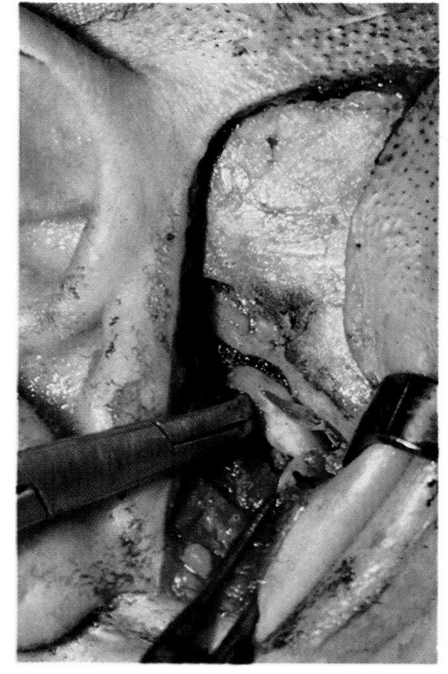

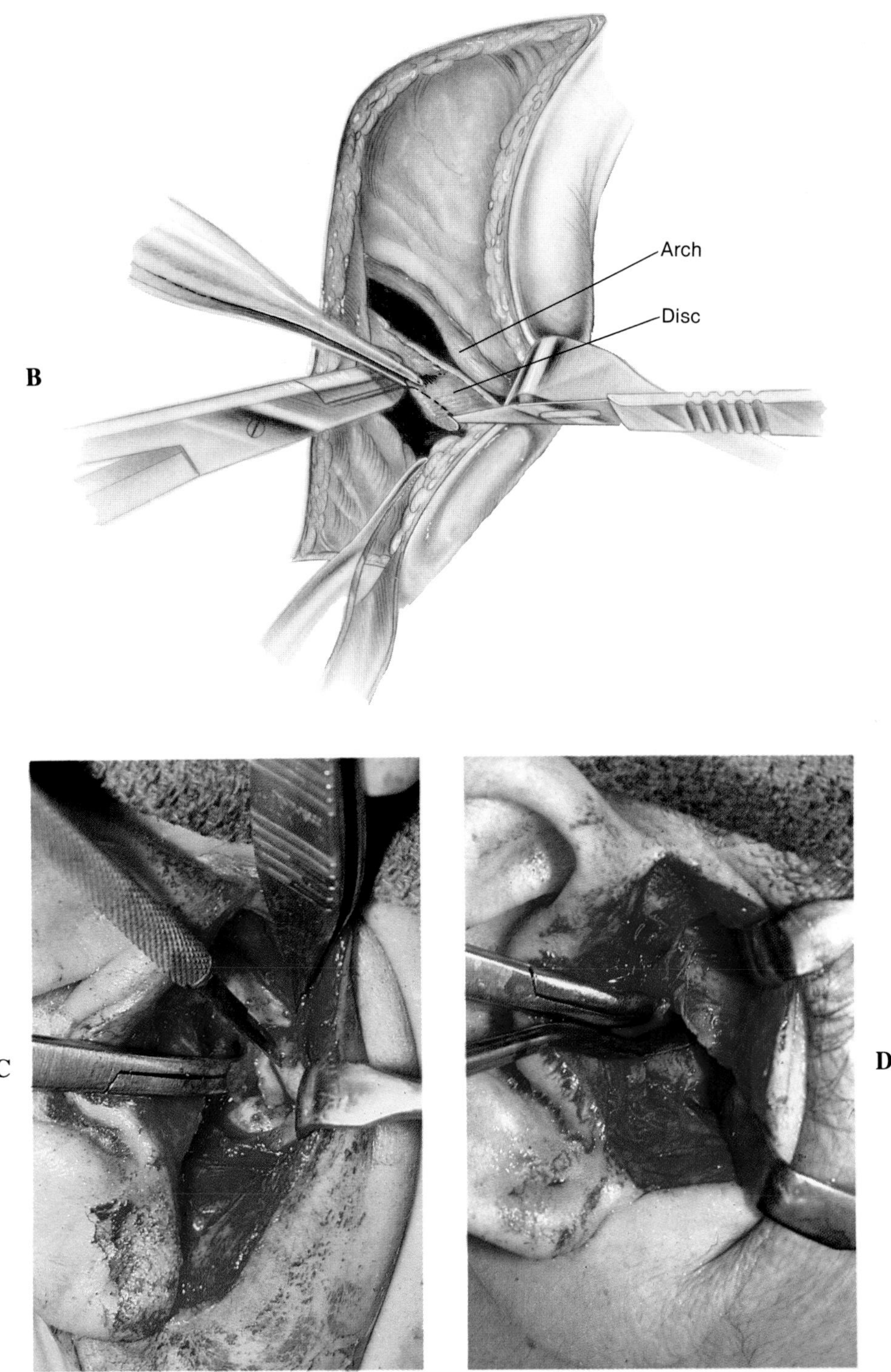
Arch
Disc
B
C
D

PLATE 5-9

A The suture is placed from the middle of the disc into the upper joint space.

B It continues through the superior surface of the posterior attachment and exits at the middle of this tissue.

C The suture is then passed from the middle of the disc into the lower joint space.

D It continues through the inferior surface of the posterior attachment and exits at the middle of this tissue.

E The knot is tied and the suture ends cut.

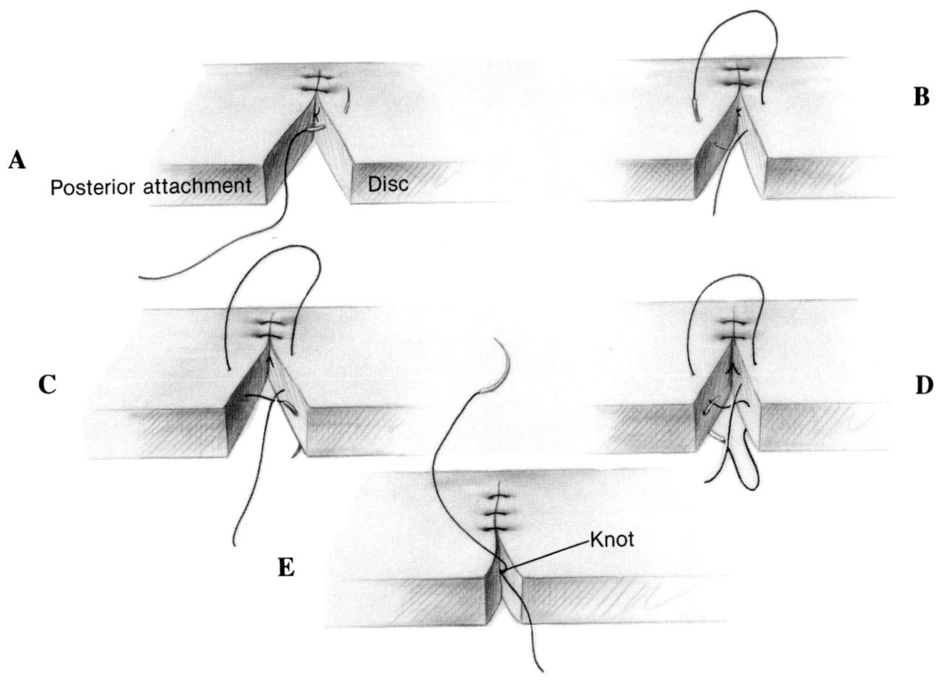
A
Posterior attachment
Disc
B
C
D
E
Knot

PLATE 5-10

A and **B** Sutures are placed until the incision in the posterior attachment is closed. The position of the disc is examined under simulated jaw movement, and there should be no clicking or folding of the disc. At rest the disc should be passively positioned above the condyle and along the posterior slope of the eminence.

A

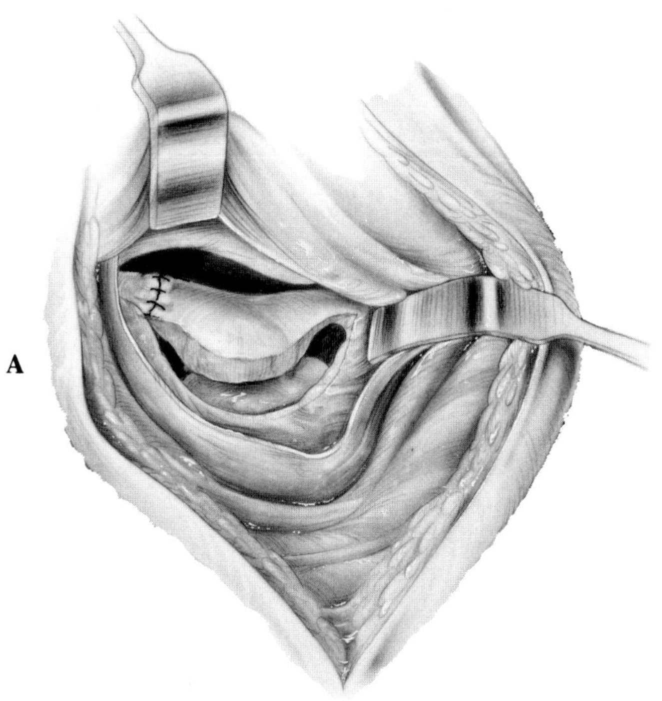

B

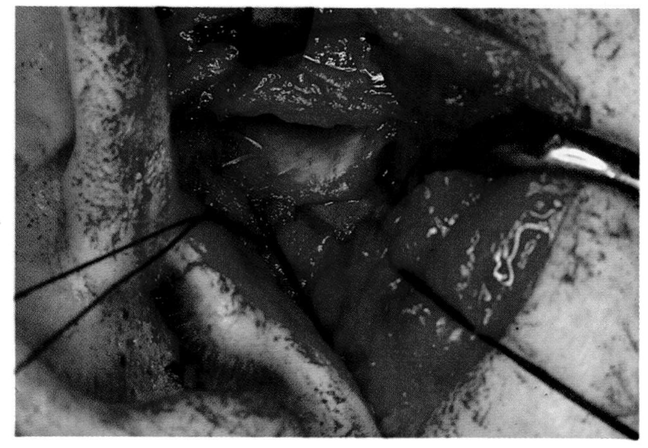

C If the disc is loose or displaced in a lateromedial direction, it is corrected by removing an appropriate strip of tissue from its lateral edge. The inset shows a frontal view of the tissue to be removed. The disc should fit tightly to the condyle so that it can rotate but not translate over the condyle.

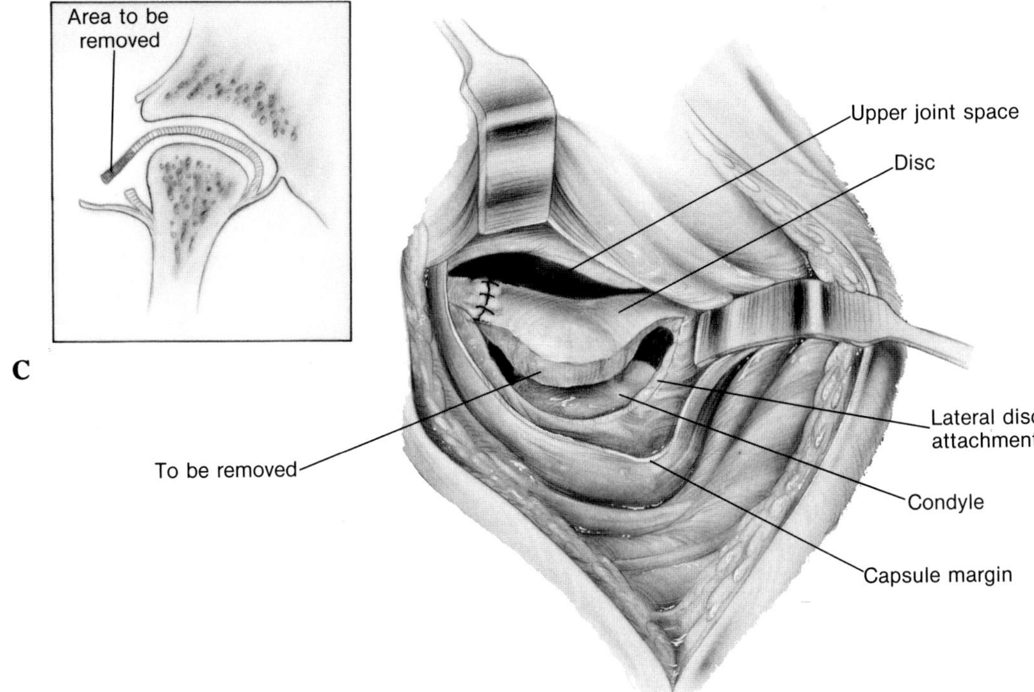

D and **E** The lower joint space is thoroughly irrigated with saline solution, and any hemorhage is controlled. The lower joint space is closed with 4-0 Mersilene by suturing the disc back to its lateral condylar attachment. The inset shows a frontal view of this. The position of the disc is again examined during simulated mandibular movements, and if clicking or disc displacement is observed, the lower joint space should be reopened and the problem corrected.

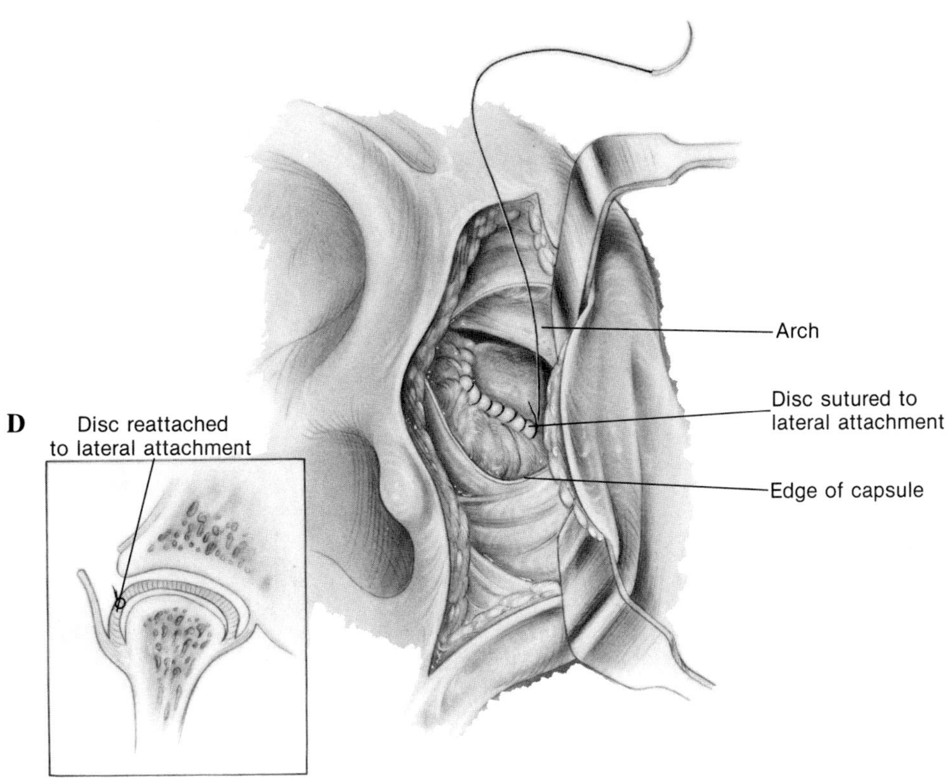
Arch
Disc sutured to lateral attachment
Edge of capsule
D
Disc reattached to lateral attachment

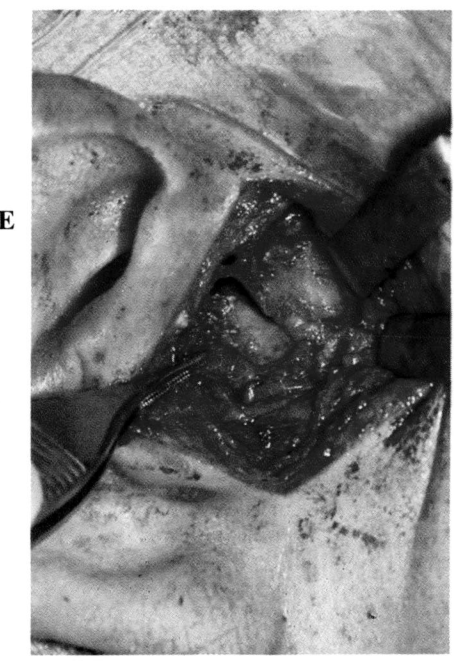
E

PLATE 5-11

A This case shows the disc displacement before surgical correction. The disc is located anterior to the condyle. The condyle articulates against the vascular and innervated posterior attachment tissues.

B Same case after surgical repositioning. The disc has been repositioned so that the condyle articulates against disc tissue during function.

A 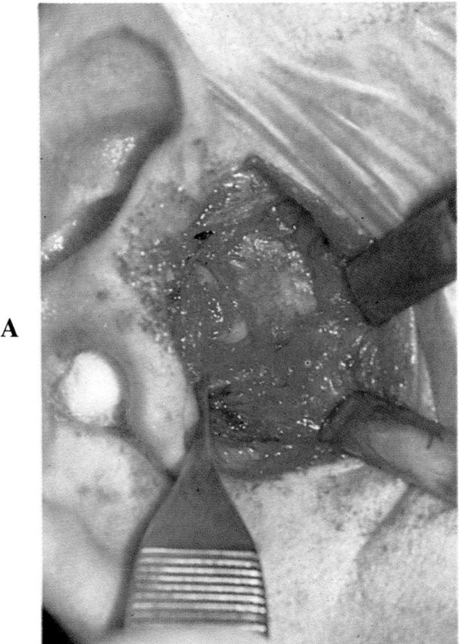

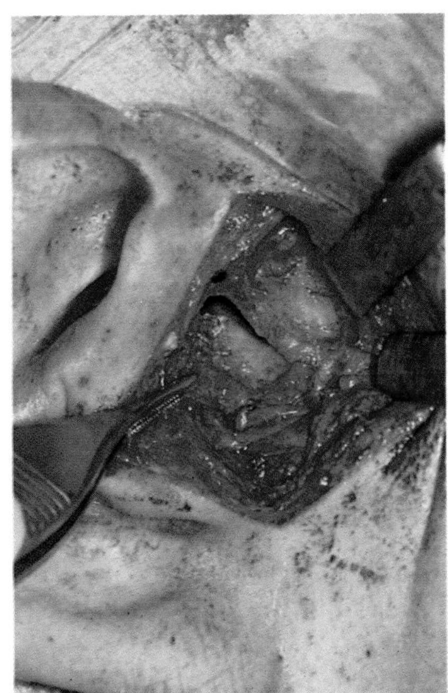 B

PLATE 5-12

A and **B** The upper joint space is irrigated with saline solution, and any hemorrhage is controlled. The capsule is closed with a continuous 4-0 Mersilene suture. The inset illustrates this in a frontal view. The towel clamp can now be removed.

A

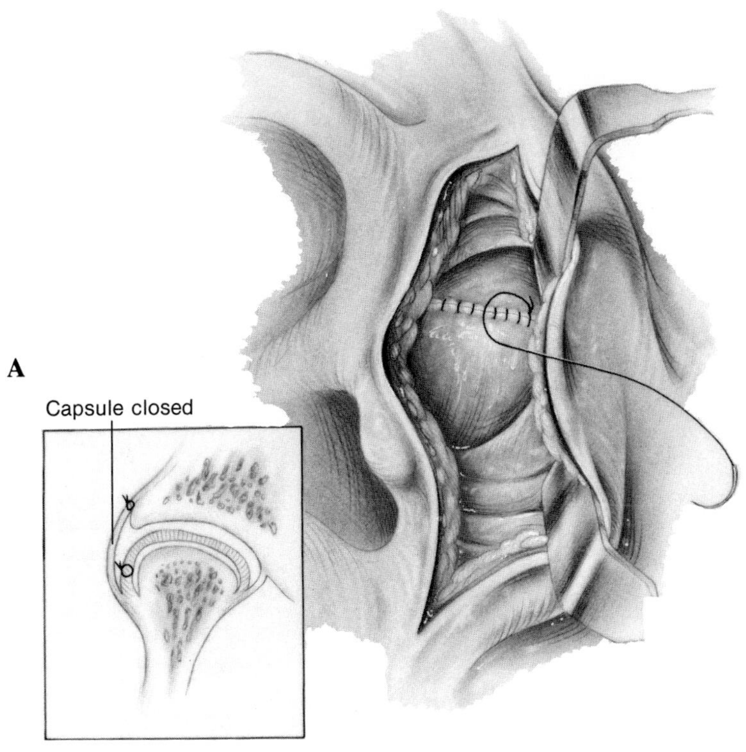

B

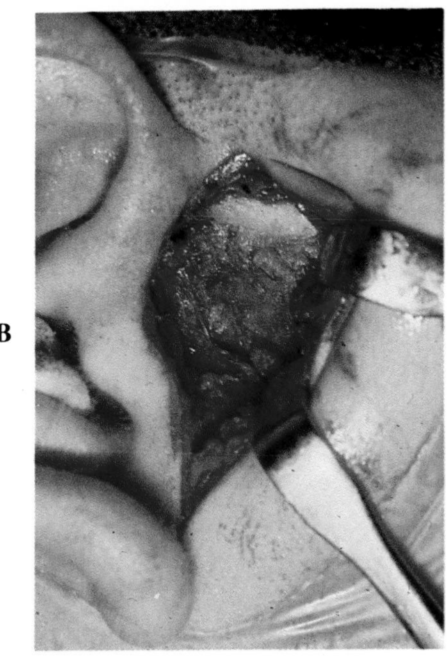

C and **D** The subcutaneous tissues are closed routinely. The skin incision is closed using a running horizontal mattress suture with 6-0 nylon.

E A mastoid-type pressure dressing is applied. The ear should be padded with gauze or cotton before placing the dressing.

C

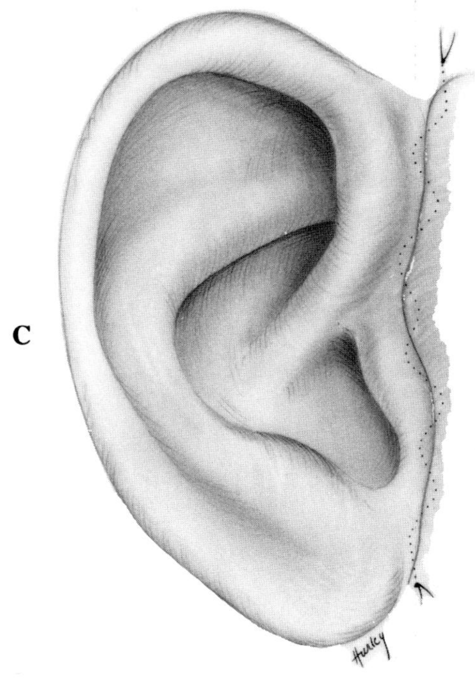

D

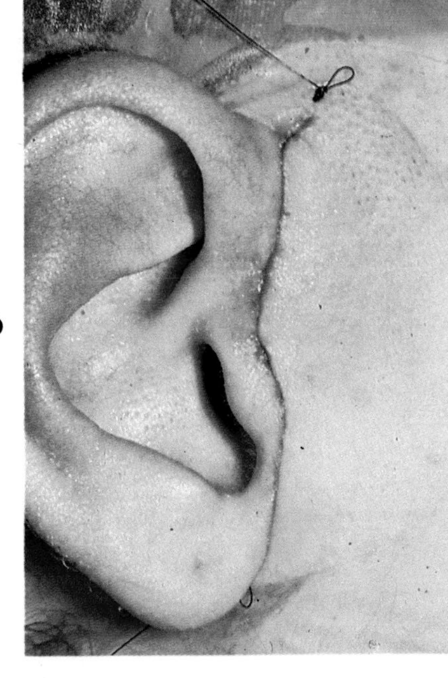

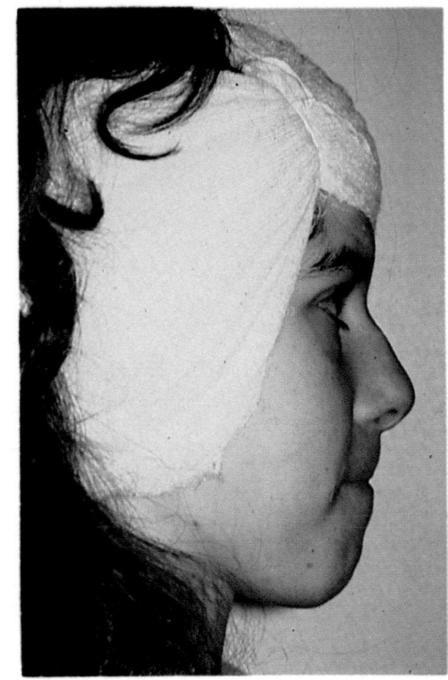

E

Meniscectomy (Discectomy) with or without Arthroplasty and Insertion of Fossa Implant

PLATE 5-13

A to **C** Meniscectomy may be necessary in cases of advanced internal derangement and arthrosis. For example, large perforations of the articular disc do not lend themselves easily to repair. Deformed discs with gross thinning or thickening, dystrophic calcifications, or extensive generalized arthrotic deterioration are candidates for excision.

A

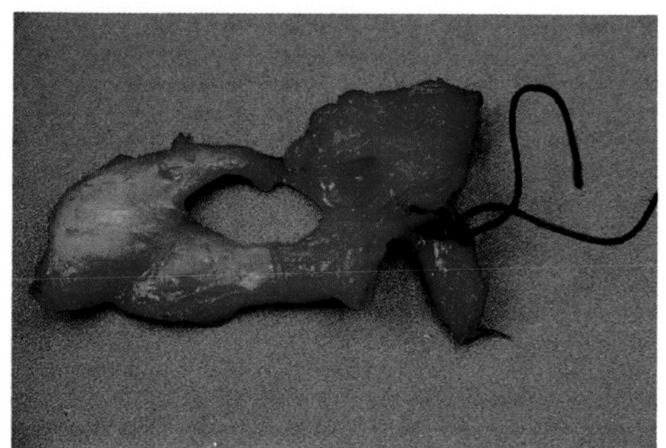

B

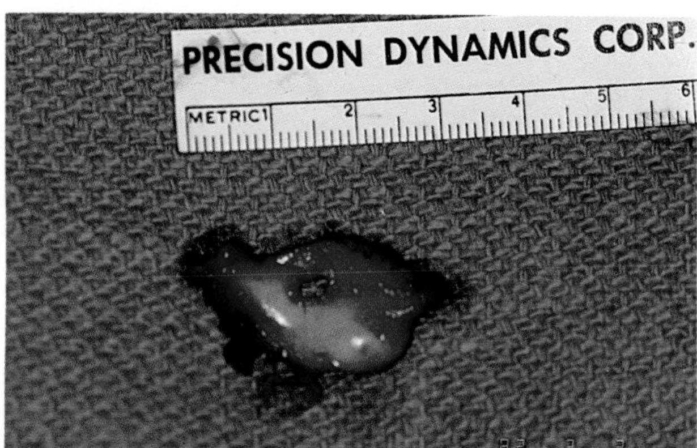

C

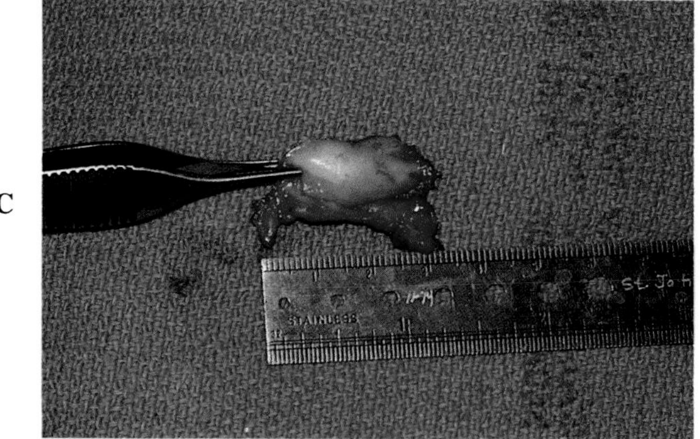

D The posterior attachment is clamped with a straight hemostat and then released after a few minutes.

E Next this compressed zone is sharply dissected with a #15 scalpel or "cutting" needle electrocautery.

F The meniscus is grasped with a pickup forceps or mosquito hemostat and pulled posteriorly and laterally. Next the anterior attachment of the meniscus is resected, cutting inferorsuperiorly against the articular eminence.

G Traction is applied to the meniscus laterally, and using a sharp dental periosteal elevator, the medial attachment of the meniscus is stripped. Finally, using a #12 scalpel, the medial meniscus attachment is resected. Hemostasis is achieved by packing a dry sponge into the area and compressing the condyle on the gauze. Obvious arterial bleeding can be controlled with hemostatic clips and/or cautery.

After meniscectomy has been completed, the teeth are placed in centric occlusion and the joint space is evaluated.

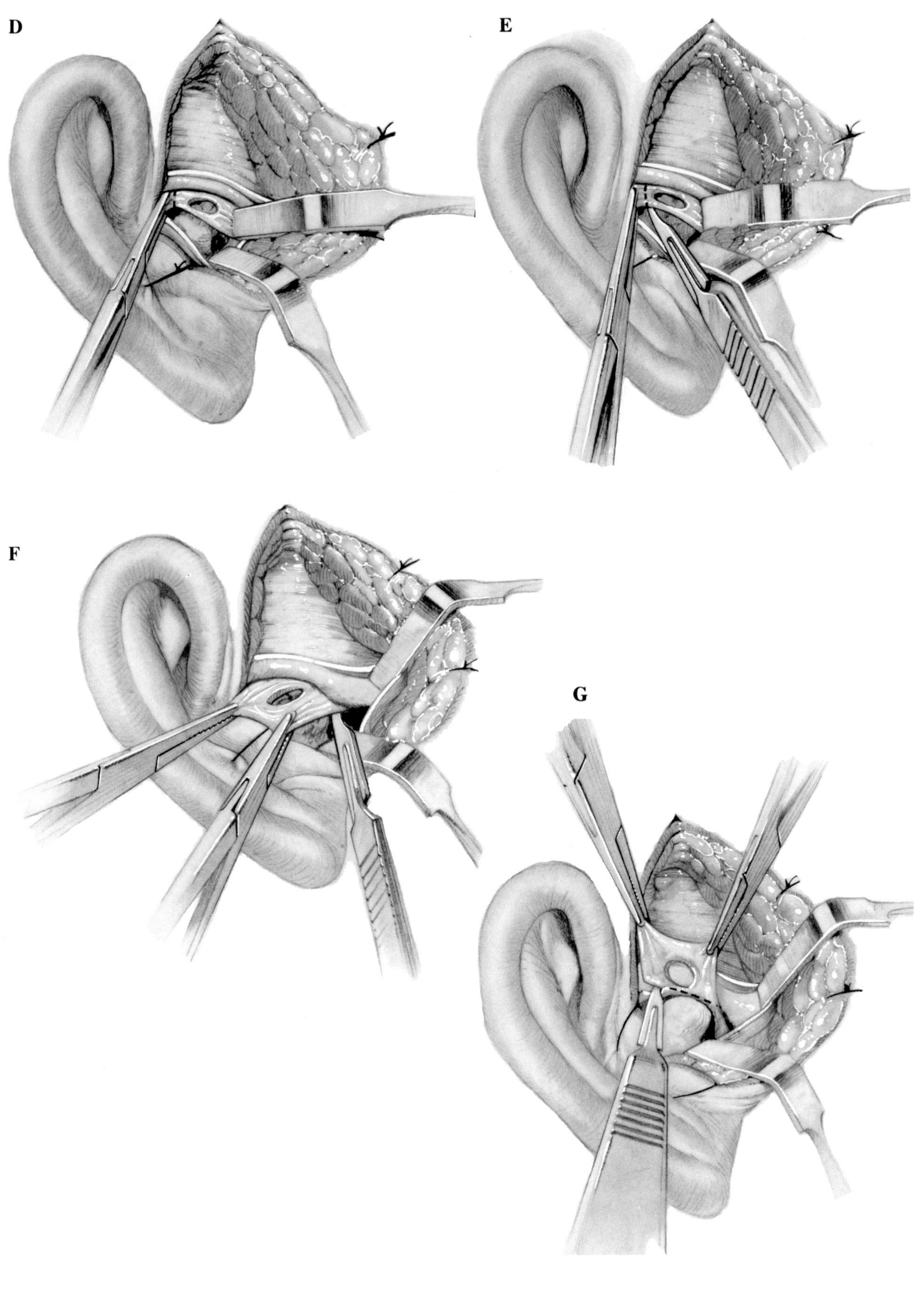
D
E
F
G

PLATE 5-14

A When there is little or no joint space, significant degenerative changes are often evident on the articular surfaces of the condyle and fossa. High condylectomy and/or eminence reduction will gain space and allow for placement of a fossa implant.

B When there is adequate joint space, no osseous surgery may be necessary. However, small articular surface irregularities may be removed conservatively to avoid excessive reduction in condylar height.

A

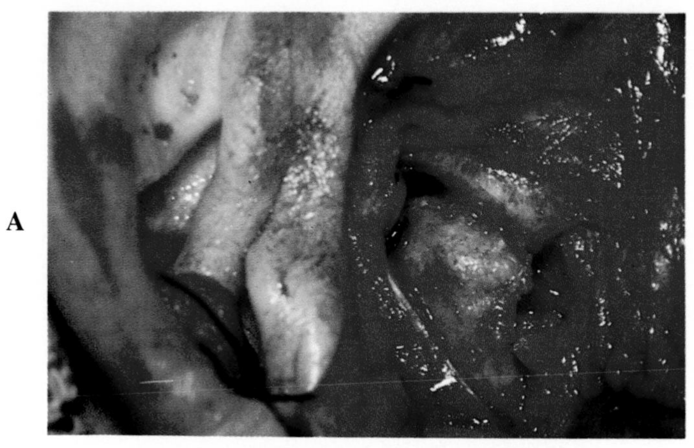

B

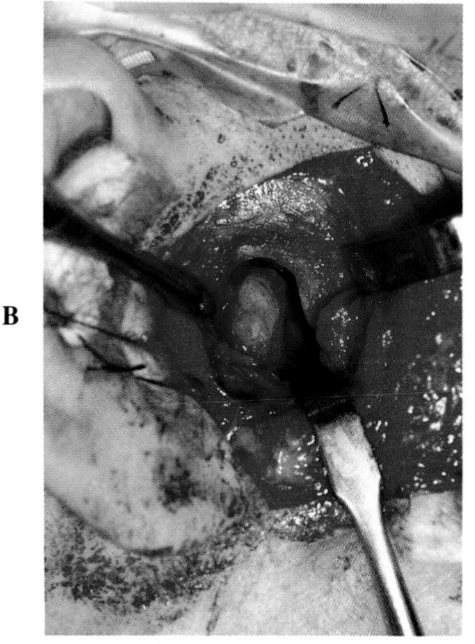

PLATE 5-15

A and **B** Note the bulbous condylar head with obvious changes in morphology. There is some lateral joint space, but the medial space is very limited.

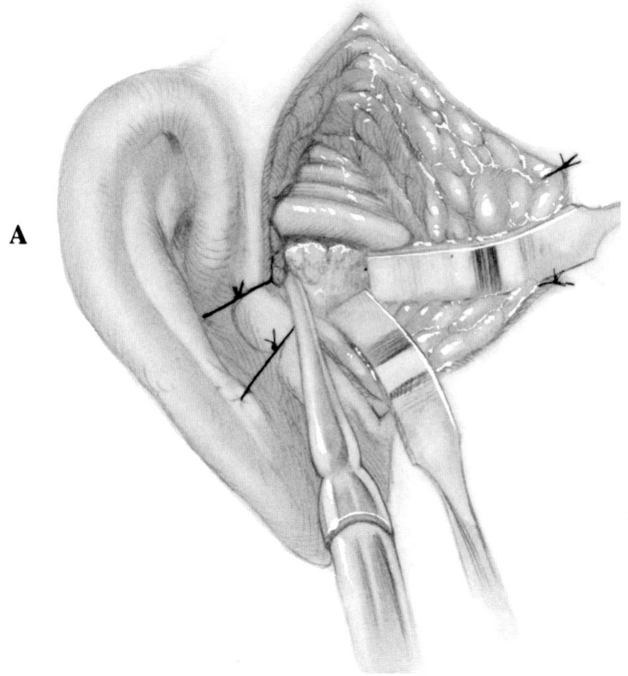
A

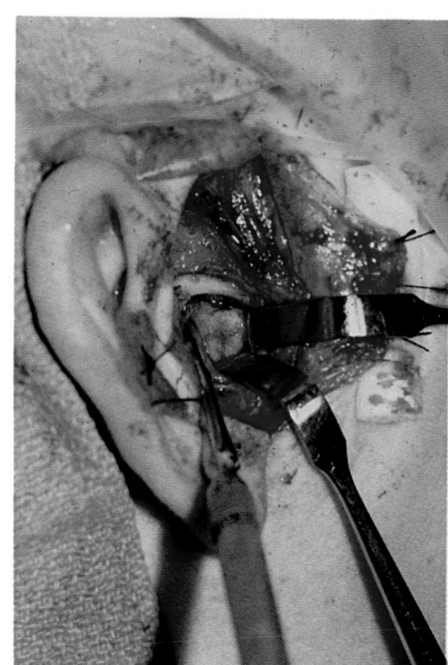
B

C Conservative recontouring of the articular surfaces with a bone file is recommended. Only areas of arthrosis are recontoured.

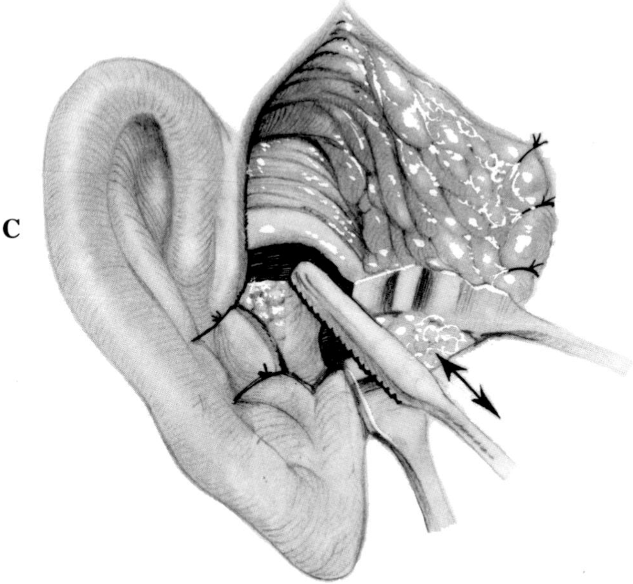

D to **F** It is important to remember that high condylectomy is done only to increase joint space; excessive bone removal can result in immediate or delayed occlusal problems. Using a reciprocating microsaw, a high condylectomy is performed. The usual height of the condylar cap excised is 2 to 3 mm. The stump is rounded and recontoured.

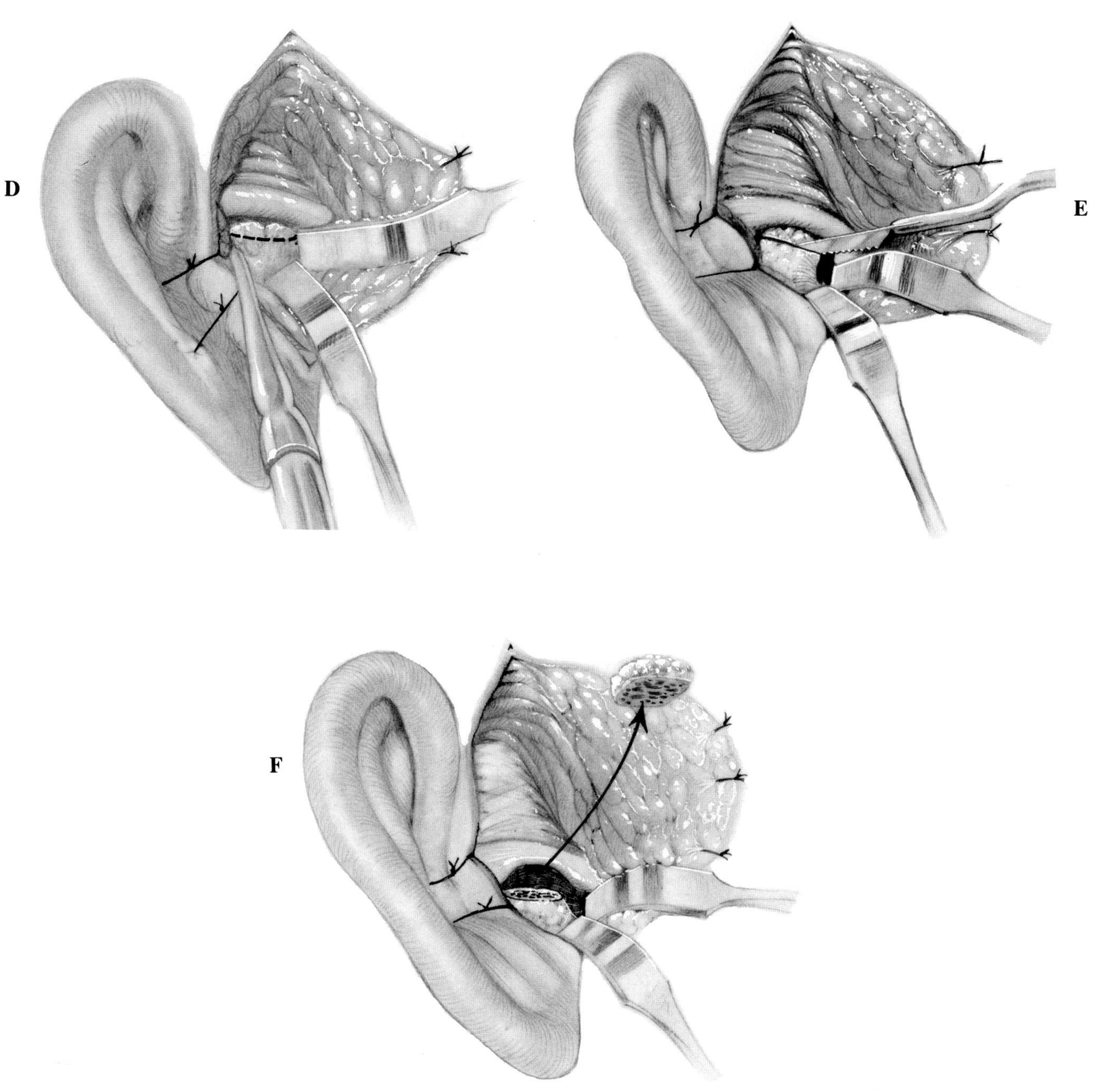

PLATE 5-16

This shows the size of the implant in relation to the excised articular disc and resected arthrotic condylar cap. Using 0.062-inch thickness Silastic sheeting an elliptic fossa implant is fashioned. The dimensions of the implant are approximately 1.5 cm mediolaterally and 1.0 to 1.2 cm anteroposteriorly. These dimensions may be even slightly smaller but are rarely much larger. An alternative is a Proplast/Teflon fossa implant. We have found both implant materials to be equally satisfactory. Placement and fixation of either implant are the same.

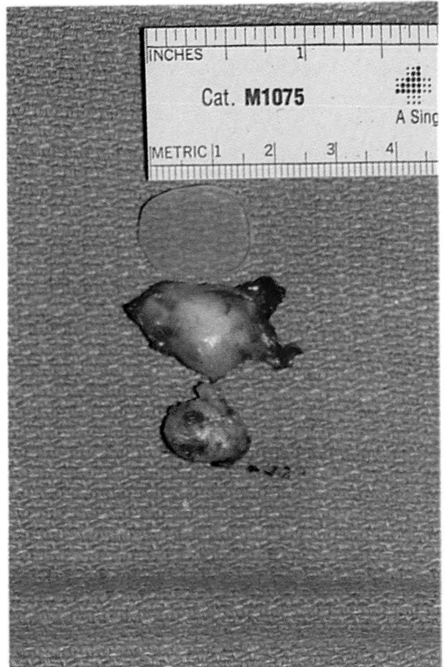

PLATE 5-17

A Using a small wire passing bur, two intraosseous holes are placed in the lateral rim of the articular fossa. The holes are angulated so that they enter the fossa at its most lateral margin.

B One 26- or 27-gauge stainless steel wire is passed through the intraosseous holes with both tails of the wire exiting just medial to the lateral rim of the fossa. The ends of the wire are placed through the lateral aspect of the implant.

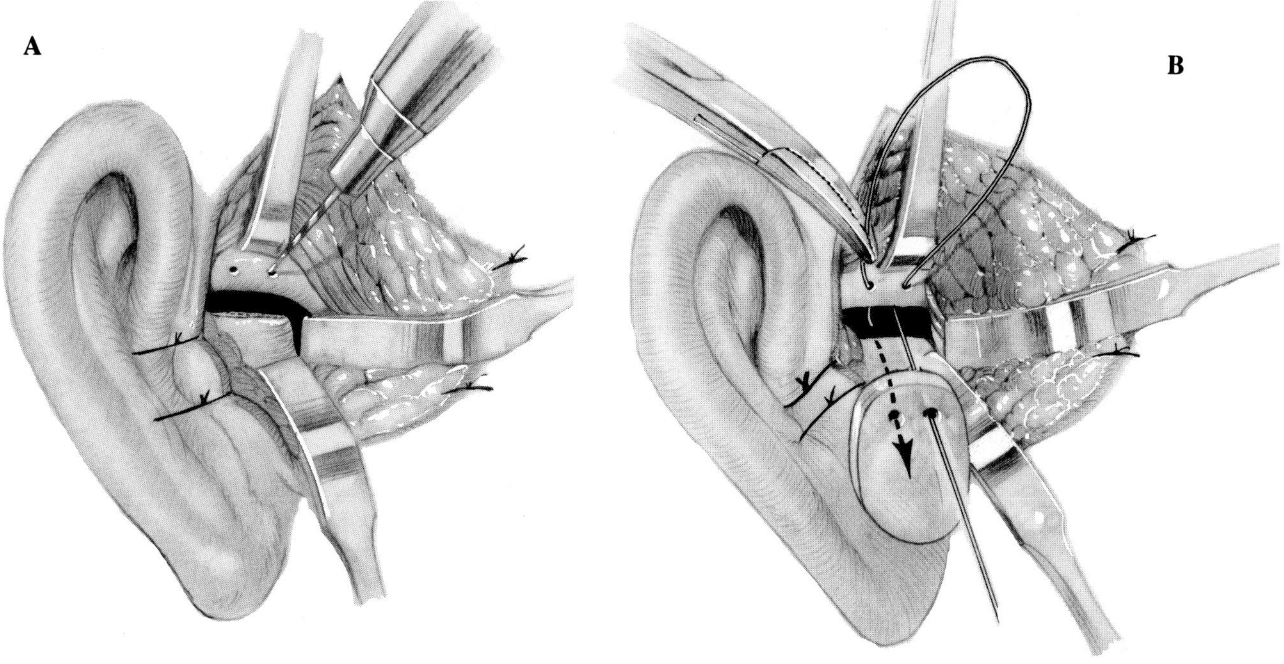

C Then the implant is placed into the fossa.

D Using a smooth Freer elevator to mold and adapt the implant to the shape of the fossa, the wire is twisted down to secure the implant.

E The wire tail should be cut to about 5 or 6 mm and then curved and gently forced into the posterior surface of the implant. This will greatly help secure the implant and prevent the medial edge from moving anteriorly.

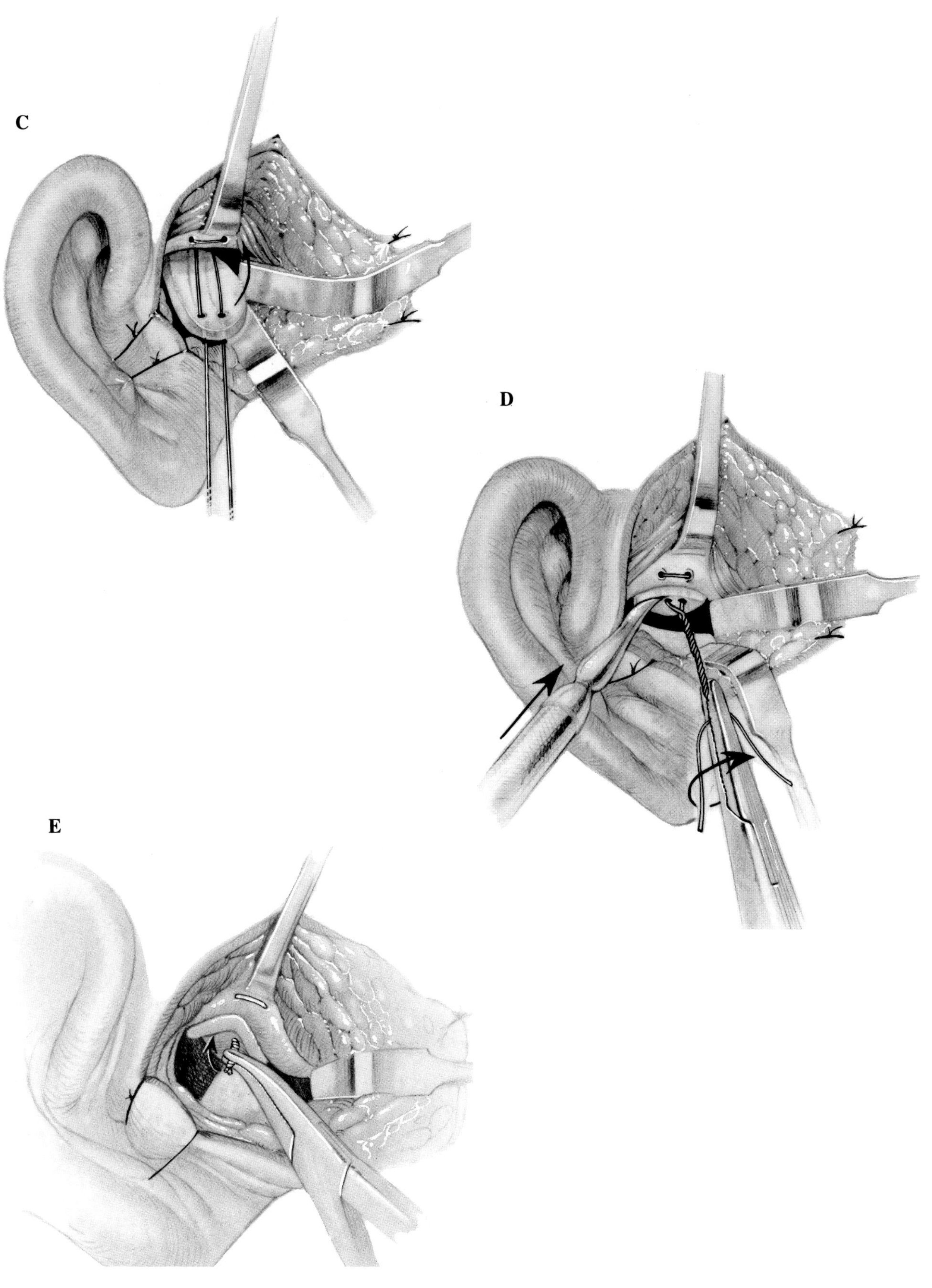
C
D
E

PLATE 5-18

A Silastic fossa implant in place.

B and **C** On manipulation of the mandible down and forward, the Silastic implant maintains its contour. Note the placement of the wire tail posteriorly; the tip has been buried in the implant.

D and **E** This is an example of meniscectomy with Silastic fossa implant and no condylar head recontouring.

F This is an example of meniscectomy with Proplast/Teflon fossa implant.

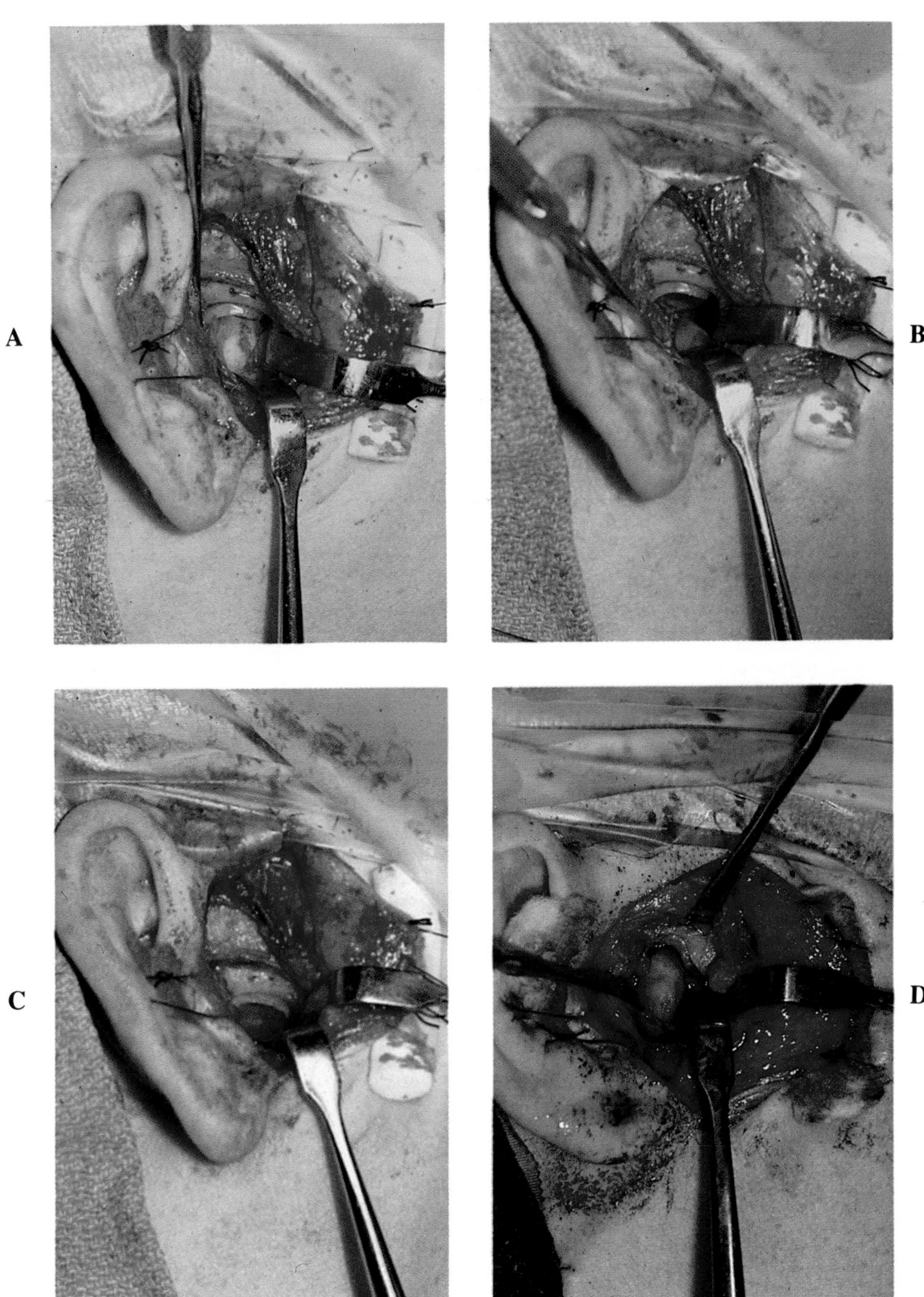

G The capsule is closed with a continuous suture. The subcutaneous tissues are closed routinely. The skin incision is closed using a running horizontal mattress suture of 6-0 nylon.

H A pressure dressing is applied. The ear should be padded with gauze or cotton before placing the dressing. This completes the case.

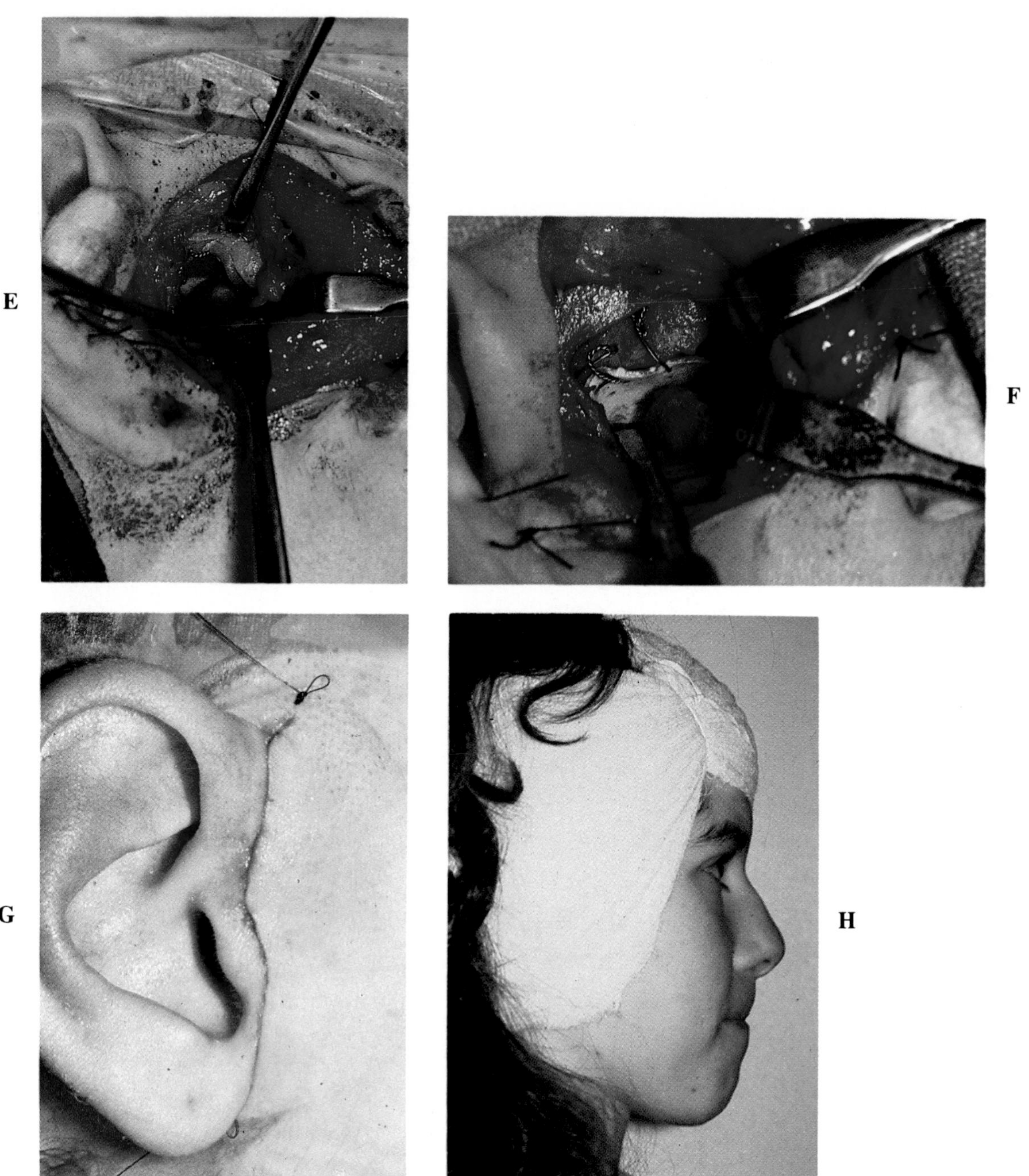

chapter 6

Postoperative Management and Results

POSTOPERATIVE MANAGEMENT

Postoperative care initially consists of minimizing facial swelling and pain. Systemic steroids may be used to decrease swelling. A typical steroid regimen is 125 mg methylprednisolone sodium succinate (Solu-Medrol) immediately preoperatively followed by 125 mg of this agent every 6 hours for 24 to 36 hours. Eighty milligrams of methylprednisolone acetate (Depo Medrol) is given intramuscularly 4 to 6 hours after the last dose of Solu-Medrol. Ice packs are also recommended during the first 24 to 36 hours postoperatively. Moist heat is then recommended until the swelling resolves. Prophylactic antibiotics are used to prevent infection. Adequate narcotic analgesics to control pain should be used during the postoperative period. However, they should be discontinued as soon as possible. They are usually administered for 1 to 2 weeks after surgery. Nonsteroidal antiinflammatory analgesic medication is also used routinely for 4 weeks postoperatively.

The pressure dressing is removed 24 to 36 hours after surgery, and the patient is usually discharged 1 to 2 days postoperatively. Skin sutures are removed a few days after surgery, completing the case.

The importance of postoperative physiotherapy cannot be overemphasized. This should be discussed in detail with the patient before the operation. Some clinicians prefer to have a physical therapist routinely participate in the postoperative physiotherapy program, and this is discussed later in this chapter.

We have encouraged early function to obtain a better range of motion. However, many orthopedists immobilize joints for about 10 days postoperatively to reduce internal bleeding and to allow wound healing to begin before the tissues move. While strict immobilization may not be necessary, the patients may benefit from minimizing jaw motion for 10 to 14 days.

Whether the jaw is mobilized immediately or immobilized for several days, it is important that a planned, supervised physiotherapy program designed to increase jaw range of motion be done. This program should include opening and protrusive movements, with emphasis on keeping the midline straight. It should also include right and left lateral movements. These exercises are done to establish symmetric movements of the condyles. Patients are encouraged to exercise at least four times a day for 5 minutes each time. Initially, the exercises are active; in other words, no forced opening with mouth props, tongue blades, etc. is done.

Patients are told to expect some mild discomfort while doing this physiotherapy. They are instructed to use moist heat for 15 minutes before the therapy and ice for 15 minutes afterward. As stated earlier nonsteroidal antiinflammatory analgesic medication is used routinely for 4 weeks postoperatively.

Patients who have inadequate opening, less than 35 mm, after 3 to 6 weeks should start a more active exercise program. This may include gentle stretching with the thumb and finger or using tongue blades. The goal of the program is to increase the opening about 2 to 3 mm each week until a more normal opening is obtained.

Load on the joint, as would occur with chewing, should be kept at a low level for 3 to 6 months. The exact time required for healing is not known, so 3 to 6 months is recommended empirically. Patients are instructed to eat a soft, nonchewing diet during this time; after 6 weeks they can slowly expand their diet. Patients are instructed to avoid foods that hurt their jaw and to avoid foods such as whole apples and raw vegetables and practices such as cracking ice and nuts *forever*.

PLATE 6-1

A and **B** The occlusion may be altered early in the postoperative period. This is manifested by a slight posterior open bite on the side of operation that frequently resolves within 2 to 3 weeks.

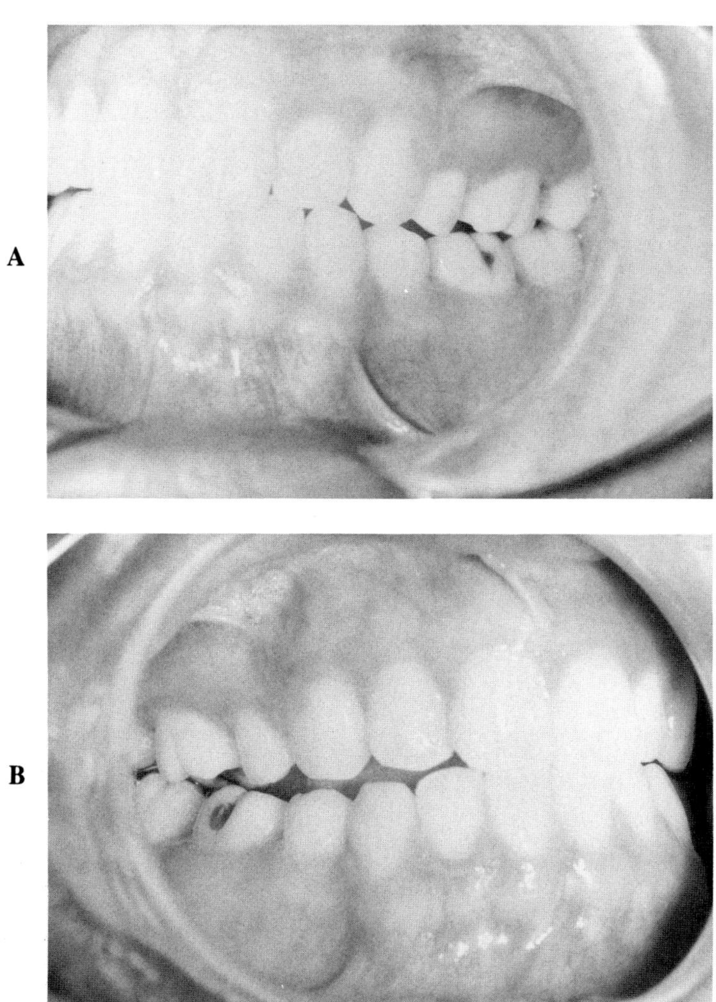

C and **D** If the occlusion remains unstable after 2 to 3 weeks a nonmanipulated bite registration is taken and an interocclusal appliance is constructed and placed to establish a stable occlusal relationship. We prefer a mandibular appliance, since the patient must wear the appliance 24 hours a day. The appliance is adjusted periodically until the bite is stable and unchanging, which usually requires 1 to 3 months. Once the bite is stable in the appliance, the occlusion is reevaluated, and treatment needed to establish a stable occlusion is planned. Active orthodontic treatment and restorative dentistry should not be started until at least 6 months postoperatively.

Bruxism seems to cause damage to the joint and has been one of the most common causes of poor surgical results. If bruxism is present, it must be controlled. Use of an interocclusal appliance at night is helpful. Other methods of control include biofeedback and use of drugs. If drug therapy is chosen, agents such as diazepam (Valium) should be used only at night and only for 2 to 3 weeks.

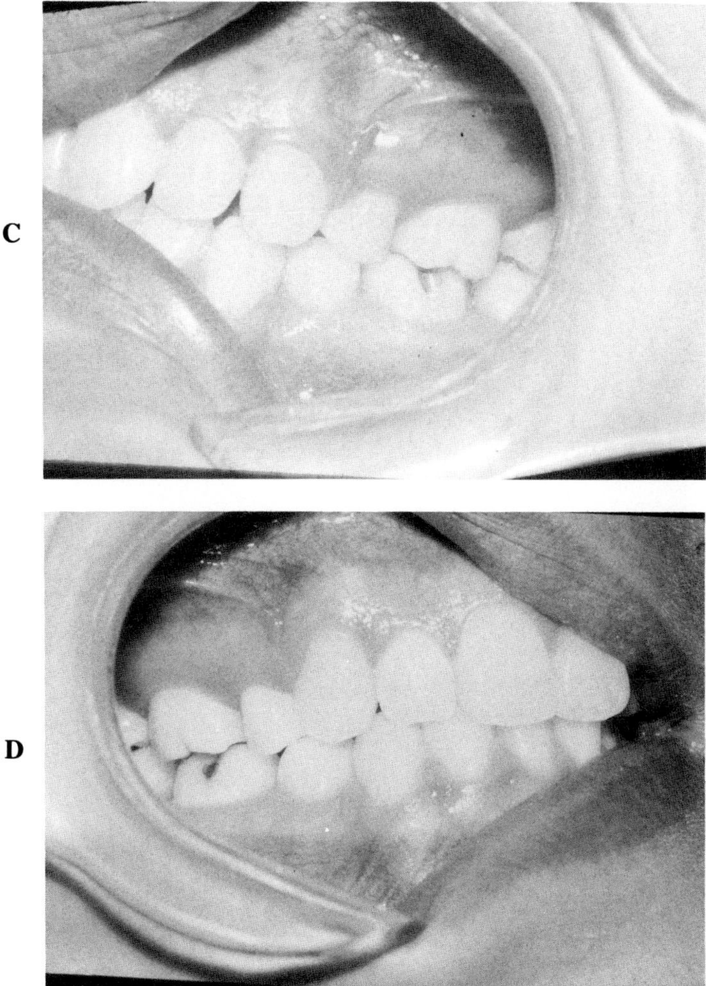

C

D

RESULTS

Criteria for success are variable and somewhat subjective. In general the objectives of the surgery are to eliminate or significantly reduce pain and to restore or significantly improve masticatory function. The extent to which these objectives are achieved determines the success of the procedure. In addition, there should be an absence of significant operative complications, for example, malocclusion or facial nerve paralysis.

DISC REPOSITIONING, RECONTOURING, AND REPAIR WITH OR WITHOUT ARTHROPLASTY

Disc repositioning procedures for the treatment of internal derangement have proven successful for the time period studied. The data cover two groups of patients. One group underwent disc repositioning with condylar reduction (Tables 6-1 to 6-3), and the second group had disc repositioning only (Tables 6-4 to 6-6).

TABLE 6-1 Clinical Material (Group I)

Patients (joints)	68 (78)
Women	59 (67)
Men	9 (11)
Average age	29 years
Duration of symptoms	4.3 years

TABLE 6-2 Surgical Outcome (Group I)

Follow-up	36 months (18-60 months)
Preoperative opening	27 mm (9-59 mm)
Postoperative opening	43 mm (35-55 mm)

TABLE 6-3 Surgical Outcome—Results (Group I)

Excellent (no symptoms)	37 patients (55%)	90%
Good (occasional symptoms)	24 patients (35%)	
Fair (improved, but continuous symptoms)	3 patients (4%)	10%
Poor (no improvement)	4 patients (6%)	

TABLE 6-4 Clinical Material (Group II)

Patients (joints)	27 (39)
Women	23 (34)
Men	4 (5)
Average age	30 years

TABLE 6-5 Surgical Outcome (Group II)

Follow-up	18 months (6-36 months)
Preoperative opening	32 mm (20-45 mm)
Postoperative opening	42 mm (30-54 mm)

TABLE 6-6 Surgical Outcome (Group II)

Excellent (no symptoms)	14 patients (52%)	85%
Good (occasional symptoms)	9 patients (33%)	
Fair (improved, but continuous symptoms)	1 patient (4%)	15%
Poor (no improvement)	3 patients (11%)	

DISC REPOSITIONING

With Condylar Reduction

Plain Films

PLATE 6-2

A Preoperative panoramic radiograph of condyle.

B During the first year postoperatively irregularities of the articular surface of the condyle and a lack of cortical outline are observed.

A

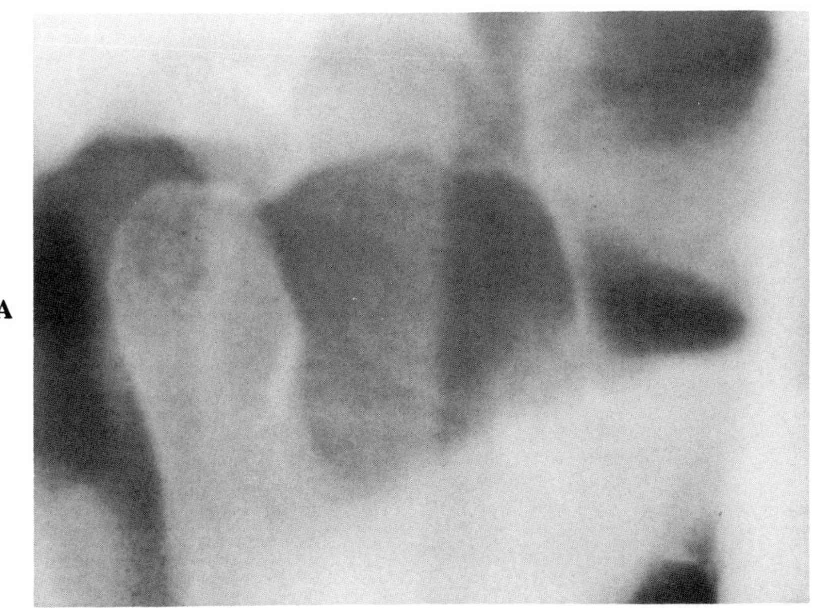

B

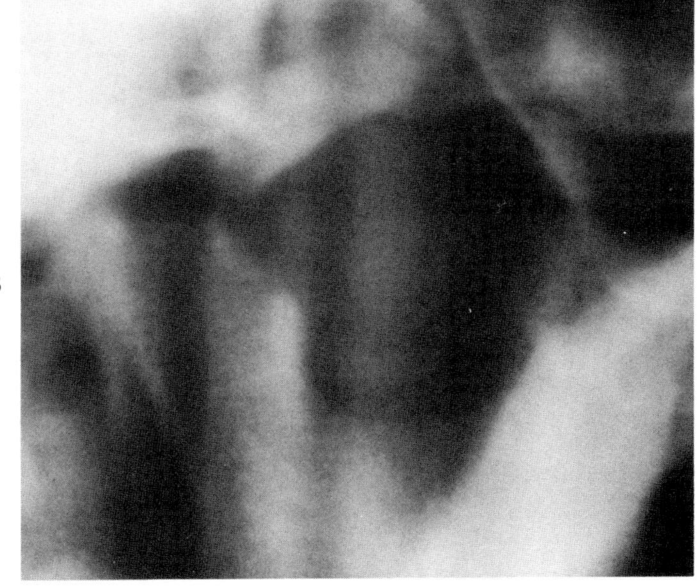

C During the second year the articular surface becomes smooth but is flattened anteriorly. During the rest of the follow-up period the condyles appear to remain stable, with only minimal changes occurring.

D Panoramic radiograph of another condyle 5 years postoperatively. There are occasional slight irregularities observed in the articular surface of the condyle. This condyle has not changed in appearance since the second postoperative year.

C

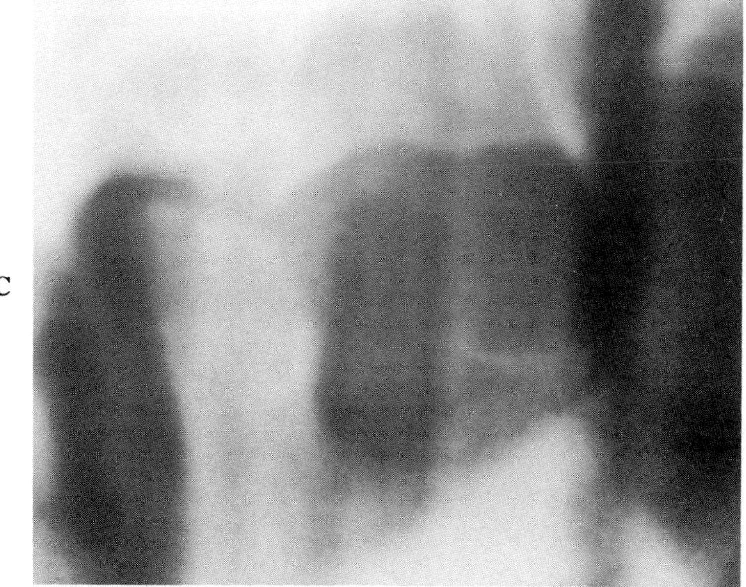

D

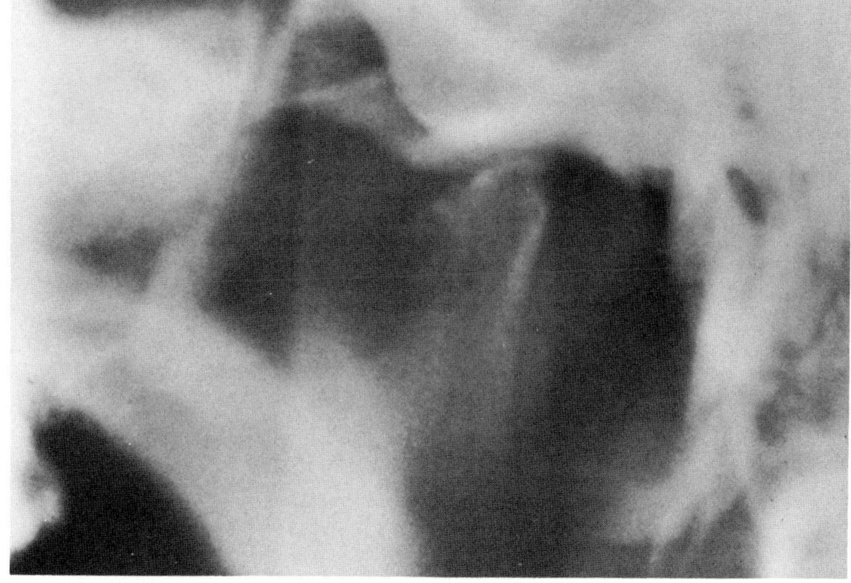

Arthrography

Five postoperative arthrograms have been done on patients who underwent successful surgery. They have demonstrated more normal-appearing lower joint spaces and normal disc function.

PLATE 6-3

A Closed-mouth preoperative arthrogram shows anterior disc displacement.
B Closed-mouth postoperative arthrogram shows more normal lower joint space.

A

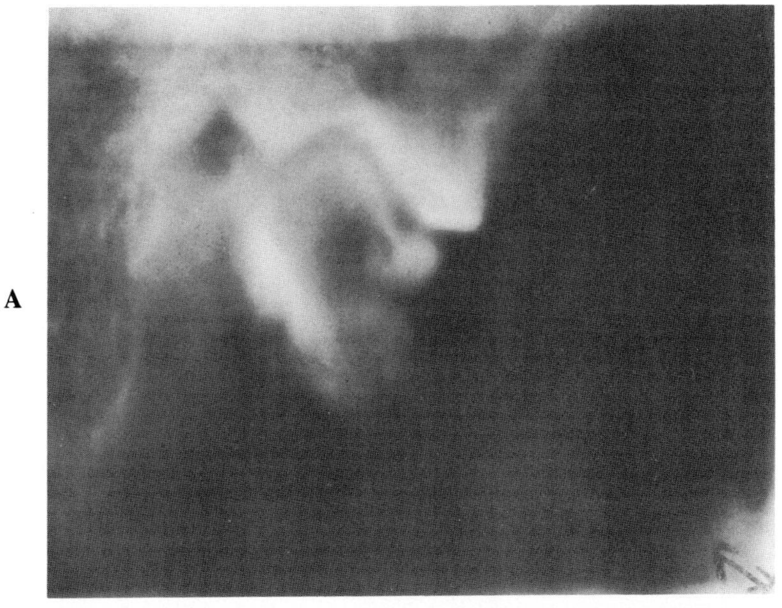

B

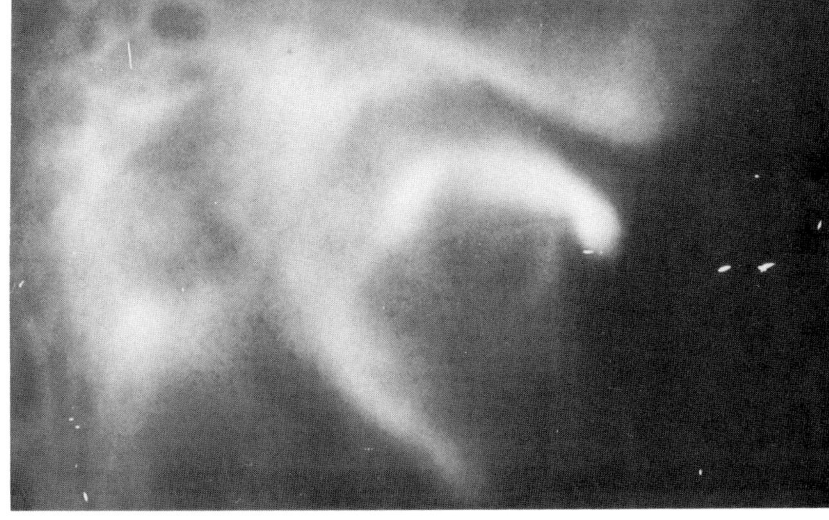

C Open-mouth preoperative arthrogram shows anterior disc displacement.
D Open-mouth postoperative arthrogram is normal.

C

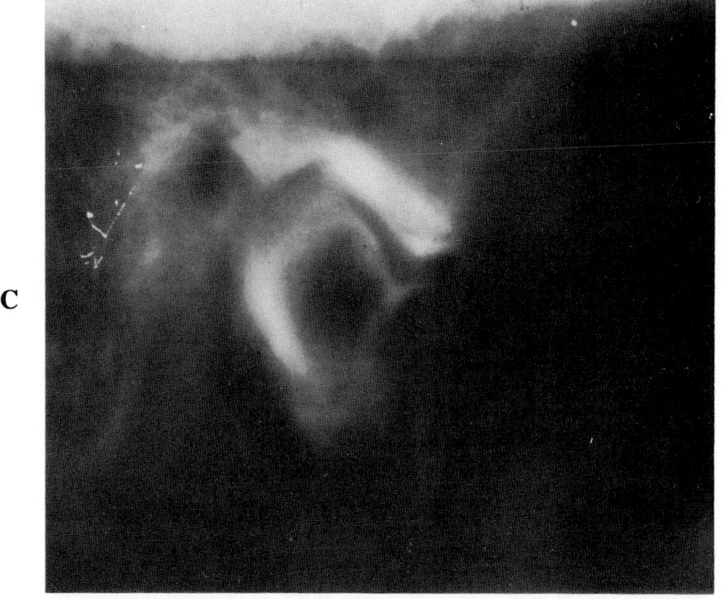

D

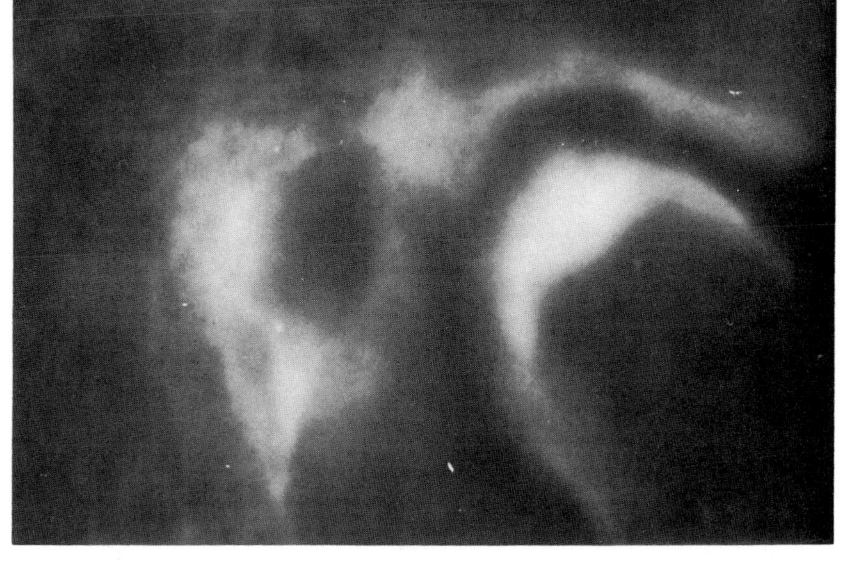

Without Condylar Reduction

Plain Films

PLATE 6-4

A Preoperative closed and open panoramic radiographs of the condyle.

B Postoperative closed and open panoramic radiographs of the condyle. This joint was operated on 3 years previously and appears unchanged from the preoperative film. This is a typical finding in cases without condylar reduction.

A

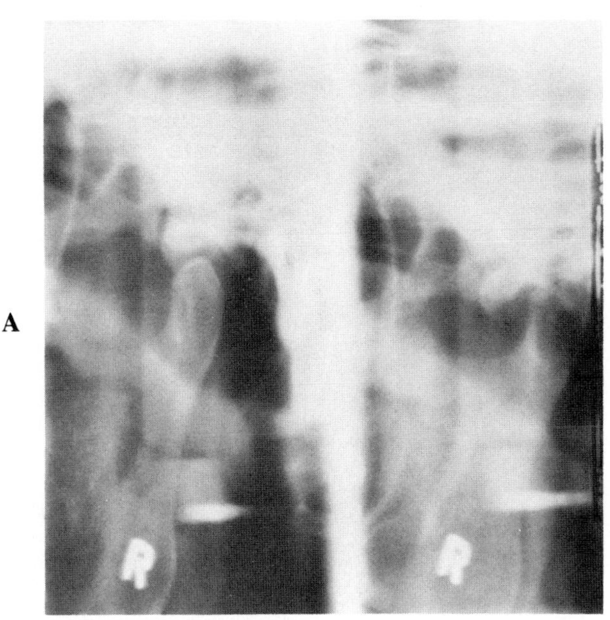

B

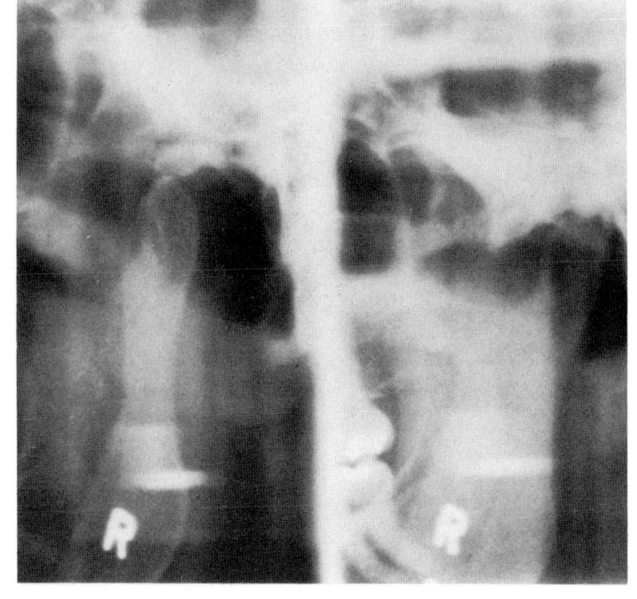

Arthrography

Three postoperative arthrograms have been done on patients who underwent successful surgery. They have demonstrated more normal-appearing lower joint spaces and normal disc function.

PLATE 6-5

A Closed-mouth preoperative arthrogram shows anterior disc displacement and perforation.

B Closed-mouth postoperative arthrogram shows normal lower joint space and no perforation.

A

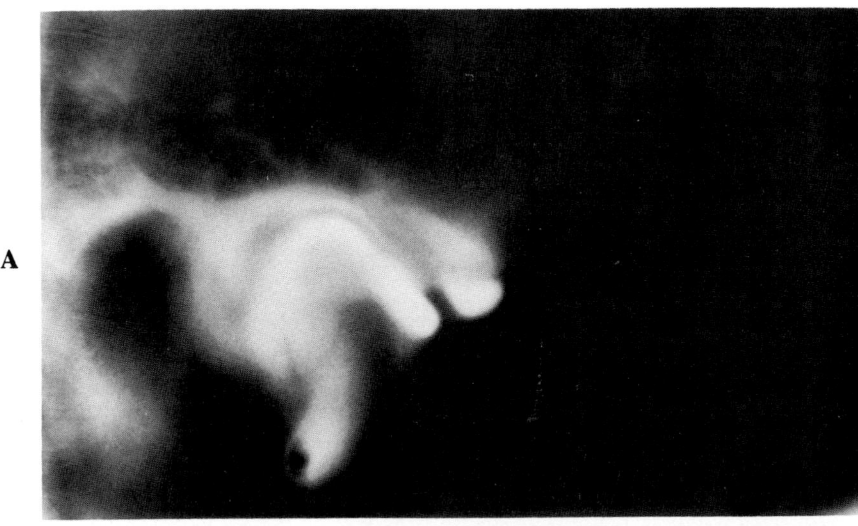

B

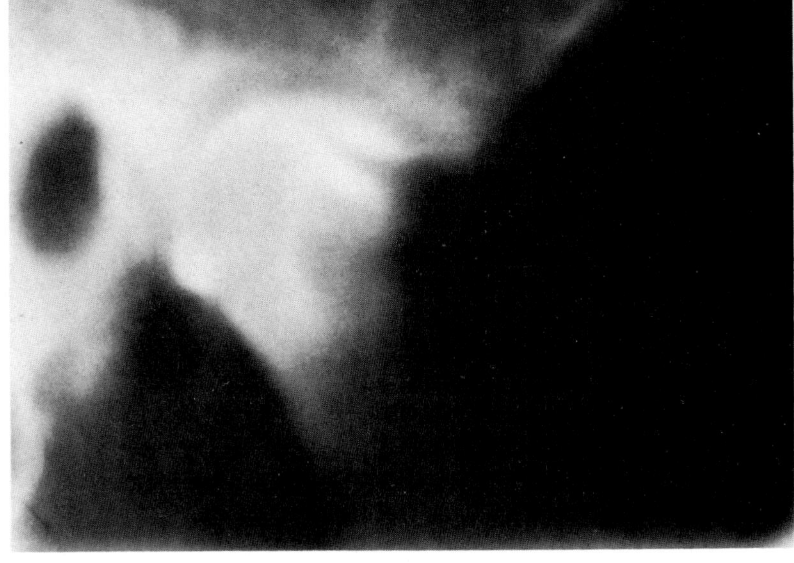

C Open-mouth preoperative arthrogram shows disc reduced to a normal position.
D Open-mouth postoperative arthrogram is normal.

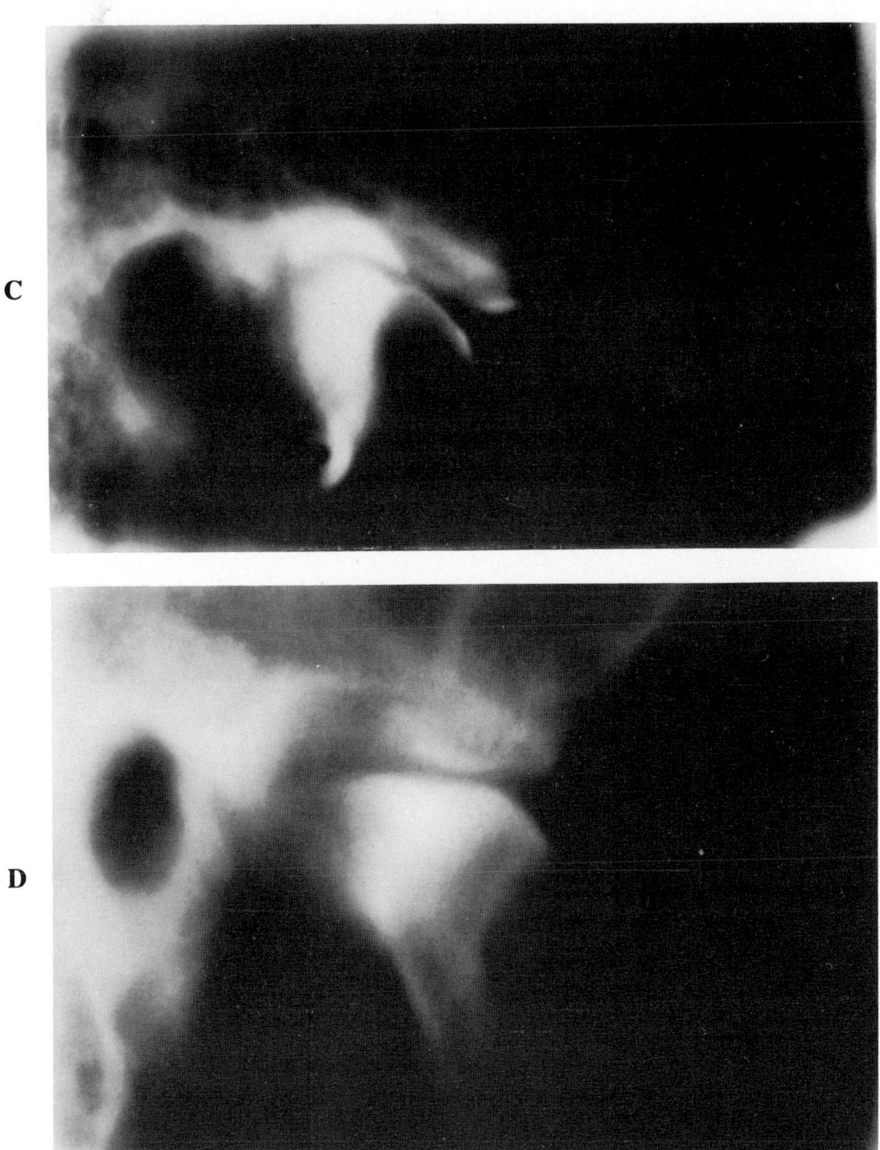

Conclusions

Both procedures have proven to be successful and results are comparable: 90% success with condylar reduction and 85% without condylar reduction. The follow-up is still relatively short for both groups of patients, and longer follow-up is needed to determine which procedure is preferred. At the present time we recommend the more conservative procedure of disc repositioning only. Each procedure has potential advantages and disadvantages.

Disc Repositioning with Condylar Reduction

Advantages

1. "Creates space," therefore allowing more surgical tolerance.
2. May accommodate the occlusion by preventing posterior open bite; in other words, makes the joint fit the teeth.

Disadvantages

1. Destroys the articular connective tissue, thereby possibly decreasing the joint's ability to remodel in response to changes in function.
2. Allows increased intraarticular adhesions with decreased joint mobility.
3. May promote unpredictable condylar resorption.

Disc Repositioning without Condylar Reduction

Advantages

1. Maintains integrity of the articular connective tissue.
2. Allows less intraarticular adhesion with better early joint mobility.
3. Promotes minimal condylar osseous changes.

Disadvantages

1. Carries fewer surgical tolerances; therefore success totally depends on correct disc repositioning.
2. May be more susceptible to recurrent disc displacement.
3. Requires greater attention to occlusion after surgery.

MENISCECTOMY (DISC REMOVAL) WITH INSERTION OF ALLOPLASTIC FOSSA IMPLANT

Disc removal procedures for treatment of advanced internal derangement and arthrosis have also proven successful for the time period studied. The data consist of one retrospective study employing patient examination and chart review (Tables 6-7 and 6-8).

TABLE 6-7 **Clinical Material**

Patients (joints)	69 (89)
Women	52
Men	17
Average age	34 years
Duration of symptoms	9.4 years
Follow-up	2-9 years

TABLE 6-8 **Surgical Outcome—Results**

Excellent (few or no symptoms)	70 arthroplasties, 78.7%	92.2%
Good (occasional moderate symptoms)	12 arthroplasties, 13.5%	
Fair (minimally improved; intermittent severe symptoms) Poor (frequent or constant severe) symptoms)	7 arthroplasties	7.8%

PLATE 6-6

These tomographic radiographs were taken 3 years postoperatively of a 25-year-old woman who underwent bilateral meniscectomies with Silastic fossa implants. Condylar recontouring was done on the right side only; note the significant remodelling as opposed to the nonrecontoured left side.

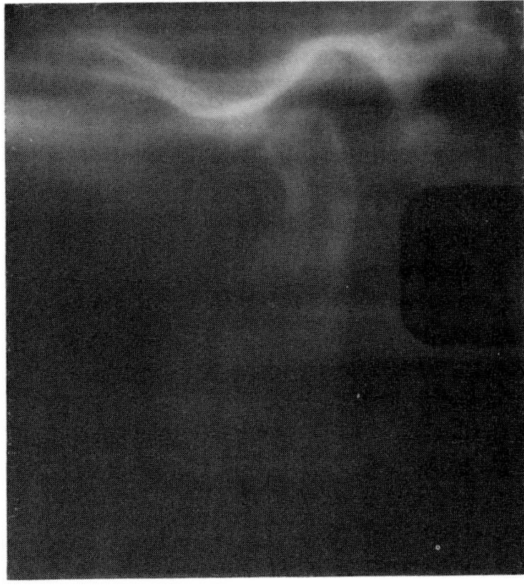

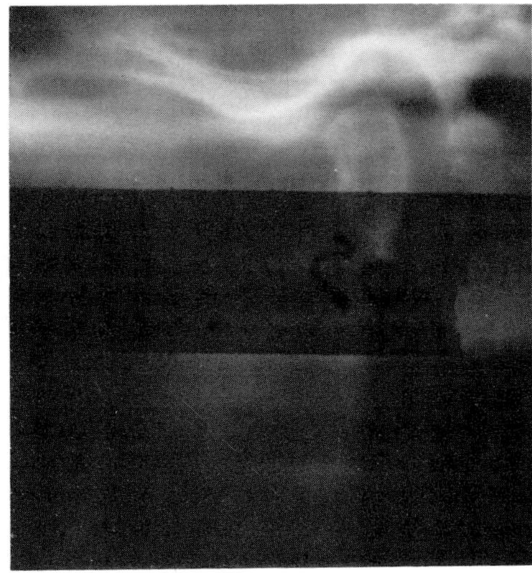

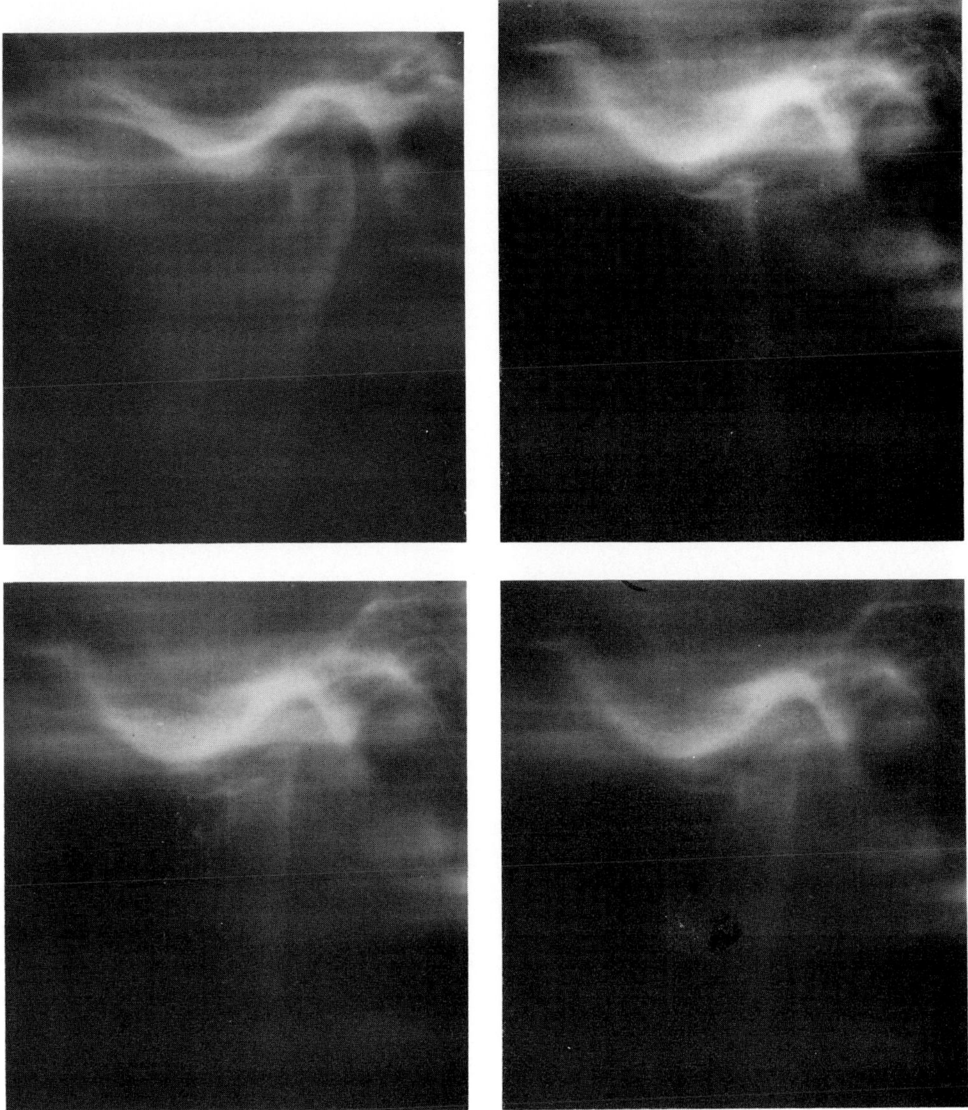

chapter 7

Temporomandibular Joint Surgery

COMPLICATIONS AND FAILURE

Before discussing the reasons for failure, criteria for surgical success must be established. Success is defined as a favorable outcome. The most important determinant of success is the effect of the surgery on the patient's pain. Joint pain should be eliminated or greatly reduced. Successful surgery should produce increased range of jaw motion without deviation and should restore the ability to masticate and to eat a normal diet with few restrictions. Additionally, there should be an absence of significant morbidity as a result of the surgery. The occlusion should be unchanged or minimally changed. There should be no permanent facial nerve damage or unsightly scars.

Failure is defined as lack of success or, in other words, an unfavorable outcome. In January 1984 the American Association of Oral and Maxillofacial Surgeons conducted a Clinical Congress that included a symposium on TMJ surgery. The general consensus at this symposium was that the surgical failure rate for various procedures was approximately 10% to 20%. The reasons for surgical failure are varied and will be discussed under the following general categories: (1) Diagnosis and patient selection, (2) surgical technique, (3) postoperative management, (4) unpredicted biologic responses, (5) postoperative trauma, and (6) unknown causes.

DIAGNOSIS AND PATIENT SELECTION

Misdiagnosis appears to be the most common reason for surgical failure. If a patient has a significant muscular component that is the source or a major source of complaints, surgical intervention will fail. The patient who is bruxing before surgery will probably continue to brux after surgery, and the muscular symptoms will therefore continue. In addition, the operated joint will be excessively loaded and most likely damaged. This would be analogous to an athlete having knee surgery and immediately running on the operated knee.

Patient selection is also an important factor in success or failure. Patients who are able to give an accurate history, describe their symptoms precisely, and have a clear and realistic understanding of what surgery can and cannot accomplish generally do well. On the other hand, patients who are poor historians, do not describe their symptoms precisely, or have an unrealistic expectation of surgery are generally likely to have failure. Patients should be able to distinguish and compare accurately preoperative and postoperative complaints.

Obviously, patients with psychologic or sociologic components to their problem are more likely to experience failure. These patients should be evaluated by a psychologist or psychiatrist before considering surgery.

SURGICAL TECHNIQUE

Incorrect choice of surgical procedure may result in failure. Disc repositioning may not be possible in all cases. Repositioning a deformed, scarred disc is likely to fail. Disc removal may be much too aggressive a procedure for many cases. In other words, the procedure must be a rational response to a specific pathologic condition.

The most troublesome intraoperative problem is excessive bleeding. Every attempt, through meticulous soft tissue dissection, should be made to prevent hemorrhage. Hemorrhage should be controlled as it occurs. If excessive hemorrhage occurs, patience must be employed in controlling it to avoid postoperative complications such as hematoma, possible infection, and adhesions.

Facial nerve injury can be a sequela of surgery. Usually only the temporal branches are involved, resulting in eyebrow lag. The injury is generally temporary, resolving spontaneously within 6 months; however, in a small number of cases it may be permanent. Rarely, facial nerve injury will be more extensive, involving other branches and at times even complete paralysis. In these cases the nerve should be evaluated immediately using nerve excitability testing to determine its functional status. If the percutaneous threshold is normal, a neurapraxic lesion exists and full recovery is highly likely. If there is evidence that the nerve has been severed, surgical exploration and nerve repair should be done. Prevention of nerve damage is best accomplished with *meticulous* soft tissue dissection and appropriate retraction.

Specific postoperative problems may be related to specific surgical procedures. Repositioned discs are susceptible to postoperative trauma. In some cases tears may develop in the suture line. A sudden increase in joint pain associated with the development of joint noise suggests that the disc has slipped anteriorly or torn. A bite appliance can be helpful managing the anteriorly positioned disc. Torn suture lines will require reoperation. The presence of joint pain without joint noise suggests the possibility of inflammation and/or compression of the intra-articular soft tissues. Physical therapy, nonsteroidal antiinflammatory medications, and a bite appliance may be helpful in resolving these symptoms.

The most common postoperative problems associated with meniscectomy and the placement of implants are related to size and fixation of the implant. Implants that are too large can result in a posterior open bite on the operated side. Dislodgement and migration of the implant or implant fragmentation can occur. This results in inflammation, possible foreign body reaction, and of course, mechanical interference. These patients should undergo reparative surgery. An implant that extends too far may irritate adjacent soft tissue, causing temporalis tenderness and pain.

Implants that are too small can also cause problems. If the implant does not adequately fill the available joint space, heavy posterior occlusal contacts may be present on the operated side. Implants that do not cover the articular surface may become dislodged by the condyle as it moves beyond the extent of the implant. These patients will have unusual joint noises and symptoms of mechanical interference as well as pain. Reoperation is usually required.

Anchorage of the implant can also be a problem. If the implant is not securely anchored, it may move during function. This movement will result in bone resorption around the wires or sutures holding the implant. Obviously, as this occurs the implant can move more, ultimately resulting in dislodgement and migration of the implant.

Arthroplasty (articular surface recontouring) should be done carefully and conservatively. Excessive arthroplasty can result in significant malocclusion in the form of heavy posterior contacts or, in bilateral cases, an open bite. The articular surfaces should be smooth without the presence of sharp projections or angles. Sharp projections of bone may tear or dislodge an implant.

The development of adhesions postoperatively is a common and significant problem. The presence of adhesions results in decreased joint mobility. This mobility is managed with physical therapy, specifically stretching exercises. Moist heat, ultrasound, and transcutaneous electrical nerve stimulation (TENS) may also be helpful. Patience and perseverance are required by the patient as well as the surgeon. Patients who do not respond to conservative efforts may benefit from forced opening under anesthesia. These patients will require continued exercises afterward if benefit is to be attained. Reoperation may help the most refractory patients. However, some patients appear to be more susceptible to adhesion formation than others and the recurrence of adhesions in reoperated joints is probable. Prevention of adhesion formation involves careful hemorrhage control and consistent postoperative physiotherapy.

POSTOPERATIVE MANAGEMENT

Some surgery fails because of inadequate postoperative management, most commonly inadequate physiotherapy. Patients must participate in a controlled postoperative physiotherapy program if a normal range of motion is to be attained. Limited motion is not only debilitating functionally but is also generally associated with pain. Marked deviation of the mandible toward the operated side will eventually result in pain and dysfunction in the opposite joint.

Postoperative occlusal management is important. The most common cause of failure secondary to occlusal problems is related to lack of posterior occlusal support. If the posterior teeth on the operated side remain out of contact, the joint will be excessively loaded and failure will frequently occur. An occlusal appliance should be used to prevent this. Likewise, the lack of posterior tooth support because of missing teeth can result in failure.

Another common cause of failure is the inability to control bruxism. Frequently this results from failure to recognize its presence, that is, misdiagnosis. Every effort must be used to control this difficult problem if surgery is to be successful.

UNPREDICTED BIOLOGIC RESPONSES

Surgery may fail because of unusual biologic responses. Unpredicted excessive condylar resorption may occur following arthroplasty with disc repositioning or meniscectomy and implant placement. This results in a deviated mandible with heavy occlusal contacts and possibly a crossbite in unilateral cases and an open bite in bilateral cases. Excessive condylar resorption appears to occur more commonly in patients with osteoarthroses who have arthroplasty and implants placed. This problem is managed by reoperation, usually requiring partial or total joint replacement or orthognathic surgery.

Foreign body response to implant material is sometimes seen following fragmentation of the implant material. The patient complains of severe joint pain and swelling, although swelling is rarely observed clinically. Nonsteroidal antiinflammatory drugs reduce the symptoms, at least temporarily, but reoperation is usually required. In reoperation the implant material should be removed and replaced with a different material or not replaced. The removed joint soft tissues show a foreign body giant cell reaction and synovitis. One case of silicone-induced lymphadenopathy has been reported.

Osseous ankylosis occasionally occurs after TMJ surgery, particularly meniscectomy. This is rare and should be managed as any other TMJ ankylosis would be managed, that is, with condylectomy or gap arthroplasty and joint reconstruction.

POSTOPERATIVE TRAUMA

Several patients have experienced recurrent joint pain and dysfunction secondary to macrotrauma following surgery. The most common cause has been trauma secondary to accidents or social altercations. Injury of the TMJ during intubation for general anesthesia has also occurred. For this reason, all patients undergoing operation should inform the anesthesiologist about their joint surgery before being given general anesthetics.

If possible, third molars requiring removal should be removed before or during TMJ surgery and not afterward, as this can be a source of postoperative problems.

UNKNOWN CAUSES

Surgeons must understand that the condition of some patients will not improve no matter how many surgeries are undertaken. Some surgeries fail because of unknown causes. Chronic pain and dysfunction management must be available. For this a team approach is strongly advocated.

• • •

The following cases demonstrate examples of surgical complications and/or failures and their management.

PLATE 7-1

This case presentation demonstrates several diagnostic and treatment problems that occurred in a 30-year-old woman who underwent left TMJ arthroplasty with meniscus relocation and repair and condylar head recontouring. The patient had a 1-year history of left facial pain and mandibular hypomobility secondary to trauma. Extensive noninvasive therapy, using splints and physical therapy, failed to release the persistent closed-lock that was present.

A Preoperative charting of pain to palpation shows moderate tenderness in the anterior external auditory meatus indicative of TMJ capsulitis. However, there is still significant myofascial pain after noninvasive therapy. This greatly complicates the postoperative stability of the joint.

B Preoperative arthrogram showing incomplete filling of the upper compartment after injecting dye only into the inferior compartment. This signifies a perforation and superior compartment adhesions. This situation would greatly complicate a meniscus repair procedure.

A

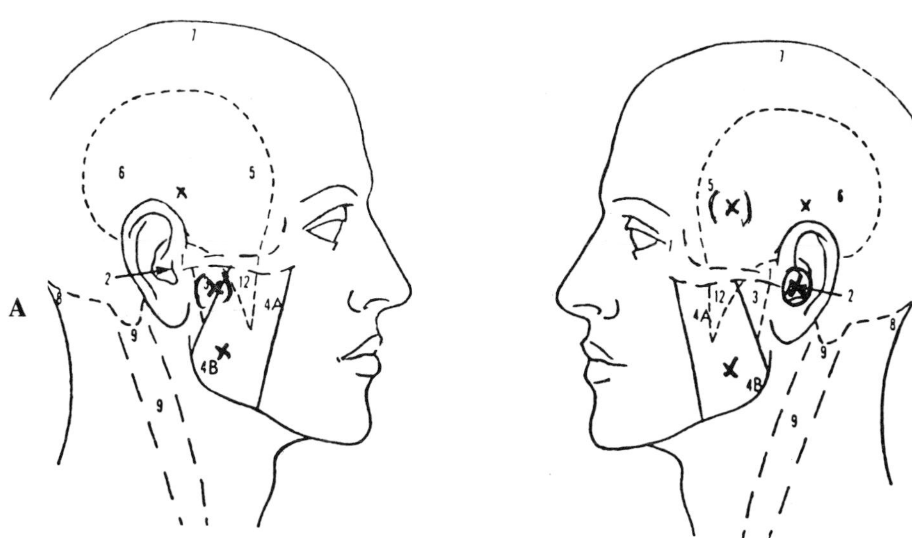

"Do you feel any difference between the two sides?"

B

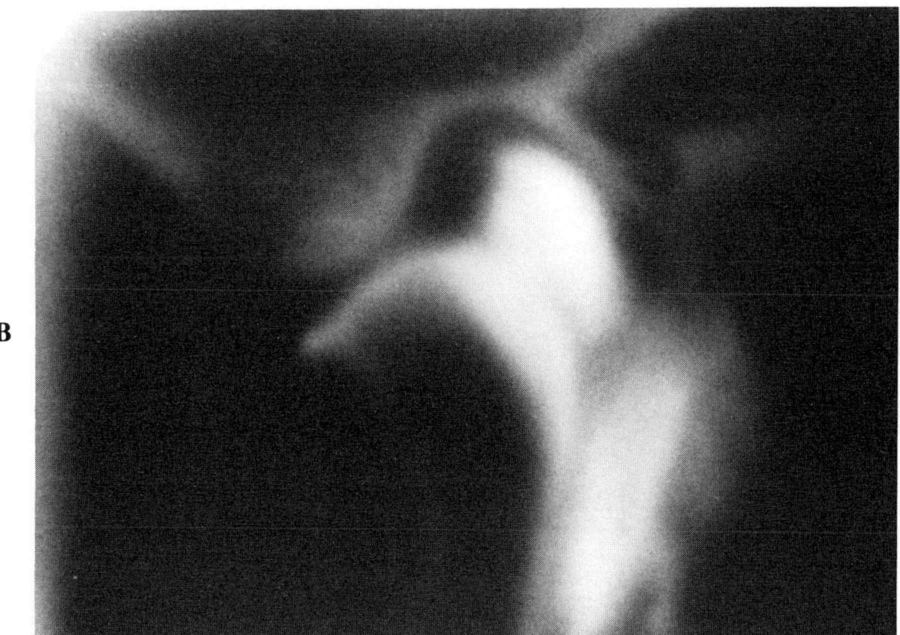

C Postoperative charting of pain to palpation shows severe preauricular pain and diffuse, severe myofascial pain on palpation.

D Postoperative opening is limited, and the mandible deviates to the operated side, indicating lack of translation of the left joint.

C

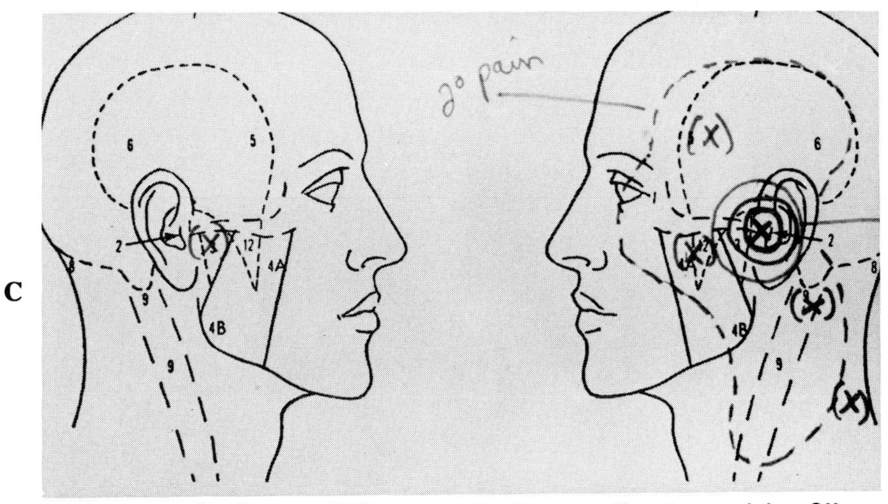

"Do you feel any difference between the two sides?"
"Does it hurt or is it just uncomfortable?"

D

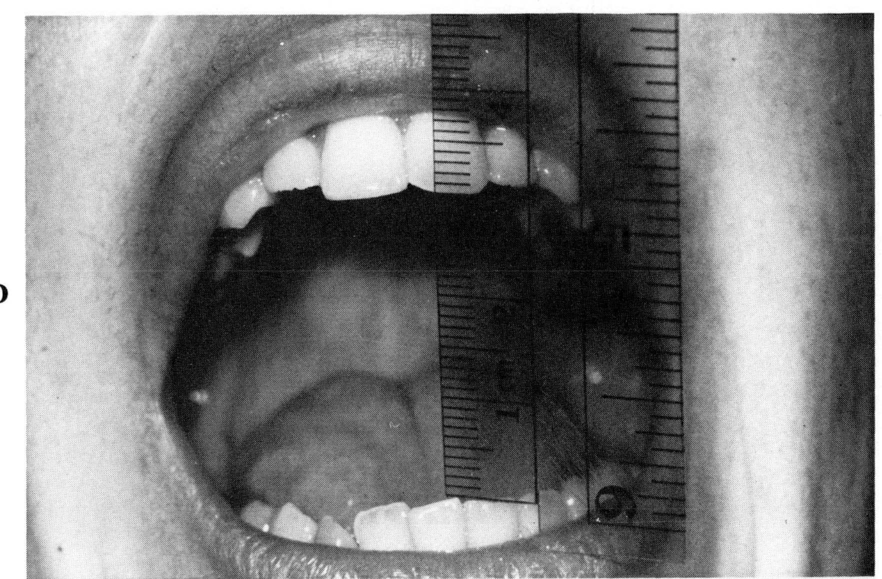

E Dental occlusion is unstable, with heavy occlusal contacts on the ipsilateral molar teeth.

F Postoperative anteroposterior tomographic views of the left TMJ taken several months after surgery show irregular lateral morphologic changes with arthrosis. This can be one of the complications of doing condylar recontouring. Double horizontal line represents high condylectomy that may have to be done. After the resection, the condylar stump must be rounded.

G Postoperative arthrogram taken several months after arthroplasty shows incomplete fill resulting from adhesions.

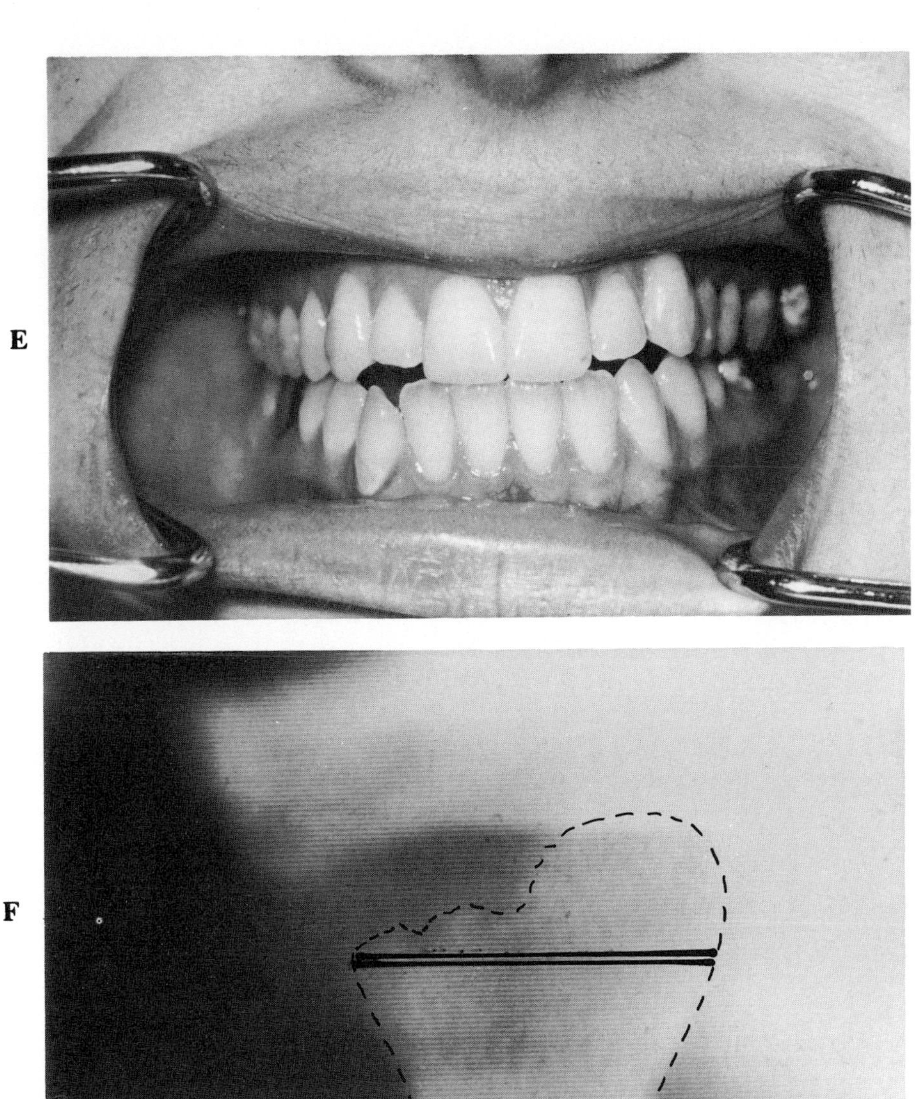
E
F

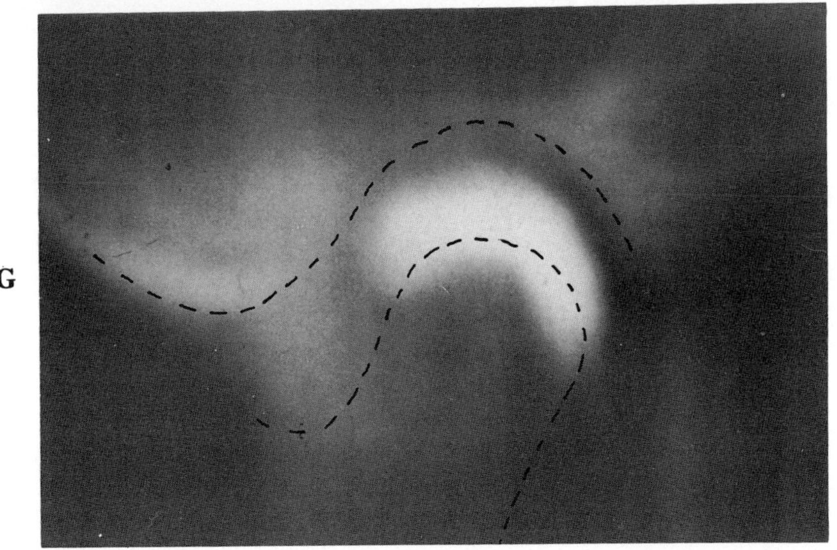
G

H Inability to wrinkle the forehead and raise the eyebrow on the ipsilateral side was an additional complication. The patient was able to close the eyelid.

I Most preauricular scars are barely visible; however, this patient developed a hypertrophic scar.

Resolution of these problems was initially accomplished by intensive, prolonged splinting and physical therapy to control myofascial pain and spasm. The patient underwent a second surgical procedure that included meniscectomy and insertion of a Silastic fossa implant. Scar revision with subcutaneous steroid injections eliminated the hypertrophic scarring. The frontal muscle weakness resolved several months after the second surgery. Four years after the second arthroplasty the patient has fair opening and relatively good function. Reported pain is minimal, with intermittent moderate pain controlled with a mild analgesic.

H

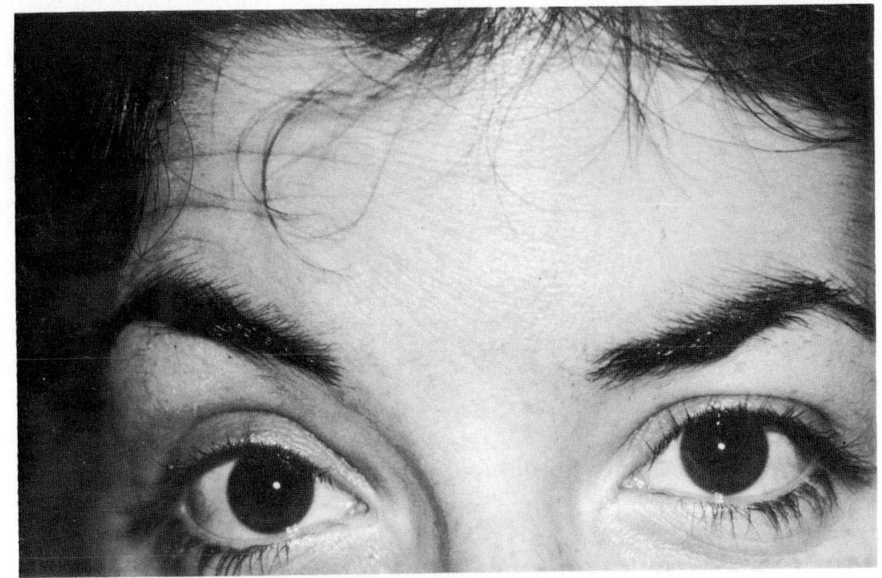

I

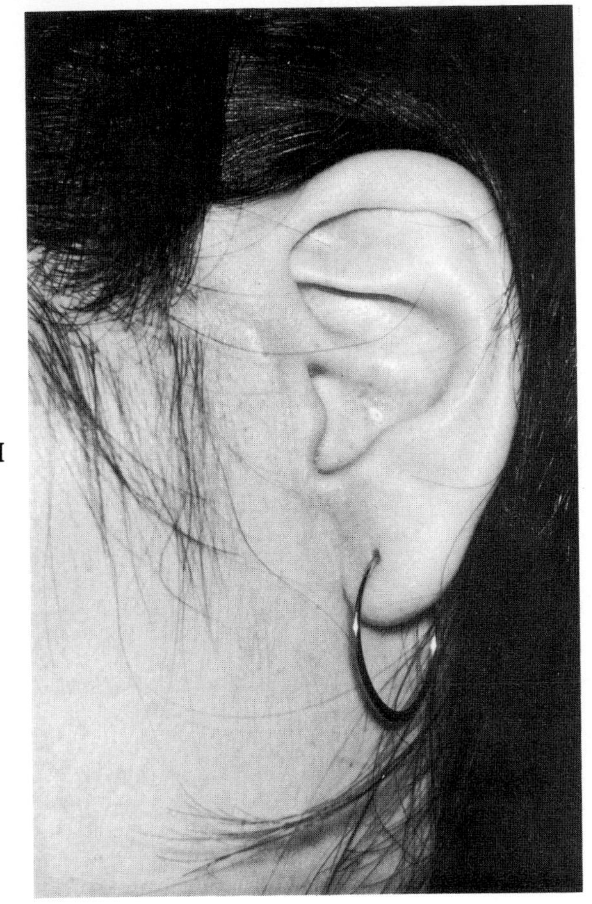

PLATE 7-2

This case presentation demonstrates technical problems associated with the use of an alloplastic implant in the inferior compartment after meniscus repair and condylar recontouring. Two years after bilateral surgery, the patient had severe pain, very limited opening and function, and very noxious, audible crepitus.

A to **C** Progressive opening and reexploration of the joints revealed large porous Teflon/Proplast implants fused to the meniscus superiorly and adhering to the condylar head. The implants were grossly overextended medially, posteriorly, and anteriorly. Much of each implant had migrated and fused with the lateral pterygoid muscle.

A
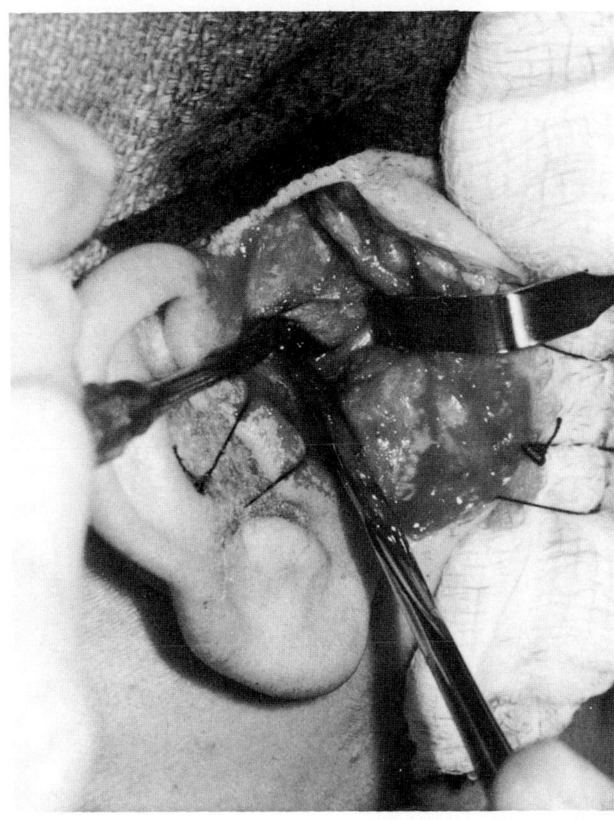

B
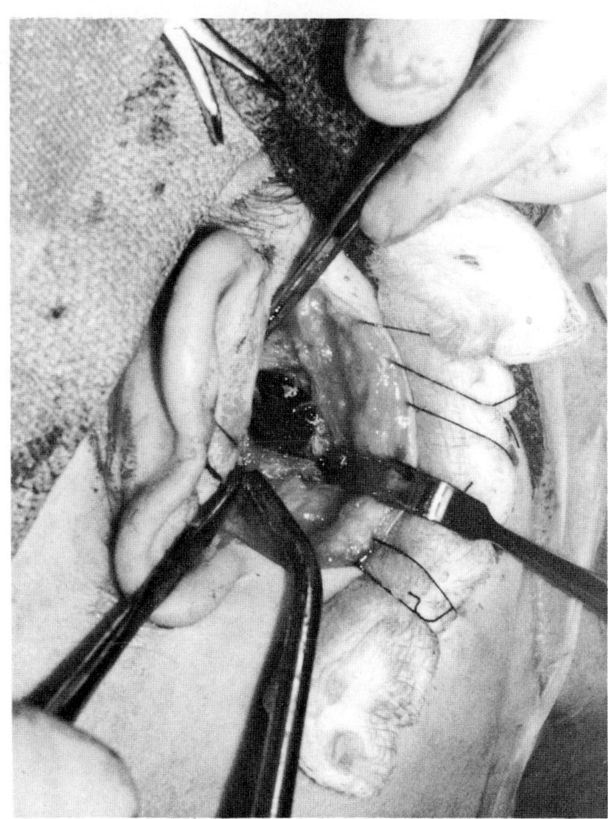

C
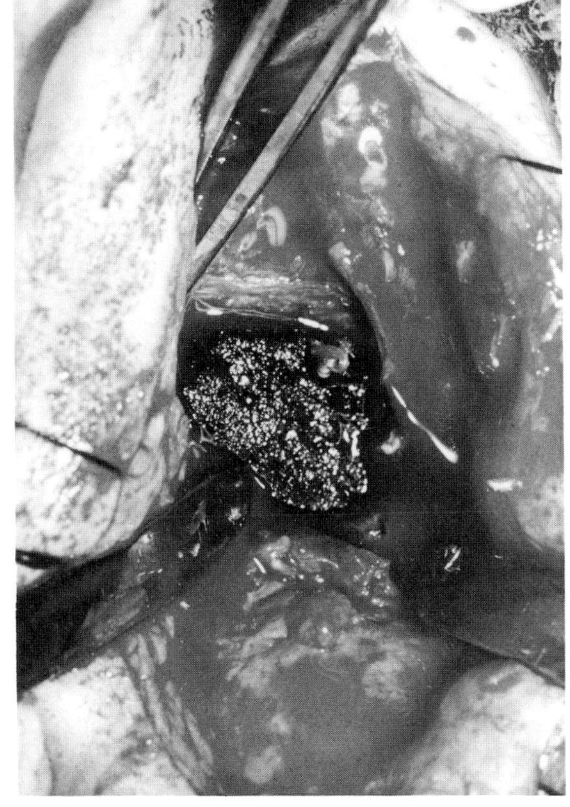

D to **F** Removal of the implants was very difficult, with resultant fragmentation of the implants. Meniscectomy and a condylar shave were necessary. The adjacent soft tissue was highly inflamed. Adjacent bony surfaces of the fossa, eminence, and condyle were stained black.

G Impregnation of the Proplast material, with foreign body reactions in the meniscus and lateral pterygoid muscle.

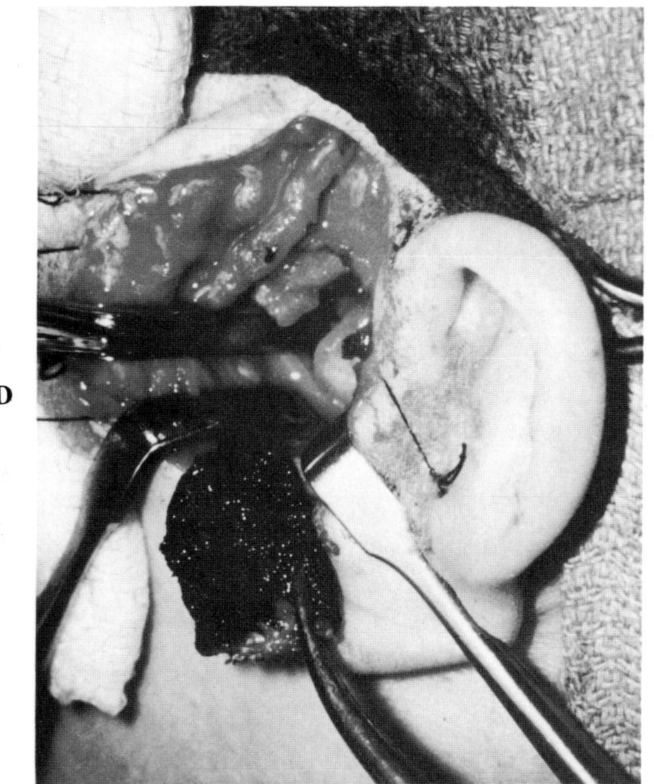

D

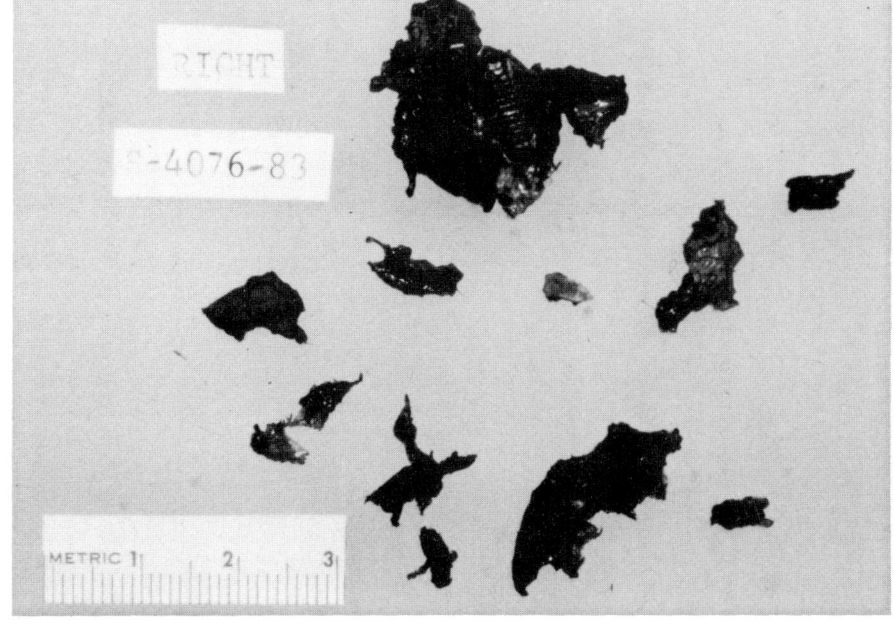

E

F

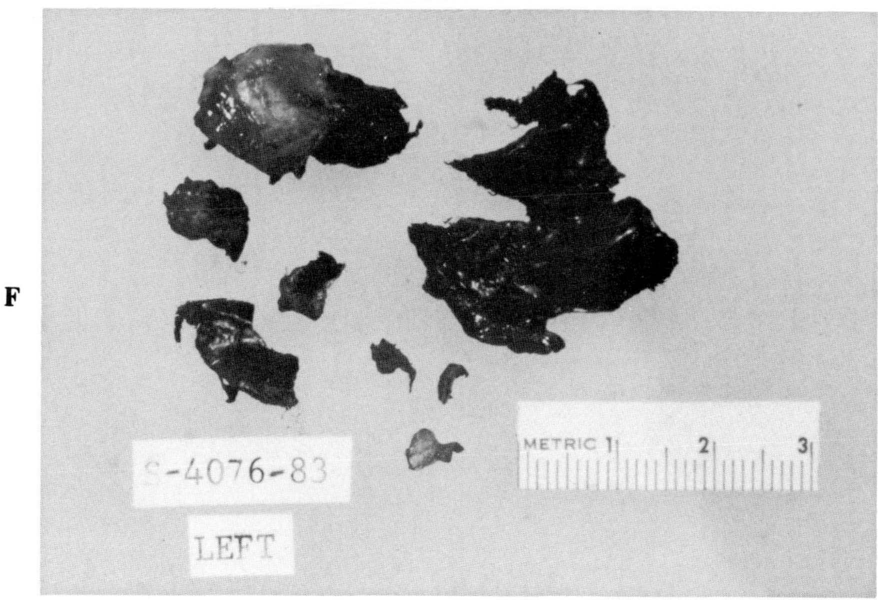

G

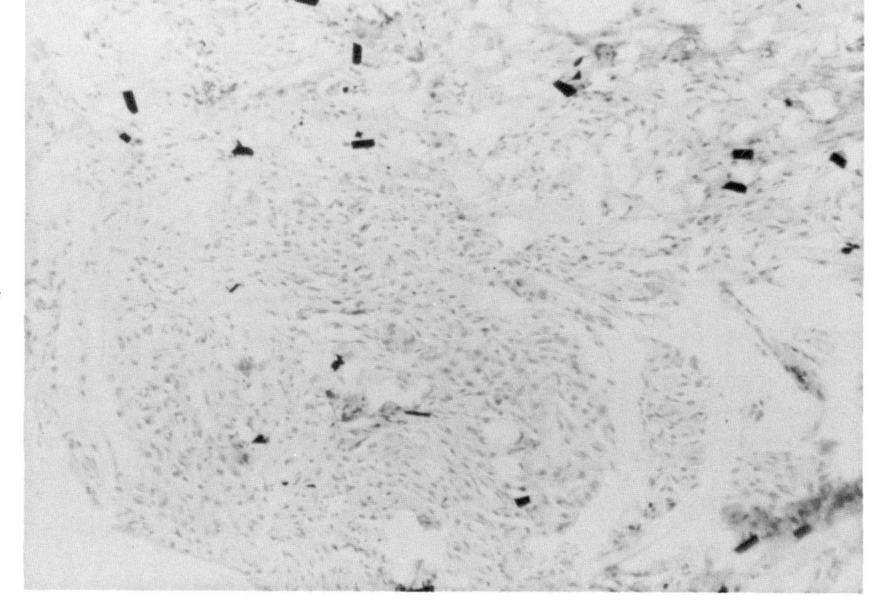

PLATE 7-3

This case demonstrates a patient who underwent right-sided meniscectomy and placement of Dacron-reinforced Silastic implant over the fossa and eminence. The patient did well for about 3 months and then began to have moderate to severe pain in the right TMJ. The patient complained of joint swelling. He also developed a very distinct ''snapping'' sound in the right TMJ. Treatment with nonsteroidal antiinflammatory medications and physical therapy temporarily reduced the symptoms but did not resolve them. The right TMJ underwent reoperation 5 months after the first surgery.

A Intraoperative photograph demonstrating that the implant had become dislodged and had slipped laterally. Movement of the condyle produced a ''snapping'' sound as the condyle moved across an edge of the Dacron-reinforced Silastic.

B Sutures were completely loose from the bone. The implant was only partially encapsulated by connective tissue, and there was an area of marked wear on the implant. The implant was probably too large and inadequately secured to the bone.

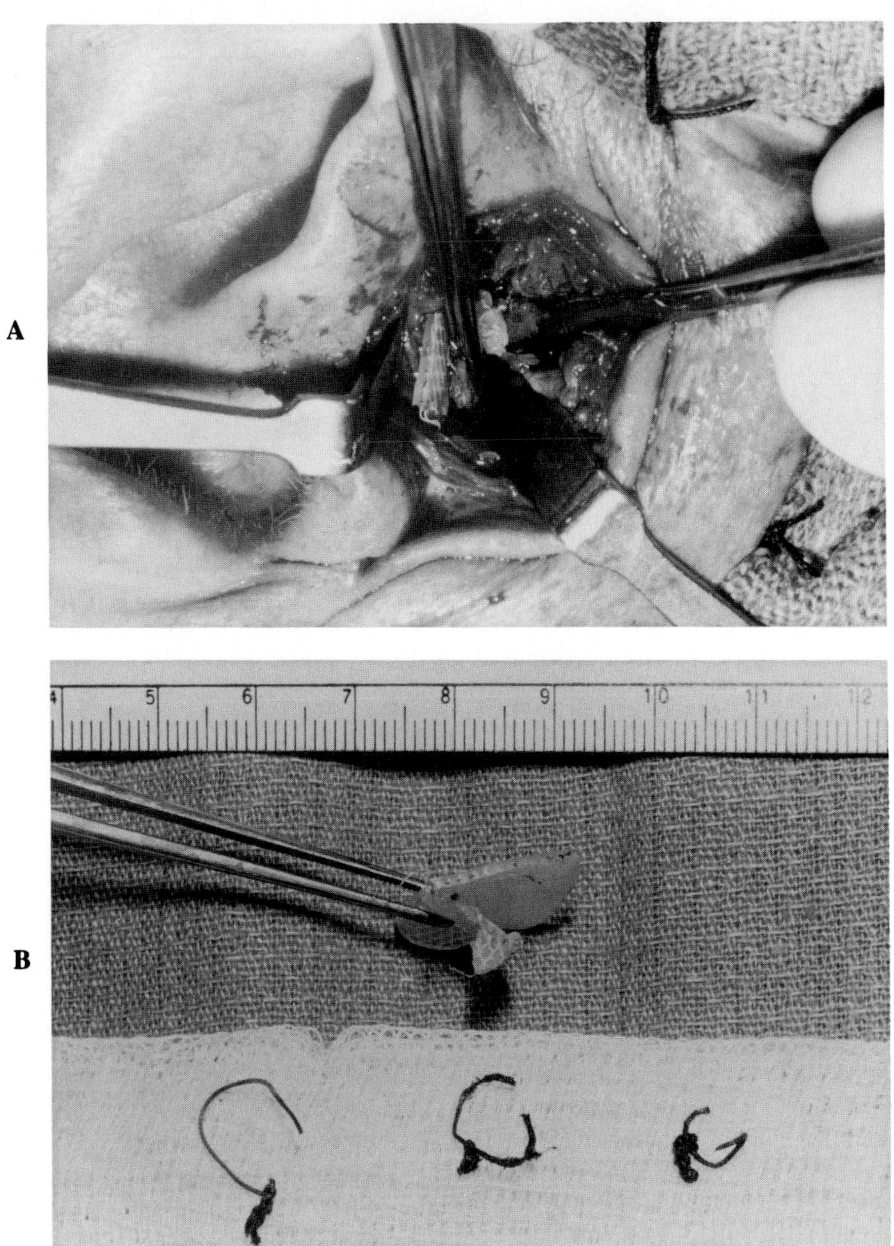
A
B
4 5 6 7 8 9 10 11 12

C Marked foreign body reaction to multiple fragments of Dacron-reinforced Silastic in the surrounding tissues. There was also evidence of detrital synovitis.

D The Dacron-reinforced Silastic implant was removed and replaced with a Teflon/Proplast implant. The patient has done well for 1 year following surgery.

C

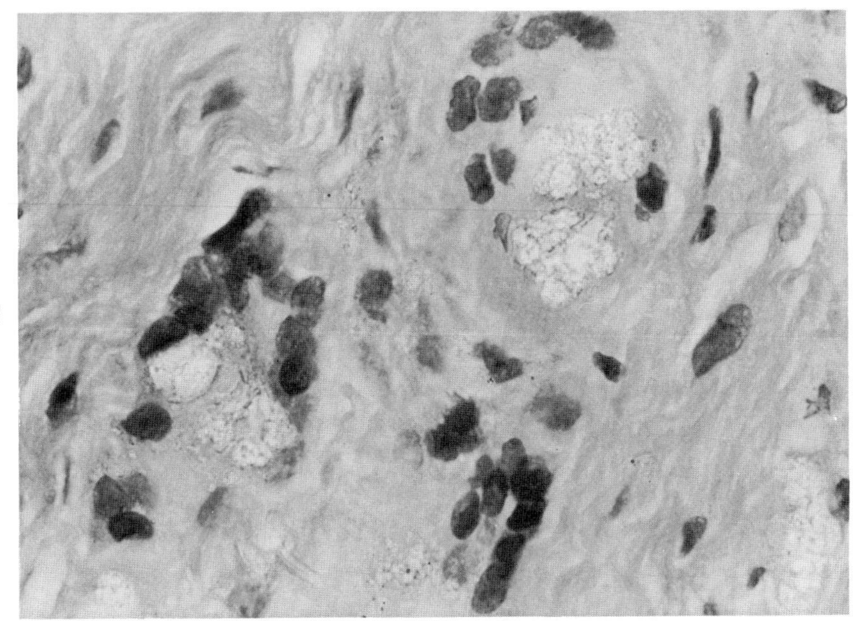

D

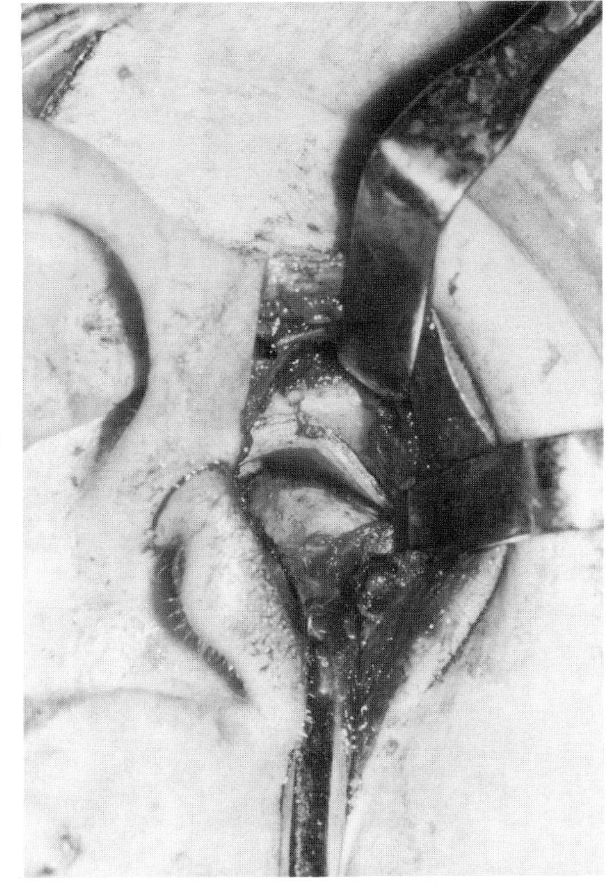

PLATE 7-4

If a patient who has undergone arthroplasty with meniscectomy and fossa implant develops a capsulitis refractory to conservative treatment, simple implant removal may be indicated. Removal is especially easy if a Silastic implant is used. Most Silastic implants will be removed intact; however, some may tear or fragment. If a smooth, thick fibrous interface (between the fossa and condyle usually) remains, no further treatment may be needed. This removed Dacron-reinforced Silastic implant demonstrates an area of wear toward the lateral aspect (side away from the ruler).

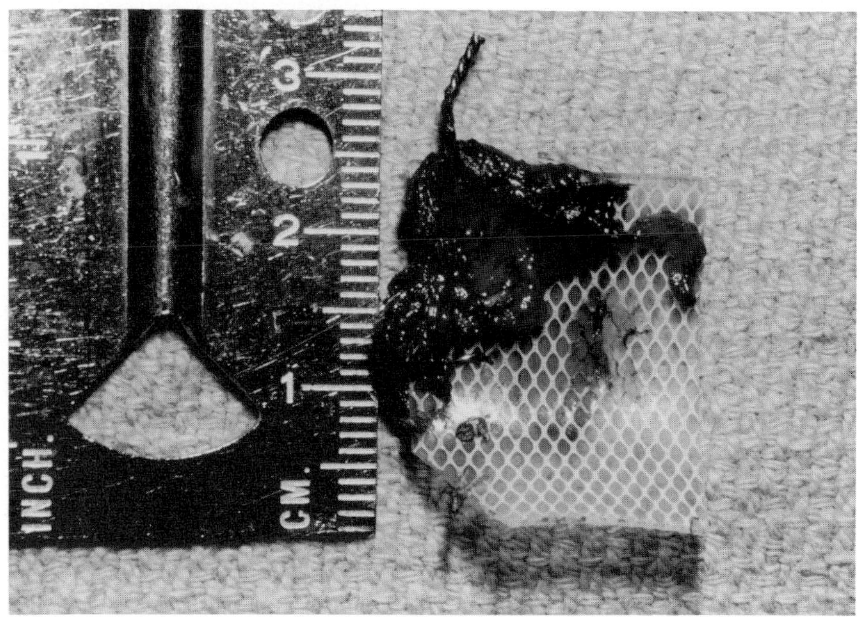

PLATE 7-5

This patient had a history of several years of severe preauricular pain and limited opening. There were no myofascial complaints or findings. Tomographic radiographs showed bilateral degenerative changes in the condyles with lack of joint space. After noninvasive therapy failed to relieve any of the pain and hypomobility, bilateral TMJ arthroplasties with minimal condylar shaves, meniscectomies, and insertion of Silastic fossa implants were performed.

A and **B** The patient did very well after surgery and routine postoperative splinting and physical therapy. Her pain was totally eliminated, and her opening was excellent.

C and **D** Serial postoperative radiographs over several months showed progressive loss of condylar height.

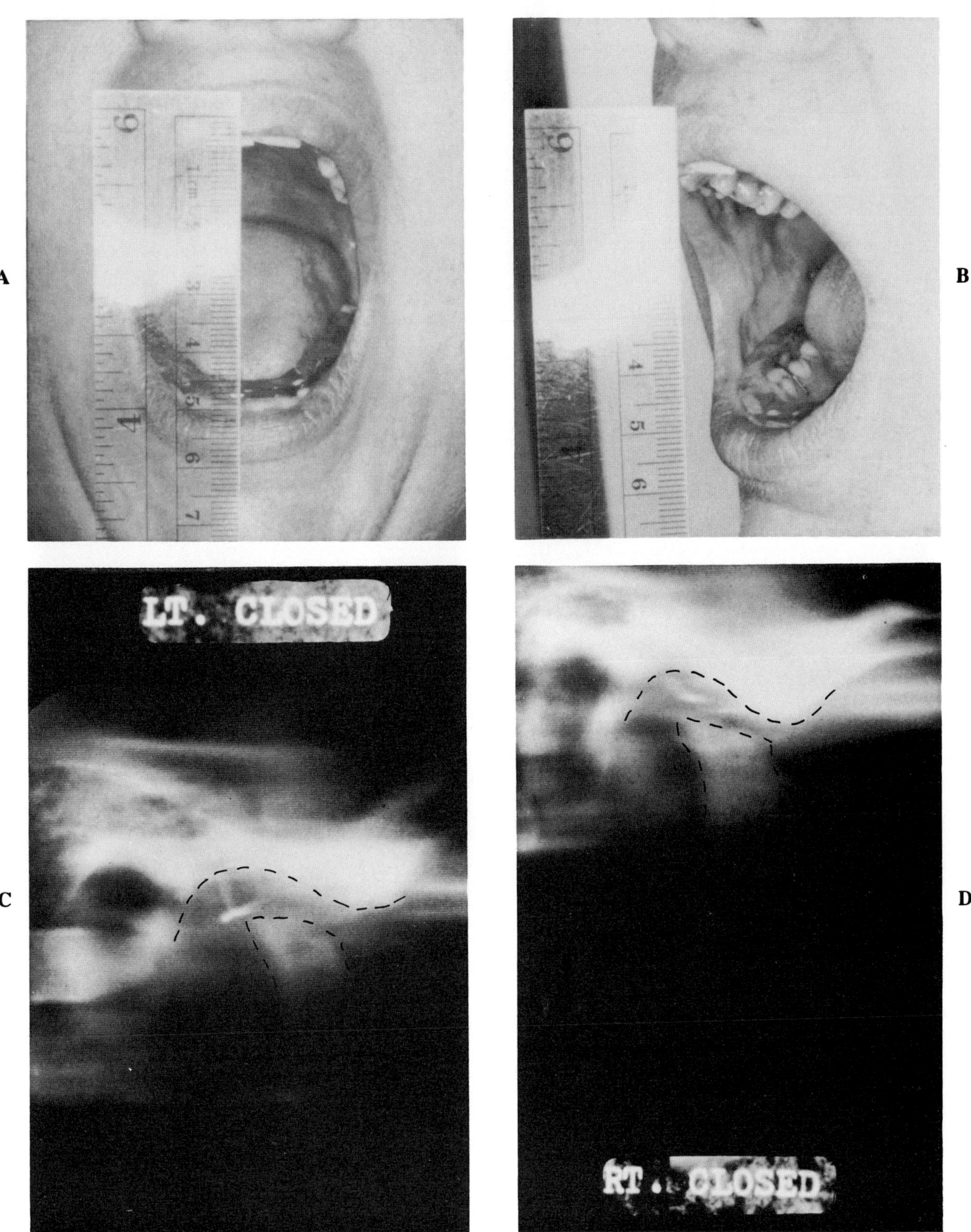

A B C D

E to **G** Clinical and radiographic examination showed development of a significant anterior open bite.

H The occlusion was stabilized with a splint. The patient was completely asymptomatic. Several months after splint therapy, a LeFort I maxillary osteotomy (with posterior impaction only) was done to reestablish the occlusion. Note that total joint replacement is not necessary in this situation.

E

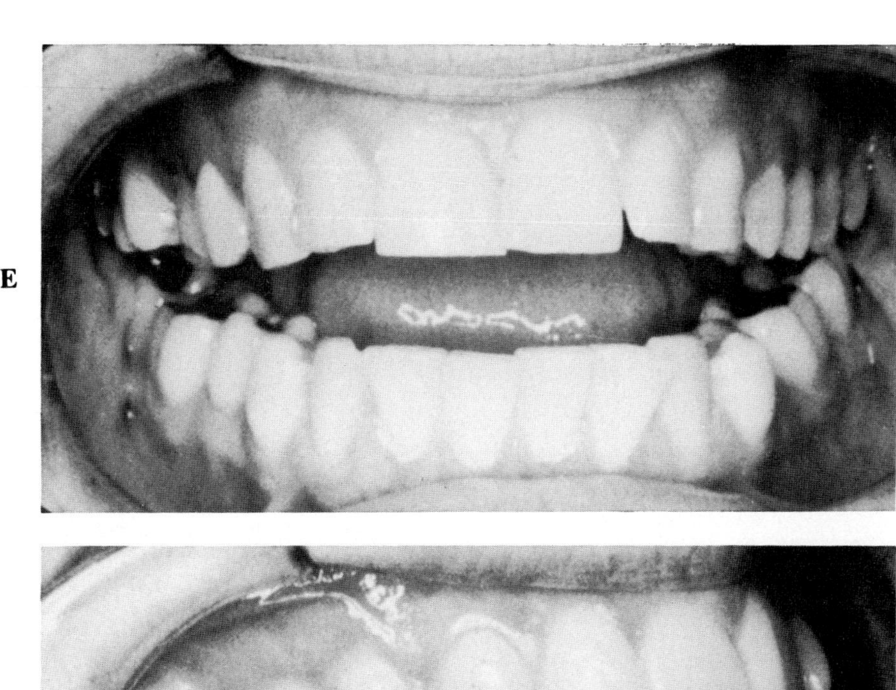

F

G
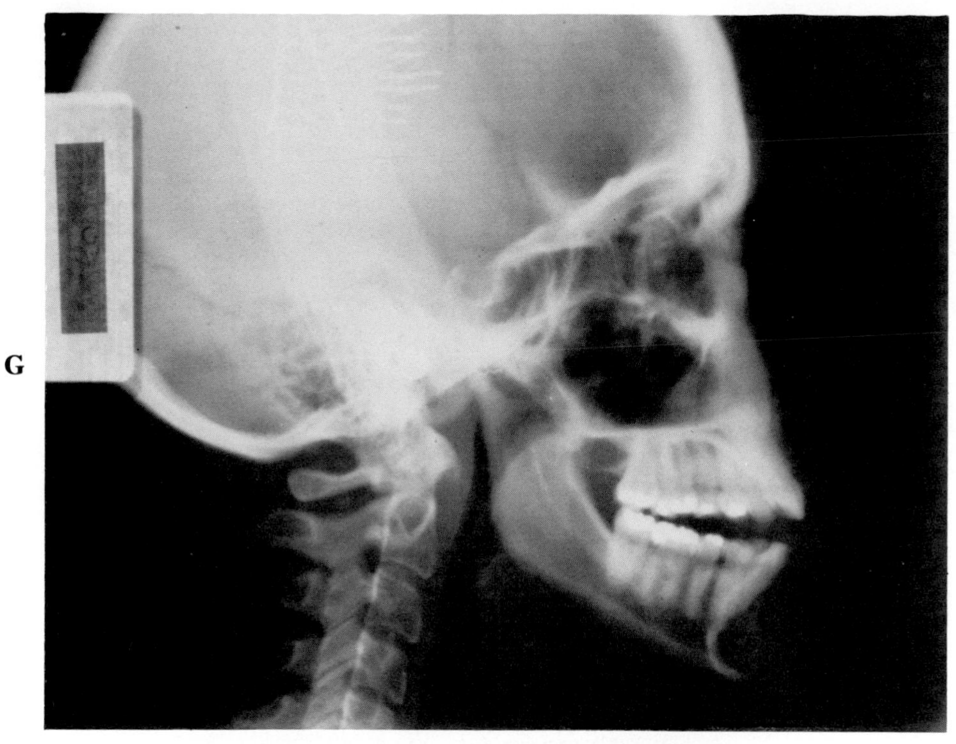

H
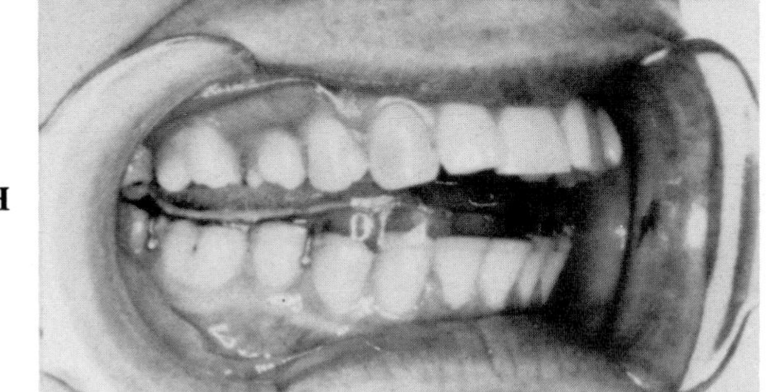

PLATE 7-6

The patient was a 30-year-old woman whose chief complaint was severe right TMJ pain. The patient's right TMJ was very tender to palpation, and crepitus was present. The patient's mandible was slightly shifted toward the right side. She had worn several bite splints, had been treated with physical therapy, and was presently taking a nonsteroidal antiinflammatory medication.

A Tomograms of the TMJ showed advanced degenerative changes of the right TMJ. The arthrogram of the right TMJ demonstrated an apparently large perforation with only a small amount of disc tissue remaining.

B At the time of surgery the disc was observed to have a large perforation. The condyle and articular eminence showed evidence of gross irregularity and advanced arthrosis. A meniscectomy and arthroplasty of the condyle and eminence were performed. A large Silastic implant was used to maintain the vertical space.

A
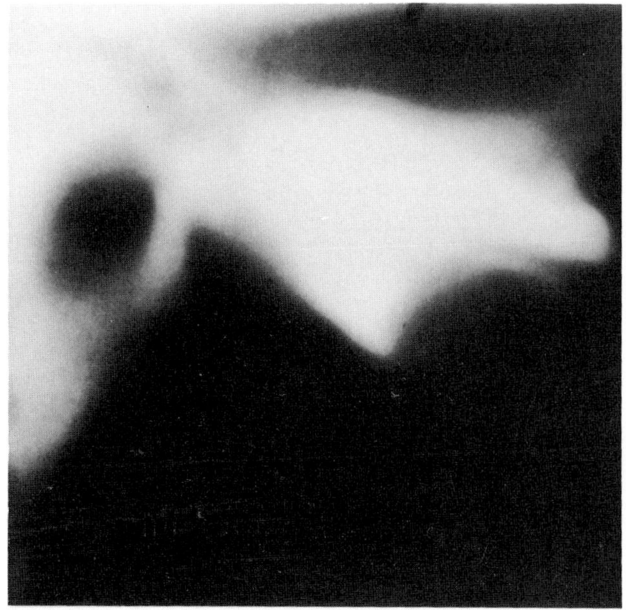

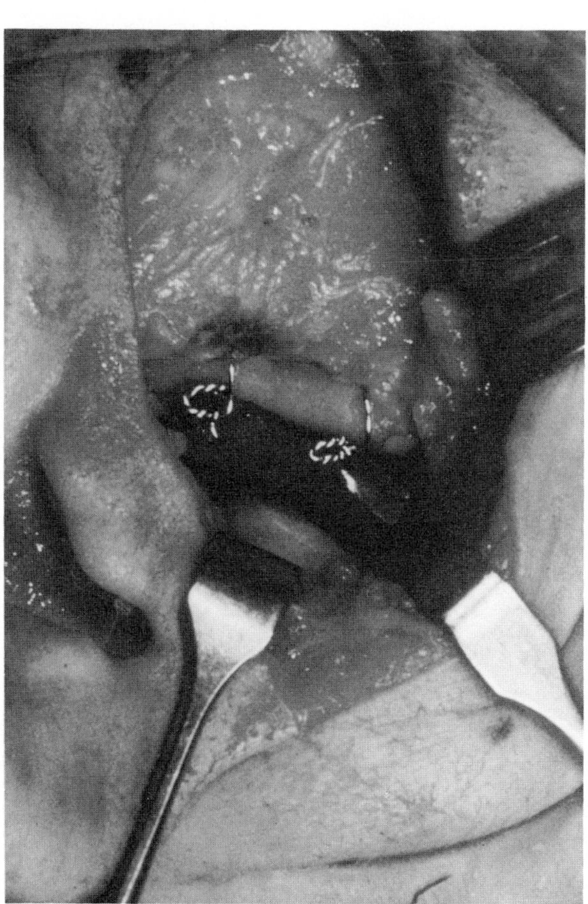
B

C Postoperative radiograph demonstrating implant. The patient did very well for 4 months.

D The patient began to complain of increasingly severe pain in the right TMJ about 5 months postoperatively. She also noted that her bite was changing. By 6 months postoperatively her occlusion had shifted grossly toward the right.

C

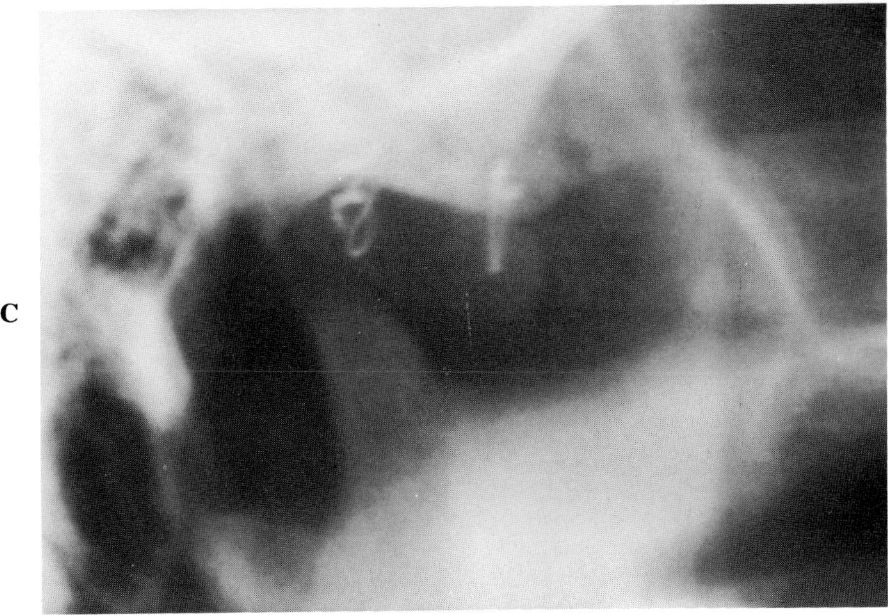

D

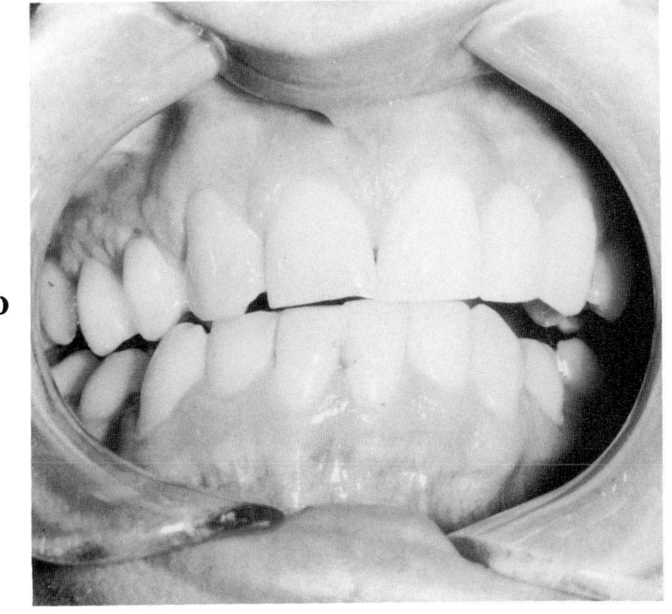

E The radiograph shows that the condyle has completely resorbed down to the level of the coronoid notch. The wires holding the implant are no longer in bone.

F The patient was maintained in a lower occlusal appliance until the occlusion stabilized. She was relatively asymptomatic during this time. A unilateral sagittal ramus osteotomy was performed to correct the deviated occlusion approximately 1 year postoperatively. The occlusion remained stable for about 4 months and then began to shift again. Condylar resorption was apparent on radiographic examination.

E

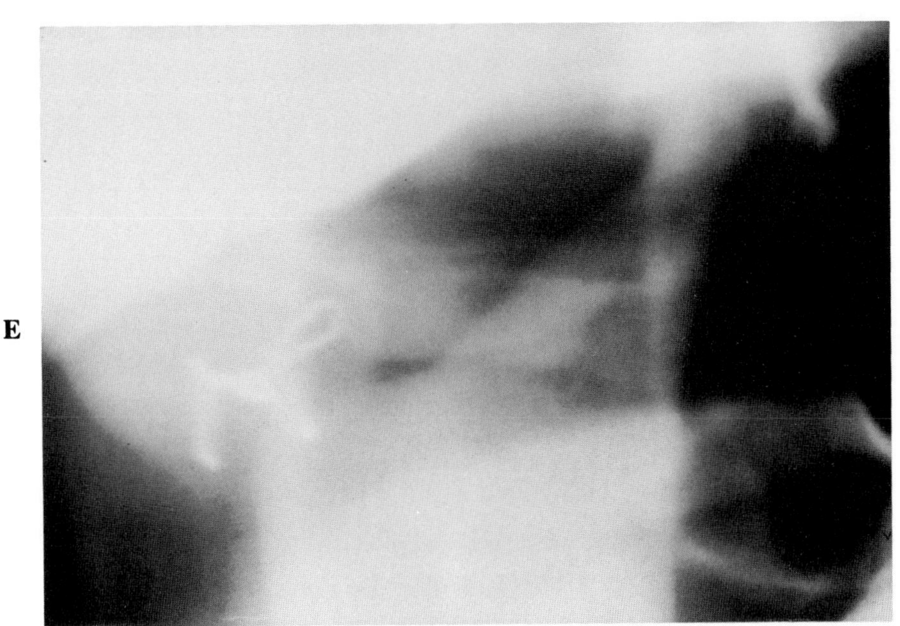

F

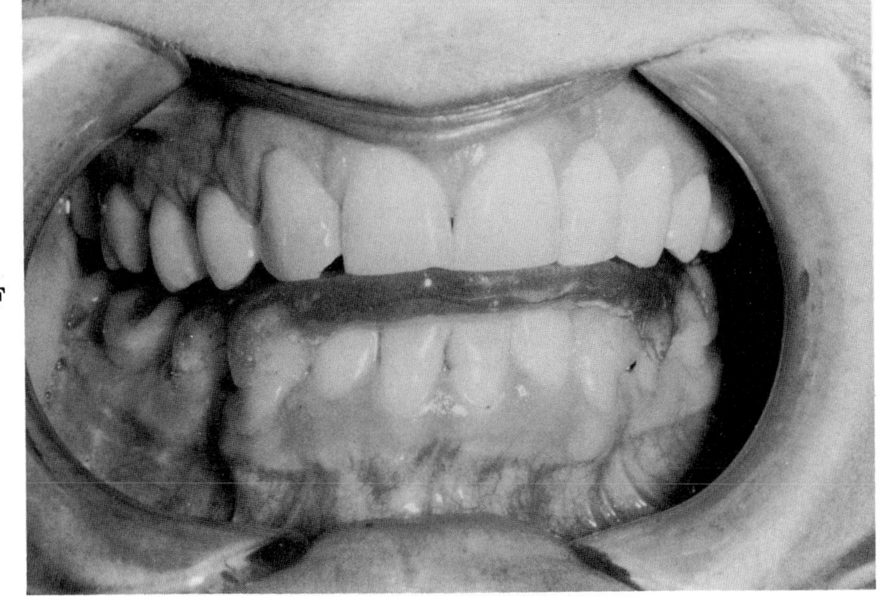

G and **H** About 1 year after the osteotomy the patient had a Kent-Vitek total joint prosthesis placed.

I Postoperative panoramic radiograph demonstrating position of prosthesis.

G

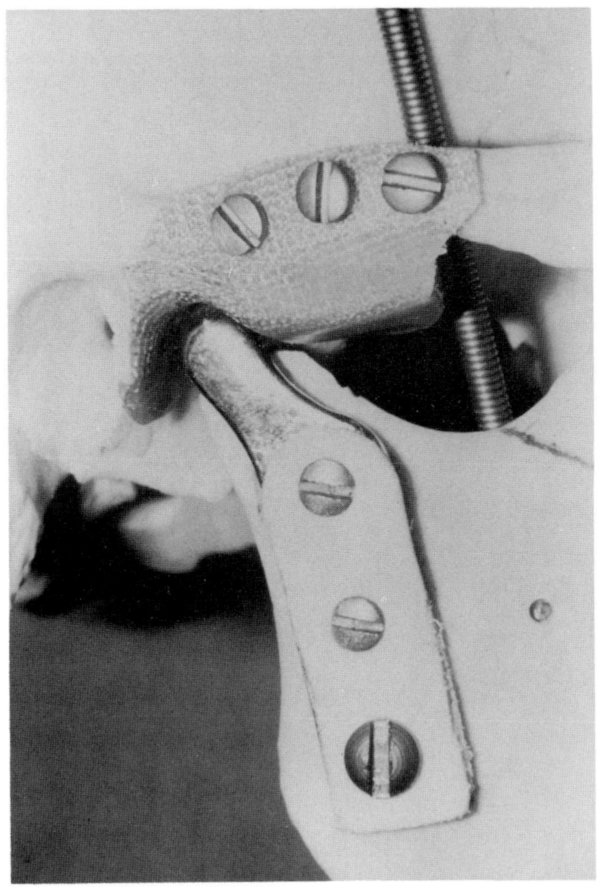

H

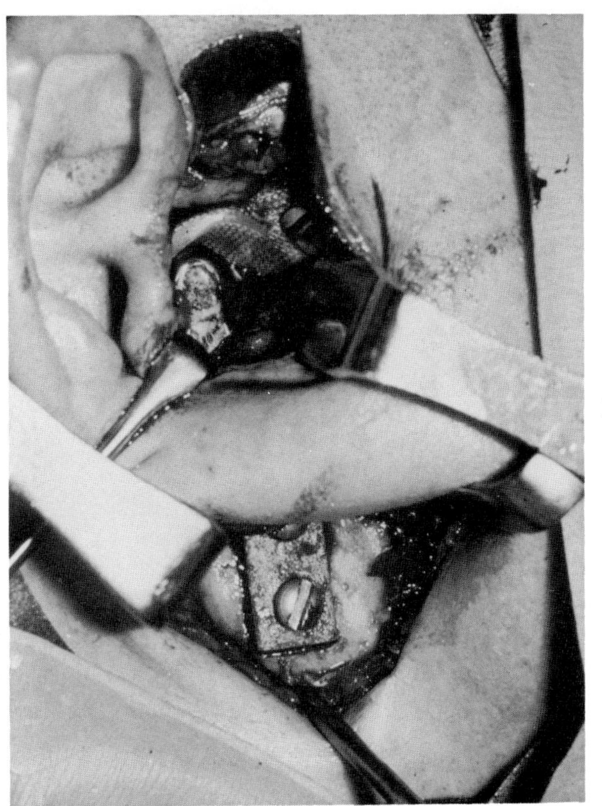

I

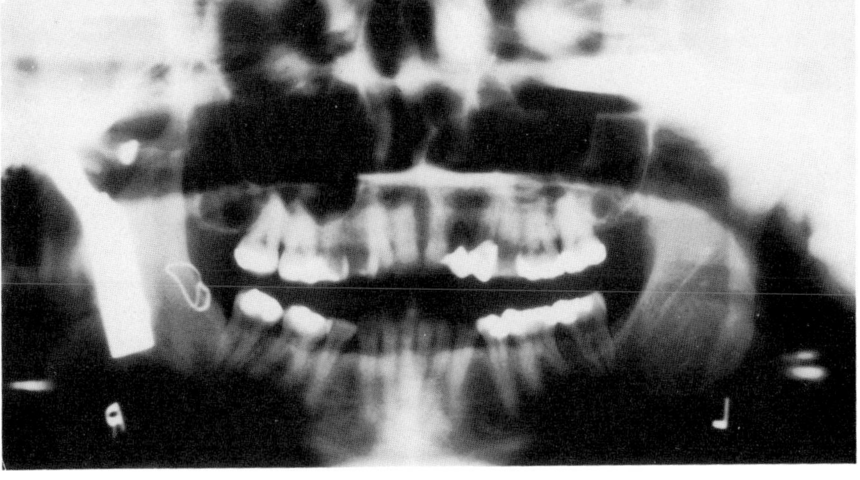

J to **L** The patient has maintained an opening of 40 mm and good occlusion for the first year after surgery. She is free of pain.

J

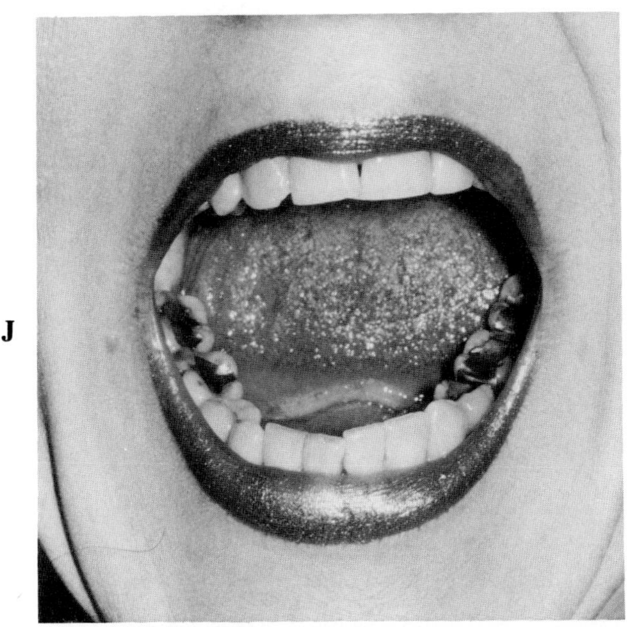

K

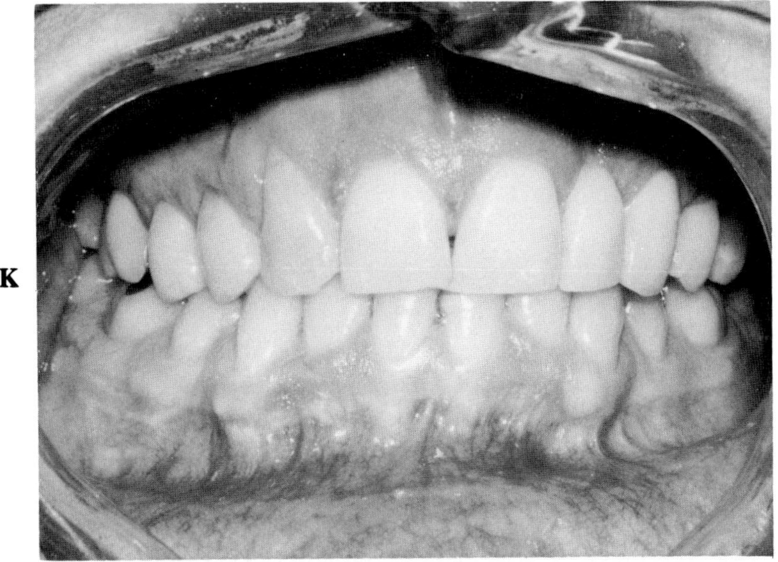

L

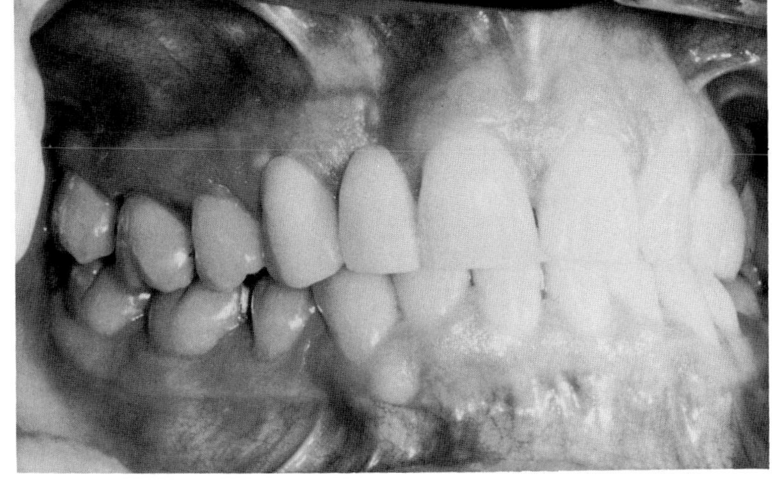

chapter 8

Case Reports

CASE 1

PLATE 8-1

Chief complaint and history of present illness. The patient was a 22-year-old woman whose chief complaint was right-sided facial pain, earaches, and temporal headaches. The problem began 3 months previously and neither improved nor worsened. The pain was poorly localized and diffuse in its distribution. She described the headaches as a tight feeling.

A The patient described her pain as being very diffuse and poorly localized.
B Likewise she outlined the location of the pain as being very diffuse.

Both the pain and the headaches were worse in the morning on awakening. The patient reported that she had difficulty getting to sleep and that she woke up several times each night. She also complained of sore teeth and thought that she was grinding her teeth. She reported that she had recently been under a lot of stress at work and that her pain may have been worse after stressful days.

Past medical history and review of systems. Negative.

Examination. The patient opened to 35 mm, with a slight deviation toward the right side, and there was a very early soft click in the right TMJ. Excursive movements were normal. There was no joint tenderness. The muscles of mastication were tender bilaterally. The dentition was Class I with wear facets on the lower left cuspid and first bicuspid. These teeth were slightly tender to percussion.

Radiographic findings. Transcranial TMJ views and Panorex were normal.

Diagnosis. Myofascial pain and dysfunction (muscle hyperactivity disorder).

Recommendations. The pain was poorly localized, diffuse, and worse in the mornings. She slept poorly, complained of sore teeth, and had a history of stress. She had no joint tenderness but severe bilateral muscle tenderness. These findings all pointed to a muscular disorder.

The patient was counseled as to the problem and possible relationship to stress. She accepted this explanation and recognized the relationship to stress. She was given diazepam (Valium), 5 mg qhs, for 7 days. Additionally, she was given a nonsteroidal antiinflammatory drug for pain and advised to use moist heat several times a day and to eat a soft diet. She improved markedly on this regimen. Because her symptoms continued she was given an occlusal appliance for muscle relaxation to be worn at night only.

A

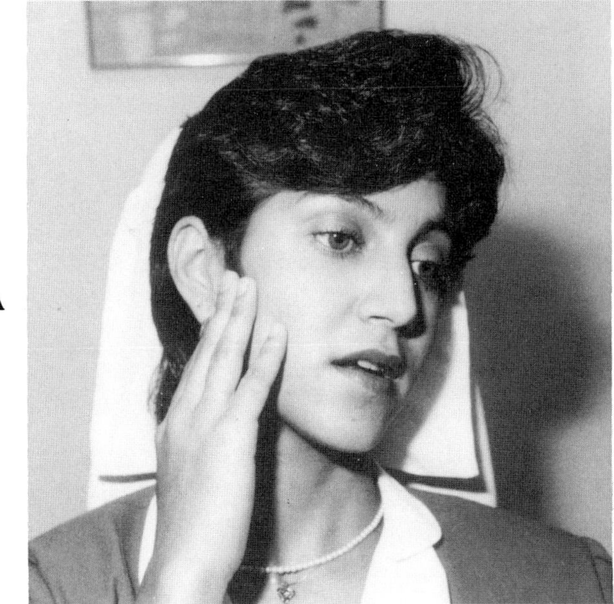

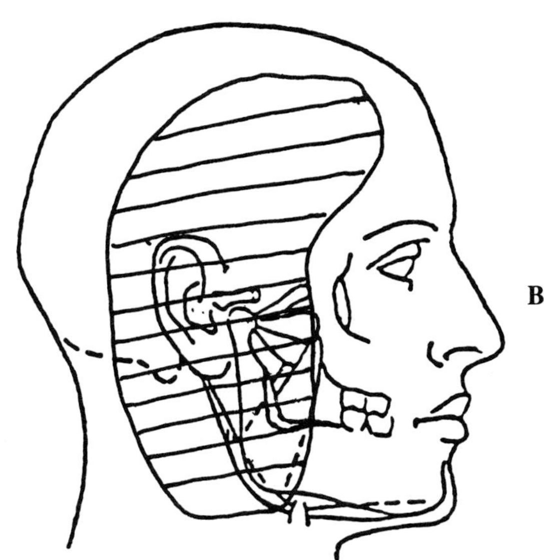

B

C The patient was given a maxillary occlusal appliance for muscle relaxation. The appliance is flat posteriorly with all teeth occluding simultaneously. The appliance has anterior and lateral guidance planes that separate the posterior teeth during protrusive and lateral movements.

Course. The patient has done very well. The symptoms resolved within 2 weeks. The patient discontinued use of the occlusal appliance after 1 month. She occasionally uses the appliance if under stress.

Comments. This case represents a classic example of myofascial pain and dysfunction secondary to bruxism.

C

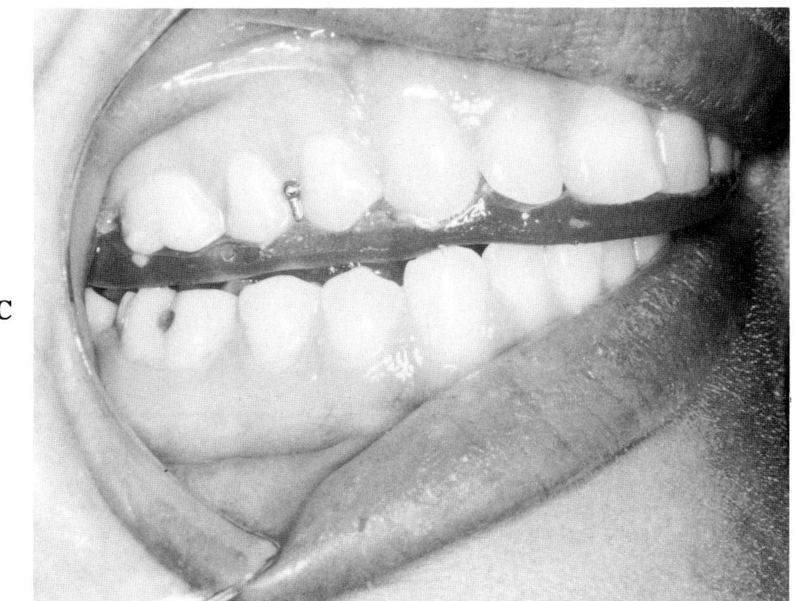

CASE 2

Chief complaint and history of present illness. The patient was a 37-year-old woman whose chief complaint was left-sided facial pain and bilateral temporal headaches for 2 years. The pain was cyclic in that there were pain-free periods of time. The pain was poorly localized and diffuse over her left side (see Fig. 8-1, *B*). The patient outlined her pain as being very diffuse and worse in the morning. Her headaches were described as a tight feeling and were worse in the morning and evening. She did not sleep well. Both joints were reported to make noise, and she occasionally had locking in the mornings. She was under stress because of her family relationships. A physician had given her diazepam (Valium), which did improve her symptoms.

Past medical history and review of systems. Negative except for a history of periodic chest pains, which had been diagnosed as esophageal reflux and spasm.

Examination. The patient opened to 30 mm without deviation. Excursive movements were normal. There were reciprocal clicks in both joints; the opening clicks were at 12 mm and the closing clicks at 3 mm. The left joint was slightly tender to palpation. The muscles of mastication were tender bilaterally. The occlusion was Class I.

Radiographic findings. Transcranial TMJ and Panorex views were normal.

Diagnosis. (1) Myofascial pain and dysfunction (muscle hyperactivity disorder). (2) Bilateral internal derangement.

Recommendations. This case is more difficult than case 1. The patient had both a muscular disorder and bilateral internal derangements. The major symptoms, however, appeared to arise from the muscular component. The patient was counseled as to the diagnosis and possible relationship to stress. She was reassured that her problem was not severe and could be treated. She was given a nonsteroidal antiinflammatory drug for pain and was discouraged from taking narcotic pain medication. Moist heat and a soft diet were prescribed.

The patient was also referred to a physical therapist for evaluation and treatment. Physical therapy consisted of ultrasound treatments three times a week that were stopped after 2 weeks. The patient also had an occlusal appliance for muscle relaxation (see Plate 8-1,**C**) made. The appliance was worn at night only.

Course. The patient improved steadily and was free of pain within 6 weeks. She continued to use the occlusal appliance periodically. Her joints continued to click but were not painful, and therefore no other treatment was recommended.

Comments. This case represents a combined problem—myofascial pain and dysfunction secondary to bruxism and bilateral internal derangements. The symptoms developed because of the bruxism. Once the bruxism was controlled, the symptoms (pain) resolved, although the clicks continued. The patient was informed about the clicks but no treatment was recommended because they were not painful.

CASE 3

PLATE 8-2

Chief complaint and history of present illness. The patient was a 23-year-old woman whose chief complaint was left-sided joint pain and clicking. The problem began 2 months previously, after the patient had been hit on the jaw. The clicking began almost immediately afterward. The pain was well localized over the TMJ area and was worse after eating or talking.

A The patient localized her pain to the left TMJ. The pain increased as she opened her mouth.

B She outlined her pain directly over the TMJ area.

The patient stated that her jaw feels very good and essentially free of pain on awakening.

Past medical history and review of systems. Negative.

Examination. The patient opened to 40 mm with deviation toward the left until the opening click occurred. The mandible then shifted toward the midline. The left TMJ was tender to palpation. There was an opening click at 16 mm in the left joint and a closing click at 4 mm. During retrusion the click occurred 2 mm anterior to maximum intercuspation (centric occlusion). There was mild left-sided muscle tenderness. The occlusion was a Class II, Division I.

Radiographic findings. Transcranial TMJ and Panorex views were normal.

Diagnosis. Internal derangement of left TMJ.

Recommendations. The patient was referred to her dentist for a repositioning appliance.

A

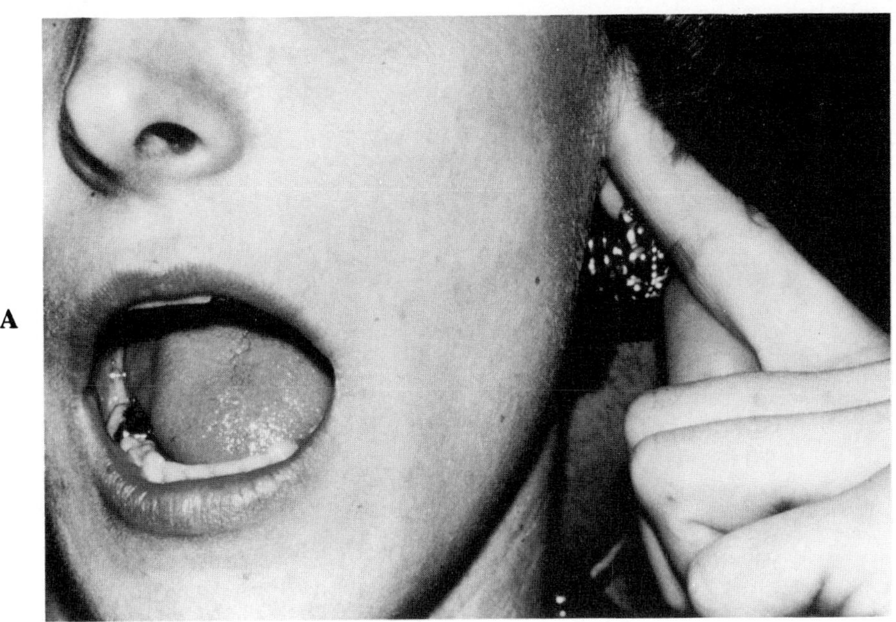

B

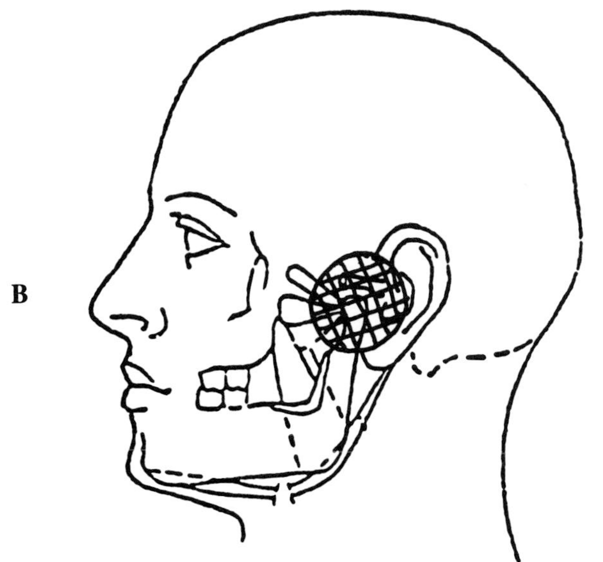

C This picture demonstrates the lower repositioning appliance. The appliance has definite occlusal stops and guiding planes to keep the mandible anteriorly positioned. The object of the appliance was to keep the discs reduced, therefore eliminating the clicks, pain, and dysfunction. The patient wore the appliance 24 hours a day.

C

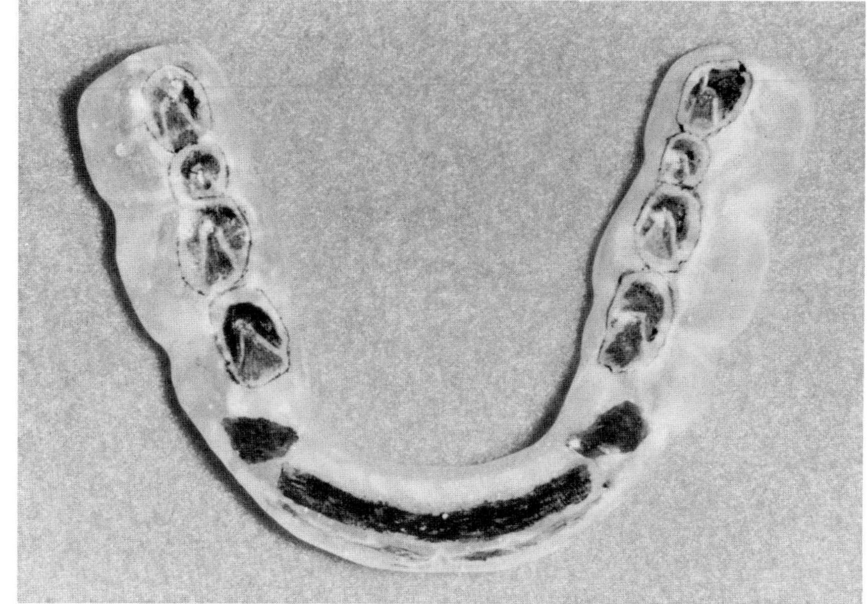

D and **E** Lower appliance is generally used because it is more esthetically pleasing and the patient can speak better than with an upper appliance.

D

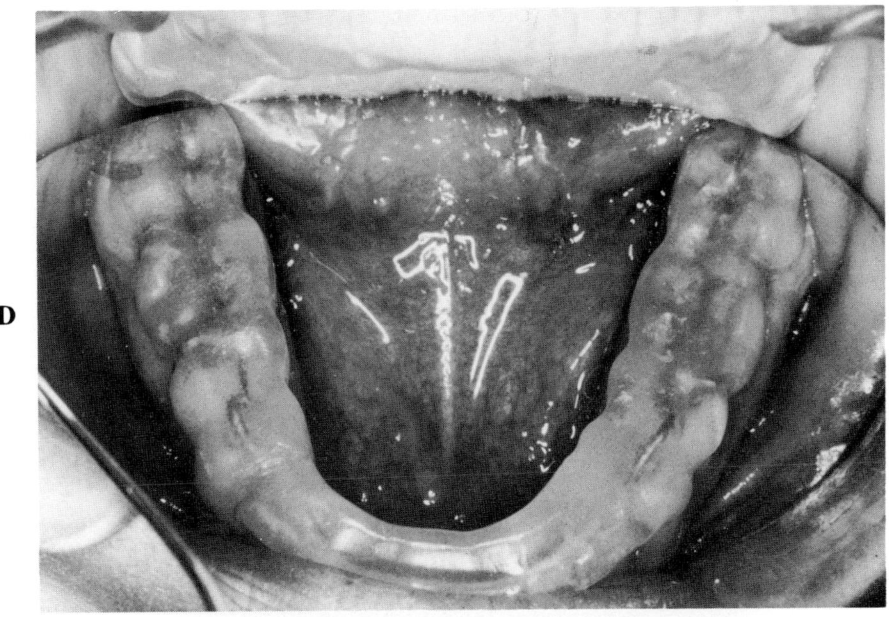

E

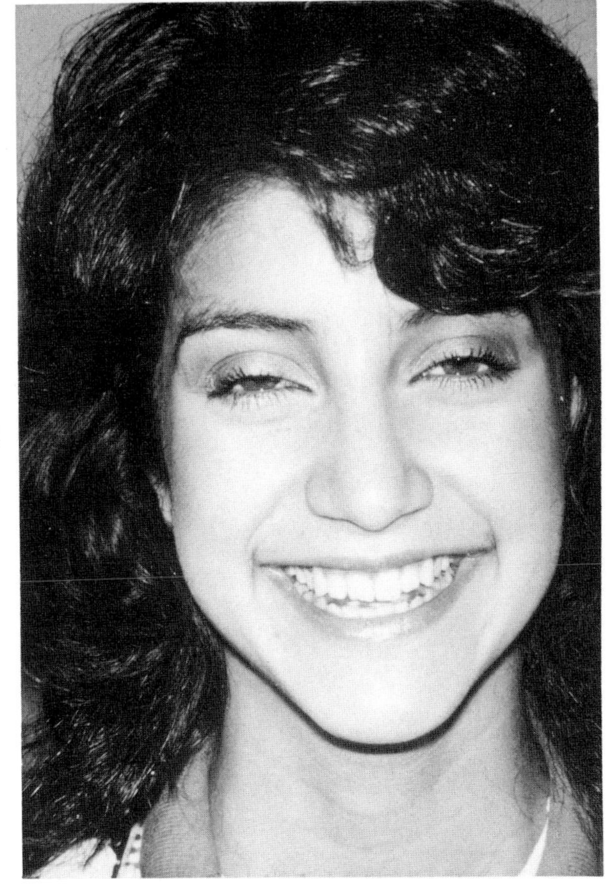

F Some patients will slip the disc off while sleeping. In these cases an upper appliance with a long anterior vamp is used at night.

Course. The patient's symptoms resolved almost immediately with use of the anterior repositioning appliance. The appliance was periodically adjusted over a 6-month period until the teeth were in occlusion again. The patient's condition was allowed to stabilize for 6 additional months, and then she was referred for orthodontic treatment.

Comments. This case had an excellent prognosis for nonsurgical treatment. The derangement was acute in onset and early to intermediate in severity. Importantly, there was an identifiable etiology—trauma.

F

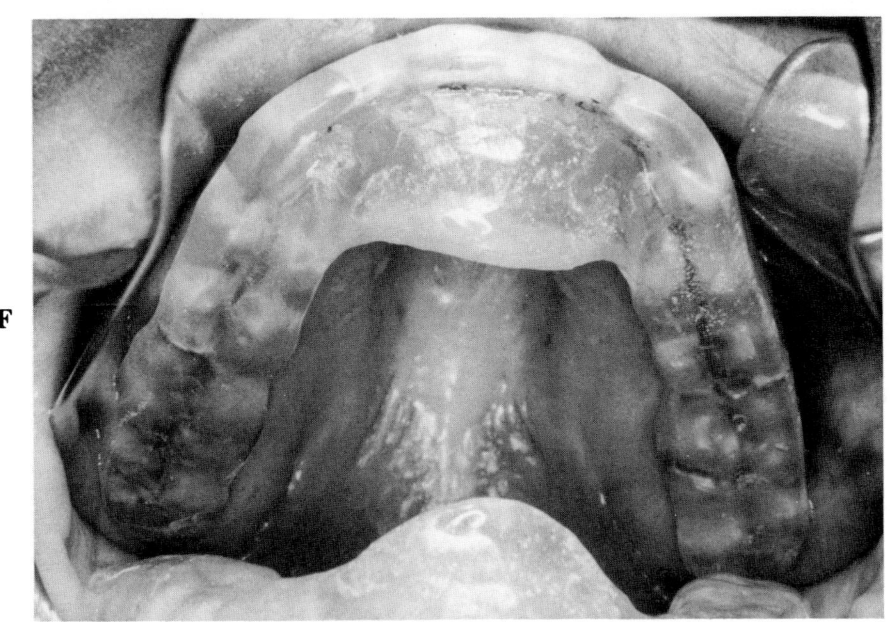

CASE 4

PLATE 8-3

Chief complaint and history of present illness. The patient was a 21-year-old woman who developed bilateral clicking and locking following an automobile accident about 18 months previously. The patient was treated with a mandibular repositioning appliance, which positioned her mandible forward 4 mm. The symptoms completely resolved; however, any posterior movement of the mandible resulted in the recurrence of bilateral clicking, joint pain, and headaches. The patient was advised to have full-mouth reconstructive dentistry to maintain her mandible in an anterior position. She wanted a second opinion.

Past medical history and review of systems. Negative.

Examination. The patient opened to 51 mm without deviation or joint noise. There was no joint or muscle tenderness. A mandibular anterior repositioning appliance was in place. Without the appliance the patient opened to 46 mm with painful, bilateral, loud opening clicks. The opening clicks occurred at 21 mm in the left joint and 19 mm in the right joint. Slight upward pressure at the mandibular angles caused the left joint to lock.

Radiographic examination. Transcranial TMJ views were normal. Both condyles were slightly posteriorly positioned without the splint. Bilateral TMJ arthrograms showed anterior disc displacement with reduction without the appliance in place.

A and **B** Closed and open transcranial views of the right TMJ. The joint was normal except for a slight posterior displacement of the condyle in the closed mouth position. The left joint was similar to the right. An arthrogram of the right joint showed anterior disc displacement with reduction.

A 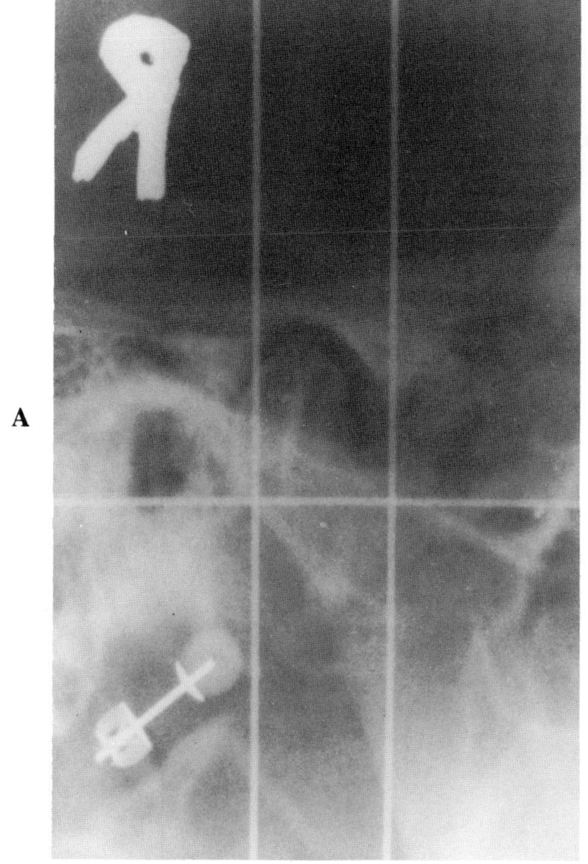

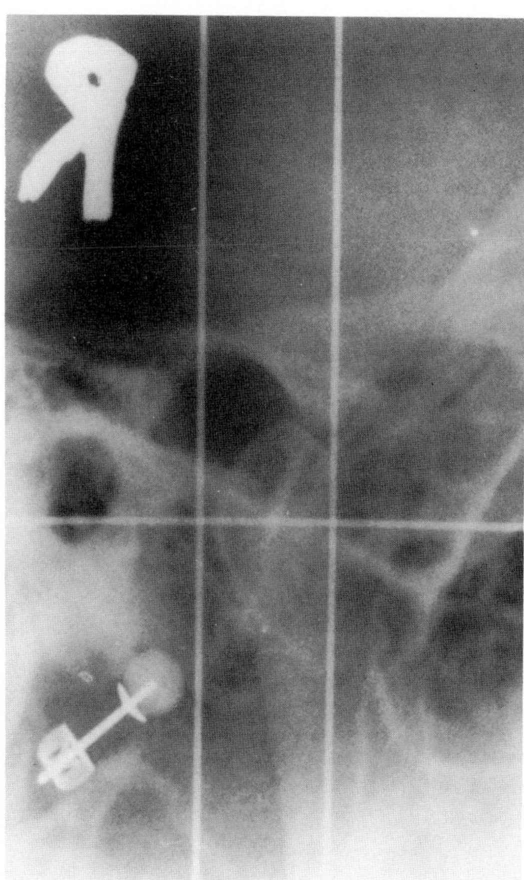 B

C Closed mouth view showing anterior disc displacement.

D As the condyle began to move forward the lower joint space changed shape. The disc appeared to fold upward.

E With continued movement of the condyle a click occurred as the disc reduced to a normal position.

Diagnosis. Bilateral internal derangements—anterior disc displacement with reduction.

Recommendation. This represents an almost ideal surgery case. The etiology is identifiable, the symptoms can be controlled with an occlusal appliance, and the patient cannot be taken out of the appliance without the symptoms returning. Although full-mouth reconstruction is an option, it would require somewhat radical treatment, which would leave the condyles anteriorly positioned and the disc attachments still abnormal. Surgery would be a more conservative treatment for this patient. Bilateral TMJ surgery was recommended.

Surgery. The patient underwent bilateral disc repositioning.

Surgical findings. The discs were found to be normal in color and texture.

Course. The patient has done very well. She had a conservative occlusal adjustment 3 months after surgery. At the present time she has full normal range of mandibular movements.

C

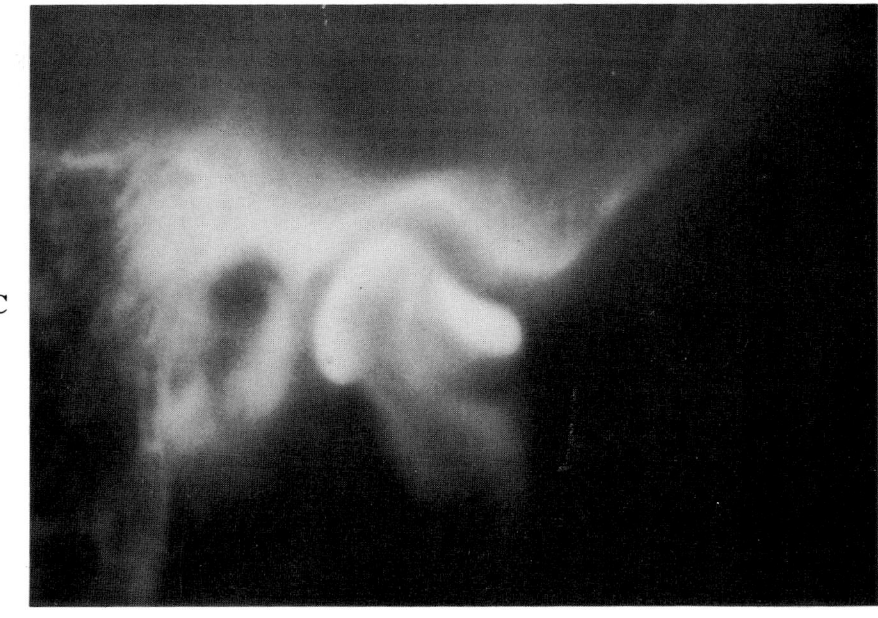

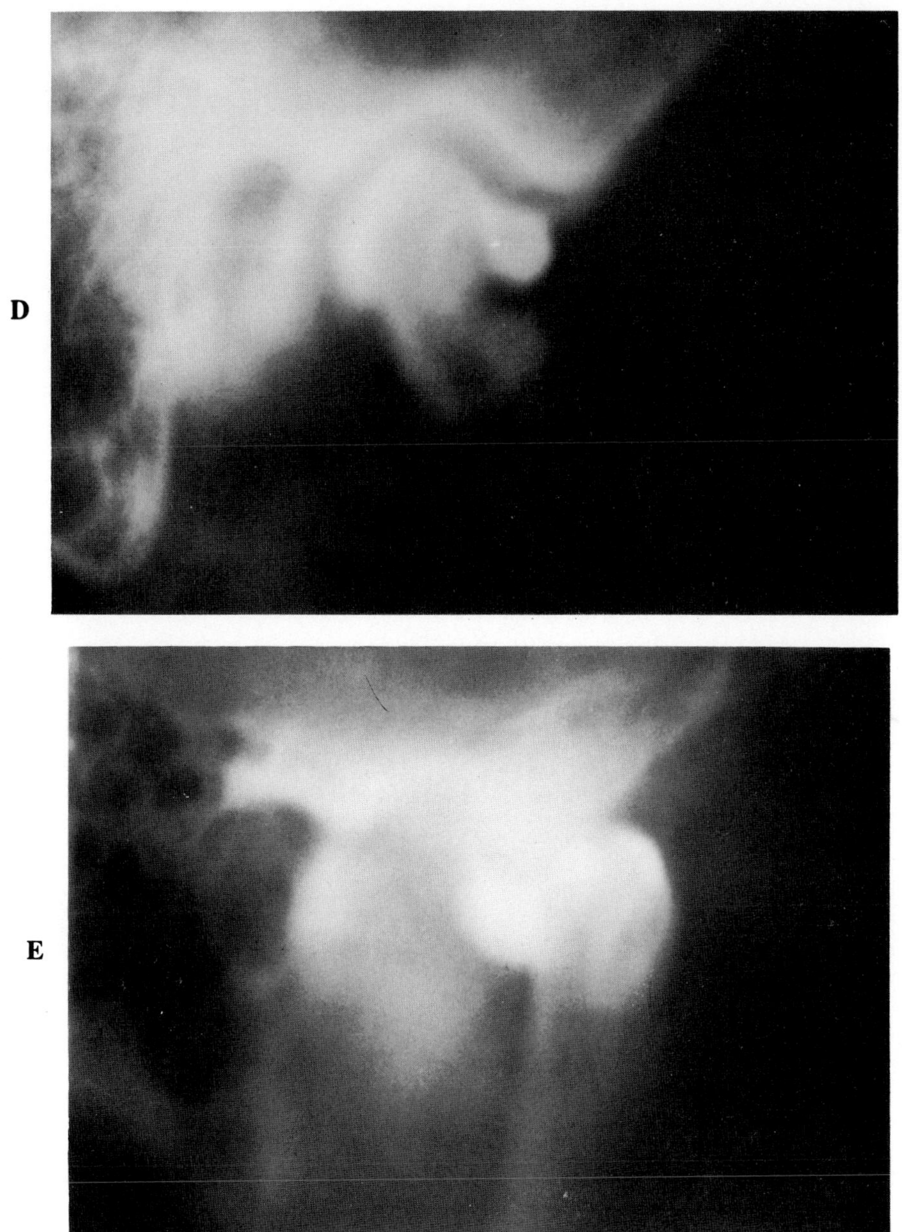
D
E

CASE 5

PLATE 8-4

Chief complaint and history of present illness. The patient was a 35-year-old woman whose chief complaint was left-sided facial pain and an inability to open her mouth normally. She had had the pain for 3 years, and it had recently grown worse. She described the pain as being diffuse over her left face and extending into her neck. She also identified an area of intense pain over the left TMJ.

A The patient outlined her pain as being very diffuse. She also drew an X over the joint, indicating a specific localized area of pain.

Her pain was severe on awakening, and she also reported increased pain with jaw function. She did not sleep well.

Her left TMJ clicked for as long as she could remember. Six months previously she began to experience occasional locking, and 2 months previously her left joint locked and stayed locked. She experienced severe pain since that time.

The patient stated that about 3 years ago she learned that her mother was ill and would need to live with her. This created some family difficulties the patient did not want to discuss.

Examination. The opening was 18 mm with deviation toward the left. Left lateral movement was normal but painful. Right lateral movement was decreased (5 mm) and was very painful. There was no joint noise. The left TMJ was very tender to palpation. The muscles of mastication were tender bilaterally, with the left side more tender than the right. The occlusion was satisfactory.

Radiographs. The Panorex view was normal. Transcranial TMJ views showed no translation of the left TMJ.

A

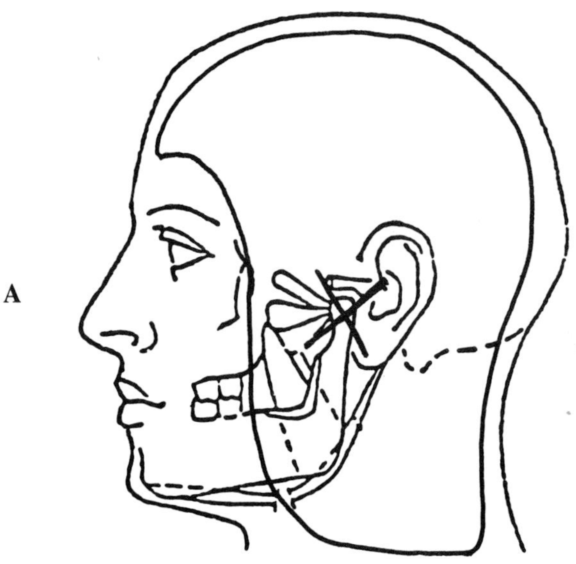

B and **C** The transcranial views of the left TMJ showed a posterior condylar position and no translation during opening.

Diagnosis. (1) Myofascial pain and dysfunction (MPD). (2) Internal derangement of left TMJ (anterior disc displacement without reduction).

Recommendations. The patient had an obvious internal derangement of the left TMJ. The patient also had a clear history of stress-related MPD. Her pain was diffuse, seemed worse in the mornings, and began about the time a significant stress was added to her life. These problems required attention. The MPD component should be managed first because correcting the disc derangement without managing the MPD would likely result in failure.

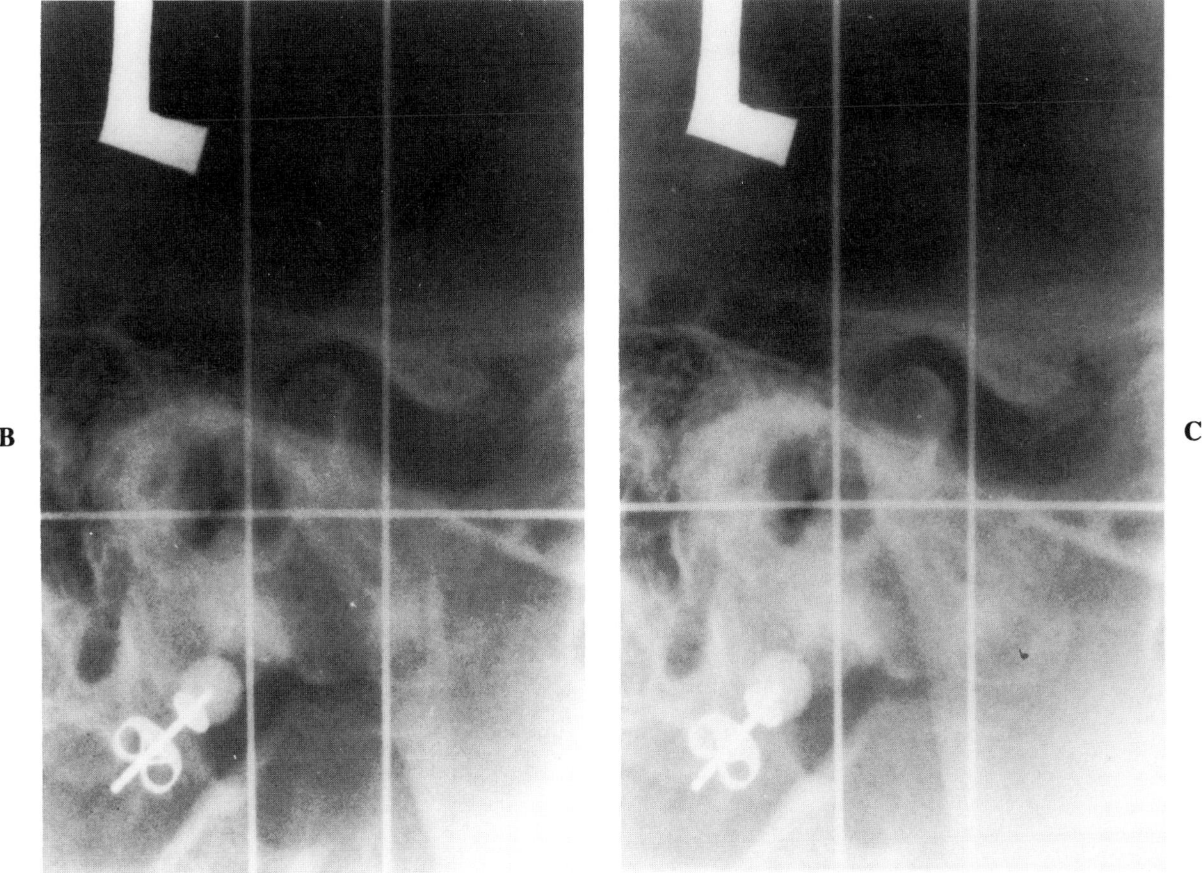

The problem was explained to the patient. She was given diazepam (Valium), 5 mg qhs, for 2 weeks. She was also given a nonsteroidal antiinflammatory drug for pain, and moist heat and a soft diet were prescribed. The patient was referred to her dentist for construction of a splint for muscle relaxation. She also was referred to a psychologist for evaluation and counseling for her family problems.

These were effective treatments for her MPD. She was a most cooperative patient, and during a 6-week period her symptoms decreased significantly. She felt better, slept better, and had a confident attitude. However, her opening remained decreased, although it had increased to 30 mm.

D The patient's opening improved to 30 mm with deviation toward the left side.

She also continued to have moderate to severe pain in her left TMJ. An arthrogram of the left TMJ confirmed the diagnosis of anterior disc displacement without reduction.

D

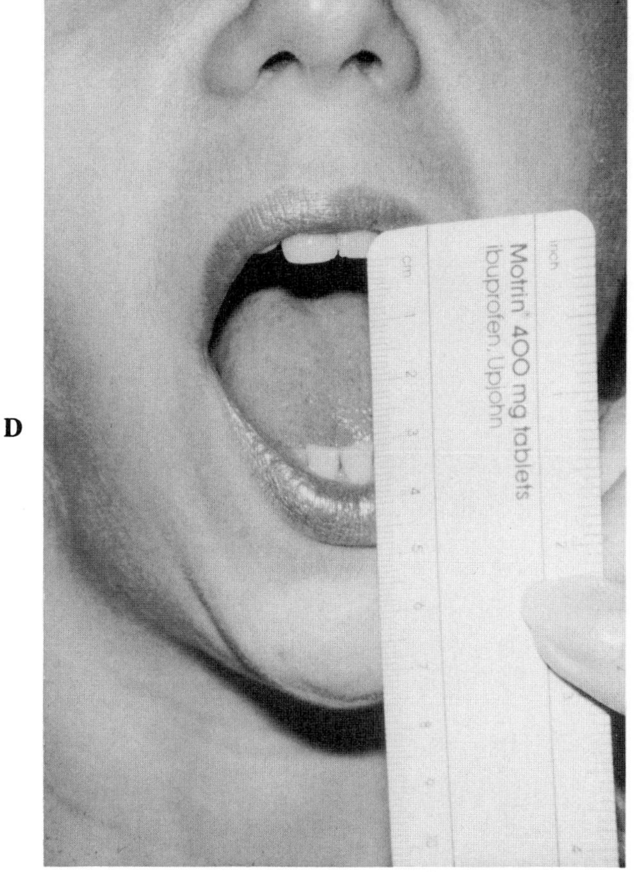

E Closed mouth arthrogram of the left TMJ showing interior disc displacement.
F During opening the condyles moved very little and the disc remained anteriorly displaced.

Surgery. The patient then underwent disc repositioning and recontouring of the left TMJ.

Course. The patient has done very well. She periodically has episodes of mild diffuse facial pain, which are managed with moist heat, aspirin, and relaxation.

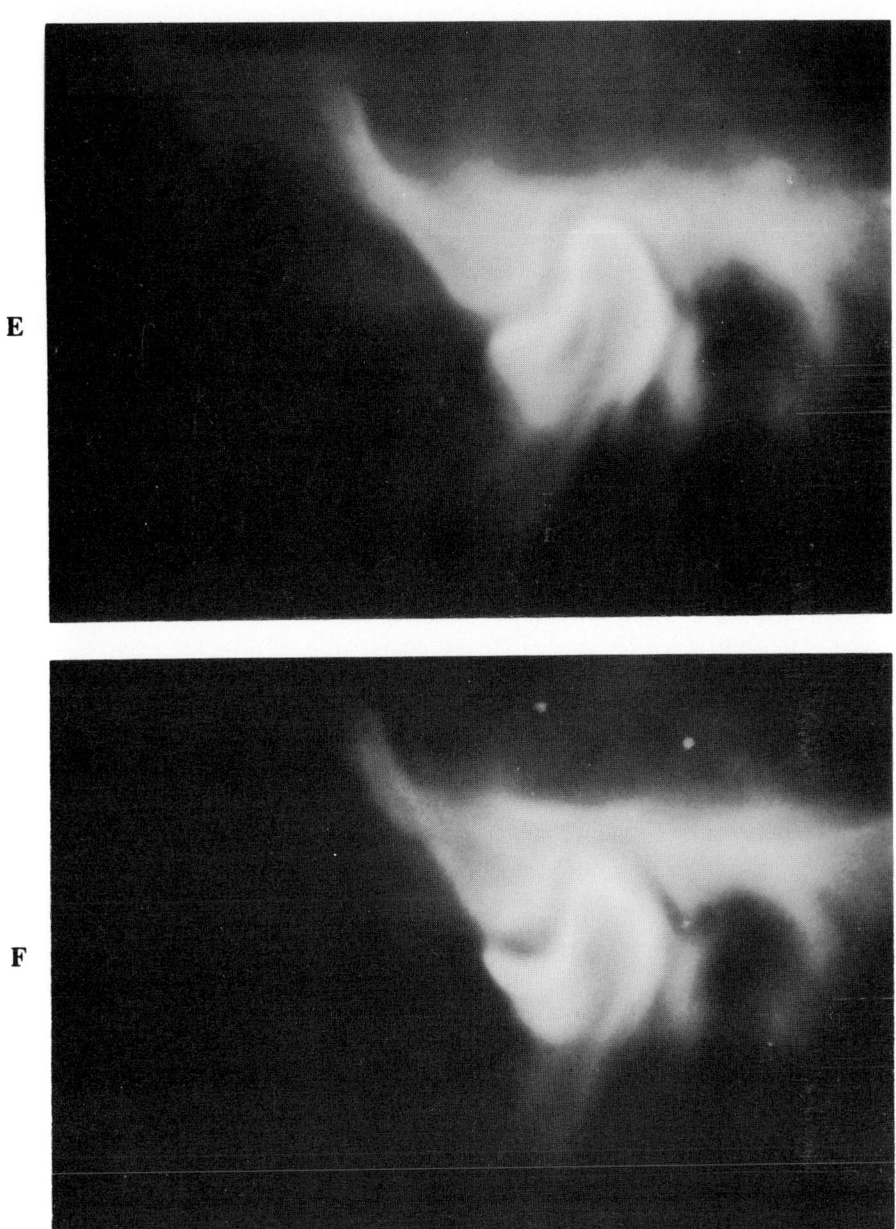
E
F

CASE 6

PLATE 8-5

Chief complaint and history of present illness. This 15-year-old girl's chief complaint was having limited left TMJ opening with a chronic closed-lock of the left TMJ and severe left TMJ pain. The patient could clearly point to the left preauricular area, and she stated that it hurt every day and that on a 0 to 10 scale it was 10 every day, with significantly increased pain while chewing. The patient stated that she had an "aching" pain with occasional sharp, lancinating extensions directly in the preauricular area. It interfered with sleep. There was some referred pain with left temporal headache, and the patient classified the pain as a disability rather than an annoyance. This was a problem for 6 months.

Past medical history and review of systems. Six months previously the patient heard very loud clicking of the left TMJ, and 2 days later she developed a persistent, very painful closed-lock. There was no history of obvious facial trauma. She received orthodontic treatment for 1½ years, and she associated this treatment with some pain development. She was seen for conservative therapy by a gnathologist, who took radiographs, did splint therapy, and performed several splint adjustments, including a pivotal splint. Jaw manipulations were tried to reduce the closed-lock. The patient had been taking aspirin and naproxen (Naprosyn). Two steroid injections into the joint were carried out with no result.

The patient was a 15-year-old high school student. She did not smoke, drink alcohol, or take social drugs. Her family history was unremarkable.

Examination. Examination showed a well-developed, well-nourished, pleasant 15-year-old girl in moderate distress resulting from left TMJ pain. Interincisal opening was 25 mm. There was a deviation to the left on opening, which was approximately 5 mm from the maxillary midline. Auscultation of the joints with the stethoscope was negative because the patient was in such significant persistent lock that no joint movement was possible to elicit noise. There was significant tenderness to palpation in the left lateral and left posterior TMJ areas, which was considered a 7+ out of 10 on an intensity level. There was no associated muscle tenderness on palpation. Maxillomandibular and dentoalveolar relationships were within normal limits.

Radiographic findings. An arthrogram was done, which showed an anteriorly displaced disc with changes in disc morphology but no reduction of the disc with jaw movement.

A and **B** Preoperative arthrograms showing anterior disc displacement without reduction.

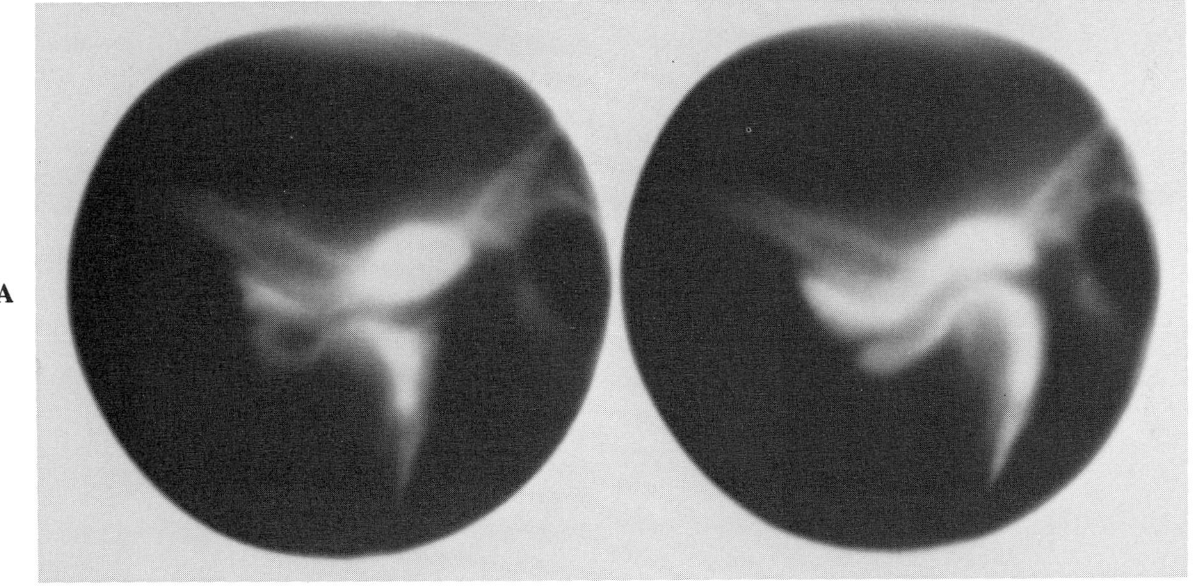
A
B

Diagnosis. Left TMJ internal derangement with persistent closed-lock.
Recommendation. TMJ arthrotomy.

C Intraoperatively the disc was found to be anteromedially displaced. It is grasped at its lateral margin and repositioned posterolaterally.
D The lateral margin of the disc is resected in preparation for the posterolateral repair.
E Posterolateral suture repair.
F Disc is in appropriate position after repair.

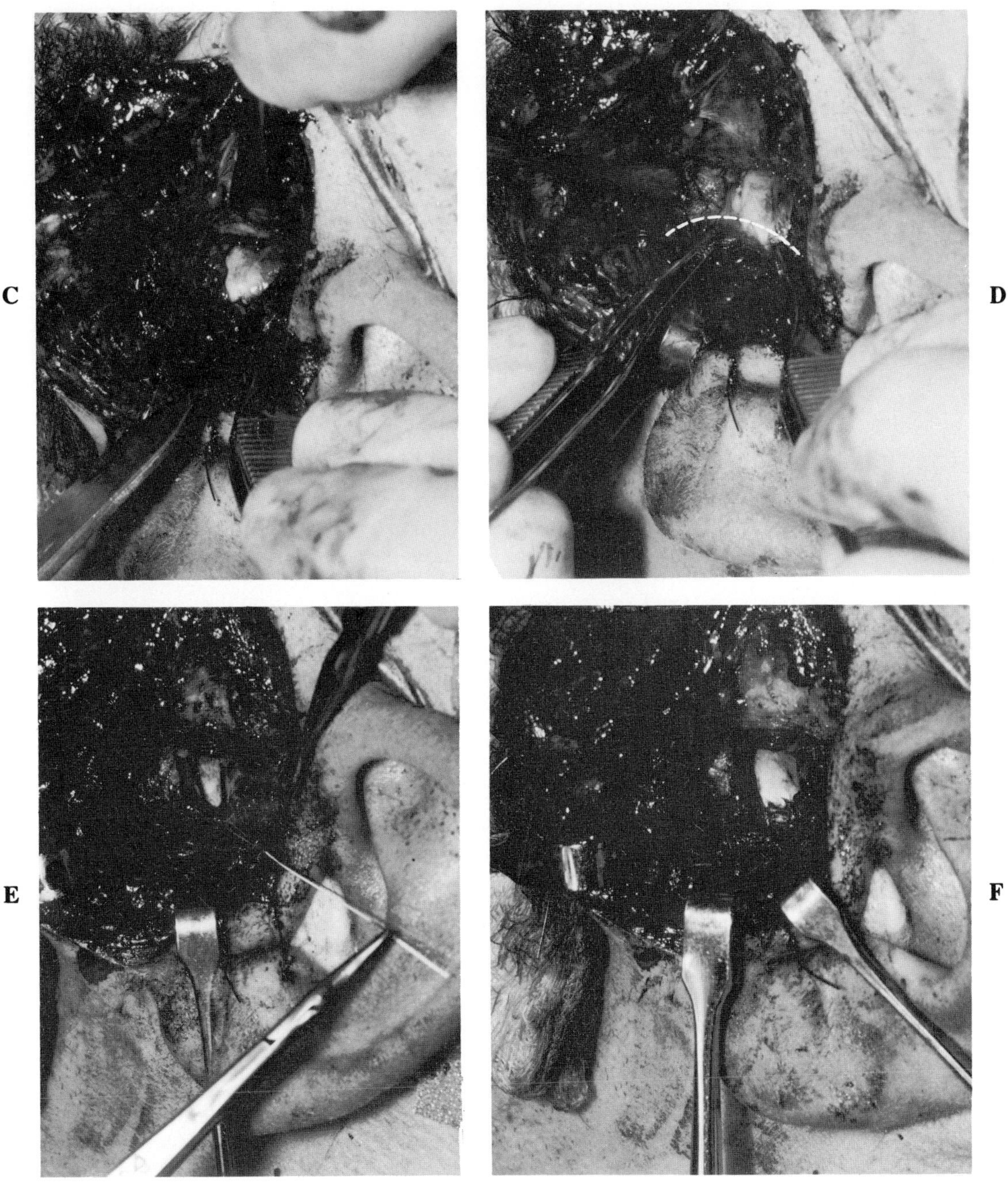
C
D
E
F

Surgery. Left TMJ arthroplasty with articular eminence reduction and posterolateral disc relocation and repair was carried out. No condylar head recontouring was done.

Surgical findings. Superior compartment adhesions were present. The very prominent deep-sloped eminence blockading the meniscus prevented it from being relocated. There was severe anteromedial dislocation of the meniscus. The condylar head had good fibrocartilage and good morphology.

Course. One year after surgery the patient is doing very well with no pain and good jaw opening and function.*

G and **H** One-year postoperative closed and open tomograms showing full translation.

*Noninvasive TMJ therapy done by Dr. Takeo Yamamoto, Santa Anna, California.

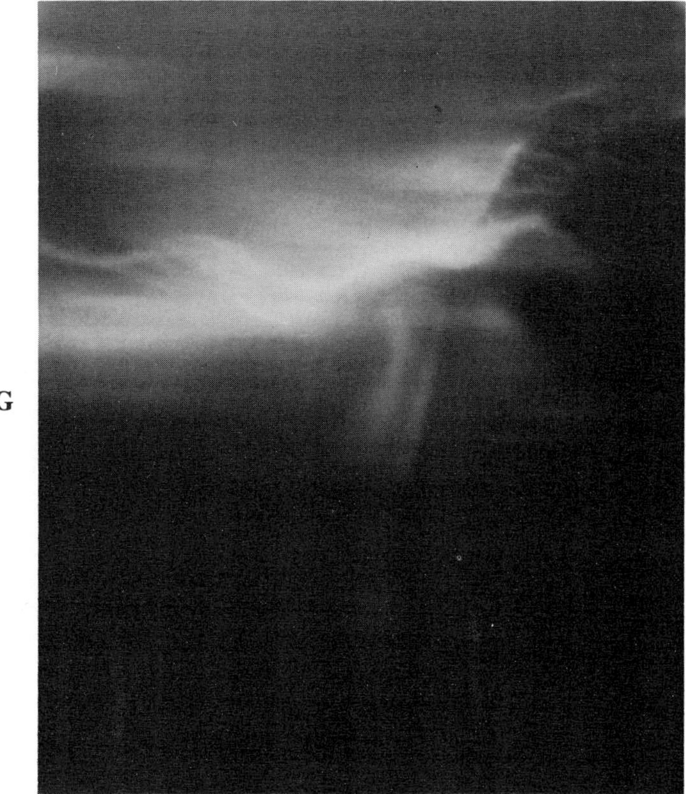

G

H

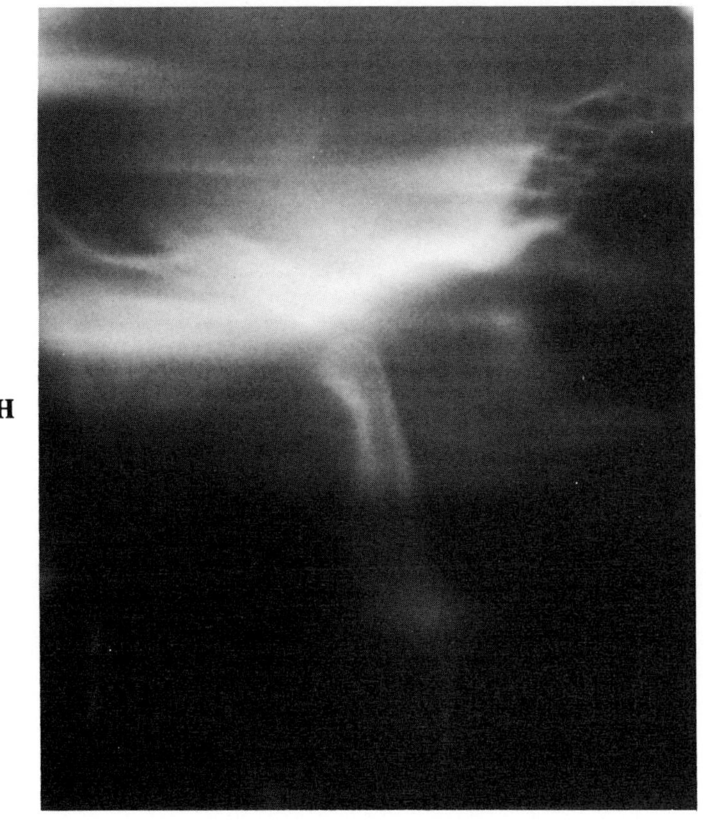

I to **K** Stable postoperative dental occlusion.

L Excellent mandibular opening. The patient is totally asymptomatic.

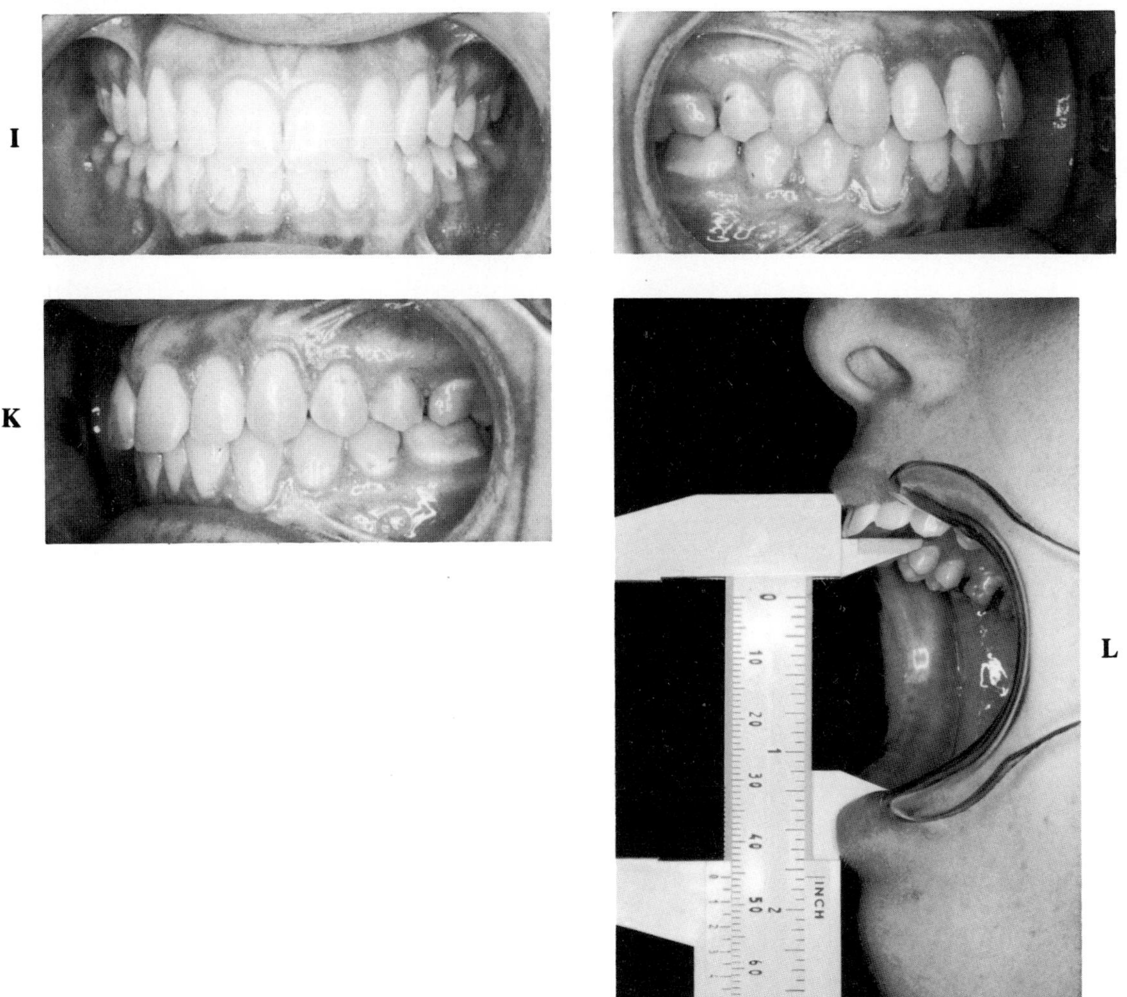
I
J
K
L
INCH

CASE 7

PLATE 8-6

Chief complaint and history of present illness. The patient was a 40-year-old man who was injured in an automobile accident 4 months previously. During the accident he hit his chin on the steering wheel and sustained a chin laceration and injury to the right TMJ. Initially his symptoms were pain in the right TMJ, limited opening, and slight separation of the posterior teeth on the right side. Radiographically there were no fractures. The patient was diagnosed as having a joint contusion. He was treated with moist heat, soft diet, and a nonsteroidal anti-inflammatory medication. Gradually his occlusion returned to normal, and his opening improved. His chief complaint was severe pain in the right TMJ, temporal headaches, and a grinding noise in the right TMJ. The noise was not present before the accident. The pain was well localized to the right TMJ and was worse with eating.

Past medical history and review of systems. Negative.

Examination. The patient opened to 32 mm with slight deviation toward the right side. The right TMJ was very tender to palpation and there was loud crepitus. The muscles of mastication were not tender, and the occlusion was good.

Radiographic findings. The Panorex and transcranial TMJ views were normal except for decreased translation of the right TMJ.

Diagnosis. Internal derangement of the right TMJ (perforation).

Recommendations. An arthrogram was recommended to confirm the diagnosis.

A The right TMJ arthrogram demonstrated an anteriorly displaced disc and a perforation.

A

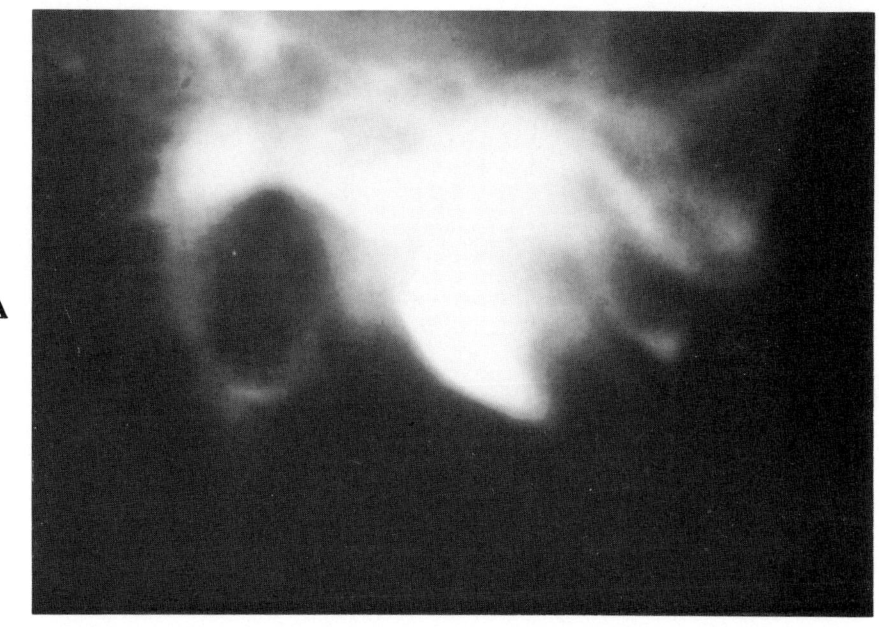

Surgery was recommended because the patient had a traumatically induced joint derangement.

Surgery. The patient was given the option of nonsurgical treatment but because of the severity of symptoms he elected to have surgery.

Surgical findings. Surgery revealed a perforation at the junction of the disc and posterior attachment. The perforation was about 1 cm long and very narrow. It was quite easy to reposition the disc and repair the perforation.

B The perforation at the junction of the disc and posterior attachment was easily repaired.

Course. The patient has done very well. His opening is 50 mm without deviation. He has no pain and no restrictions as to diet. He does have some very soft crepitus in the right TMJ.

B

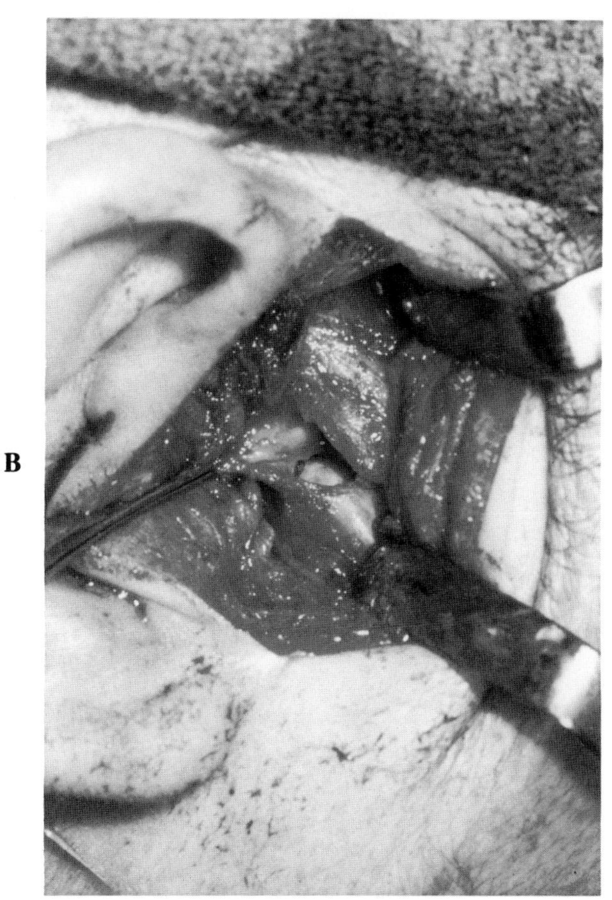

CASE 8

PLATE 8-7

Chief complaint and history of present illness. This 26-year-old woman reported a constant dull ache in the left preauricular region. She pointed clearly to the left TMJ. She said, however, that this distinct pain radiated to the neck and left temple area. She reported that she had had this problem for several years and that she also had limited opening and painful limited opening. She reported that her joint had been persistently in a closed-lock, and there was no longer any clicking because of the limited opening and lock.

A The patient indicated the location of her facial pain.

Past medical history and review of systems. Relating to the TMJ, the patient stated that she had a very long history of TMJ problems on the left side, a long history of clicking going to intermittent locking, and a persistent lock since October 1982. She had orthodontic treatment for 4½ years (from ages 9 to 13), and she had problems persistently. She was diagnosed as having a TMJ problem by her dentist. She saw a gnathologist for several months, who treated her with physical therapy, splint therapy, manipulation to try to reduce the displaced meniscus, and injections into the muscles and joint. He recommended home exercises in addition to thermal therapy. The patient had taken acetaminophen (Tylenol) and diflunisal (Dolobid) for her pain. Rheumatologic workup was negative. The patient enjoyed generally good health all of her life. She denied a history of any significant cardiovascular, pulmonary, hepatic, renal, gastric, or hematologic disorder; diabetes mellitus; anemia; neoplastic disease; severe infectious disorder; rheumatic fever; rheumatic heart disease; heart murmur; congenital heart disease; pulmonary problems; tuberculosis; asthma; bronchitis; dyspnea; chest pain; shortness of breath; thyroid disorder; or seizure disorder. The patient reported occasional sinus trouble, which she related to seasonal allergies.

The patient had had a lumbar disc removed in 1979. She reported a history of penicillin allergy.

The patient was a housewife. She reported smoking 10 cigarettes a day. She did not drink alcohol. The only medications she took were her pain medications pertaining to the TMJ problem. In the past she had taken Percodan for pain as well as acetaminophen and diflunisal.

She stated that multiple people in her family have arthritis.

The patient reported difficulty in opening the joint widely and pain in doing so. There was a left TMJ lock. She reported left TMJ pain and habitual posturing of her jaw forward.

Examination. The patient was a well-developed, well-nourished, pleasant 26-year-old woman in moderate to severe distress because of left TMJ pain. Maximal interincisal opening was 28 mm. Auscultation of the TMJ area with a stethoscope was negative because of the extremely limited rotation and lack of translation of the TMJs. On opening, the patient's jaw deviated to the left significantly. There was tenderness to palpation in the left lateral TMJ, the retrodiscal posterior aspect of the TMJ joint, and the anterior wall of the ear canal. All of these signs indicated adhesive capsulitis. Palpation of the muscles of mastication and facial expression was completely negative, indicating no myofascial component. Maxillomandibular relationship showed a significant forward posturing of the mandible, especially on the left. There was mandibular retrognathism, mandibular asymmetry, and an open bite when the patient was placed into centric relation.

In reviewing dentoalveolar status, there were occlusal interferences because of this relationship of the mandible and a significant slide from maximum retruded position to intercuspal position.

A

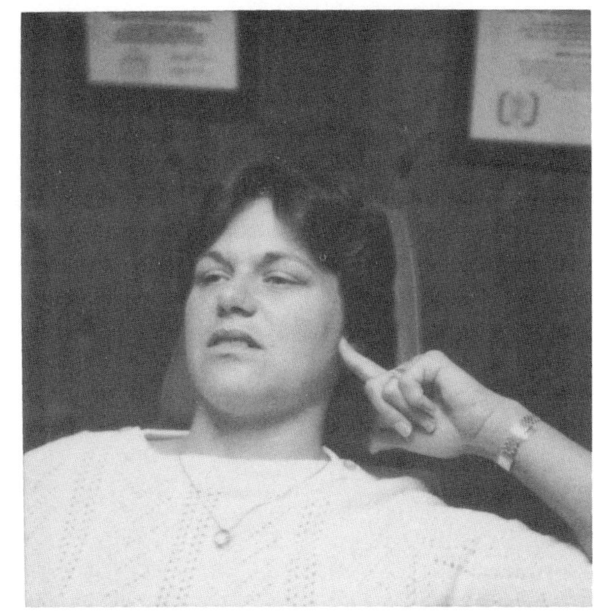

Radiographic findings. The tomographic x-ray films showed no evidence of severe degenerative change. However, arthrograms showed anterior displacement of the disc without reduction. The disc had lost its normal morphology and was hypertrophic. With condylar translation the disc was compressed anteroposteriorly. The retrodiscal tissues were elongated anteroposteriorly, indicating a chronically displaced disc without reduction.

B Preoperative arthrogram in closed position.

C Preoperative arthrogram in open position. Arthrogram shows anterior disc displacement without reduction.

Diagnosis. Left TMJ internal derangement with persistent closed-lock and occlusal deformity with an open bite and mandibular asymmetric retrusion.

Recommendation. Temporomandibular joint arthrotomy.

Surgery. Left TMJ arthroplasty with condylar head recontouring and meniscectomy with placement of Silastic fossa implant were carried out.

Surgical findings. Superior and inferior compartment adhesions were revealed. The meniscus was displaced anteriorly with small anterolateral perforation, and there were gross changes in morphology. The disc was elongated anteroposteriorly and grossly thinned, with thickening in the anterior aspect. The condyle was seated in the posterior attachment hernia sac. The disc was displaced anteromedially. The condylar head was grossly deformed.

There was a large osteophyte on the superolateral surface of the condylar head and eburnation of the condylar articular surface. The eminence was grossly arthrotic, with a very hyperplastic steep eminence, which would seem to be contributing to the closed-lock position. The TMJ capsule appeared to be thickened laterally and chronically inflamed.

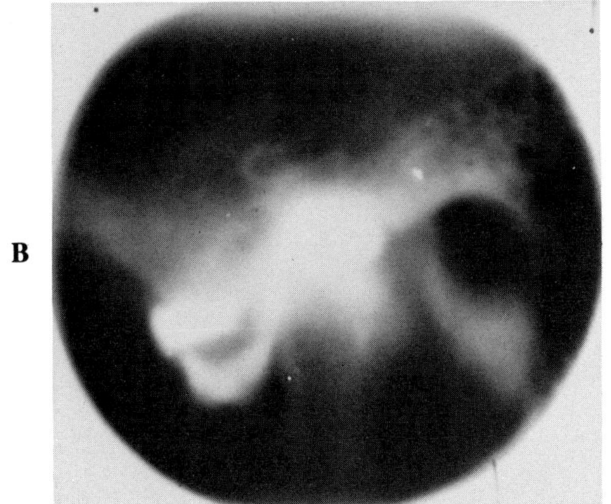
B

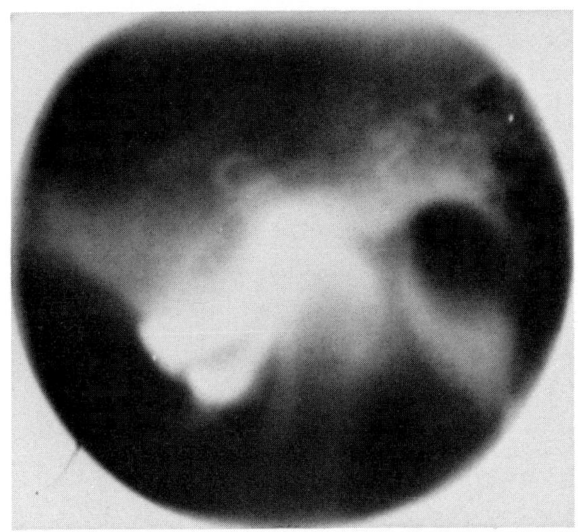
C

Postoperative course. Approximately 1 year postoperatively the patient is totally free of pain. She has excellent opening (45 mm interincisally) and very good function with a splint. Occlusal stability will include equilibration, restorative dentistry, and possible orthodontic and orthognathic surgical treatment.

D One year postoperative tomogram of left TMJ in closed position. Note condylar remodelling.
E Open position.
F Excellent mandibular opening 1 year postoperatively.

D

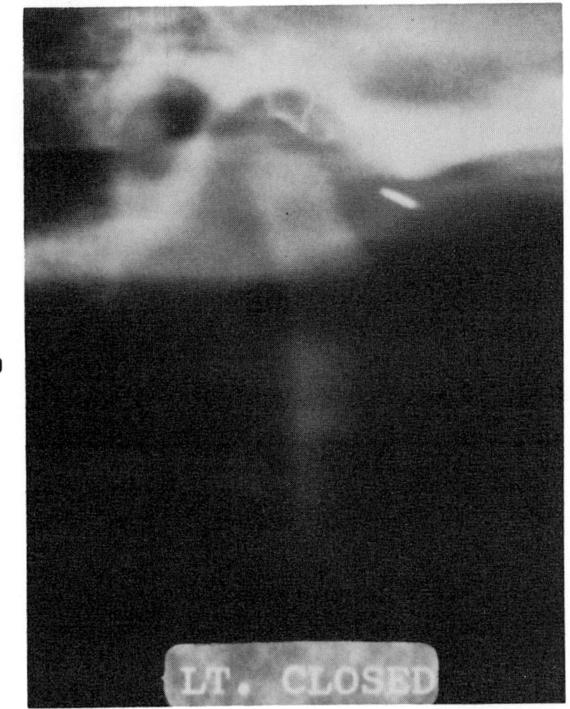

E

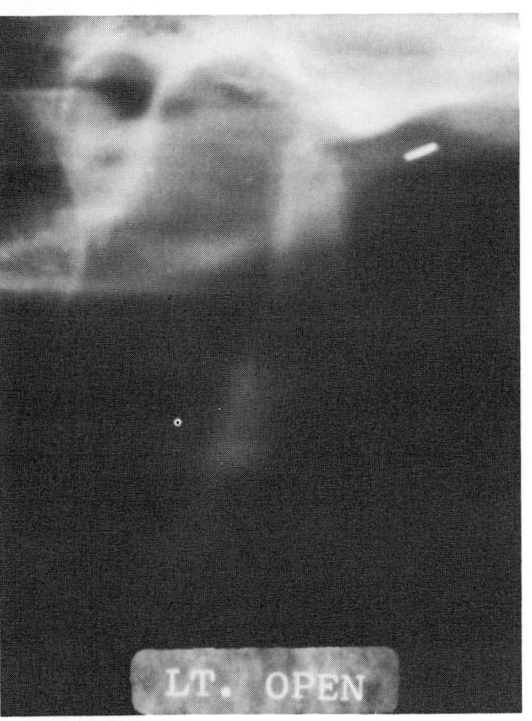

F

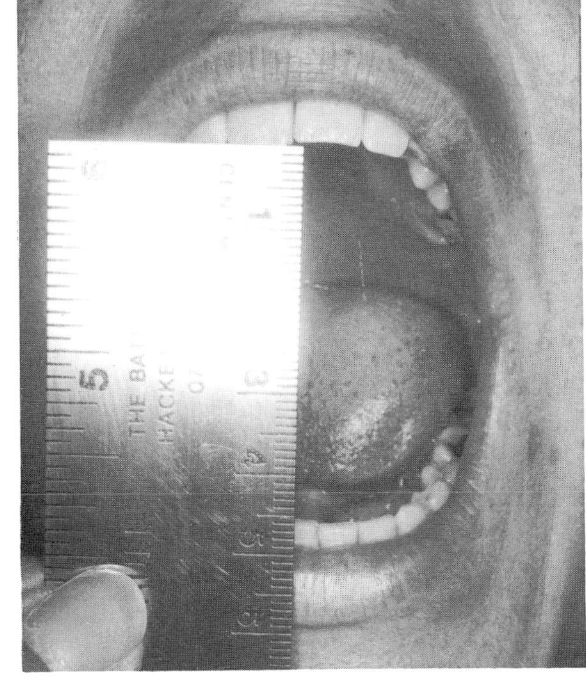

G to **I** Occlusal deformity is stabilized with splint. Eventual equilibration, restorative dentistry, orthodontics, and possible orthnognathic surgery (LeFort I osteotomy) will be necessary to reconstruct the occlusion.*

J The patient is pain free and satisfied with the surgical outcome.

*Noninvasive TMJ therapy done by Dr. Greg Arnett, Encino, California.

B

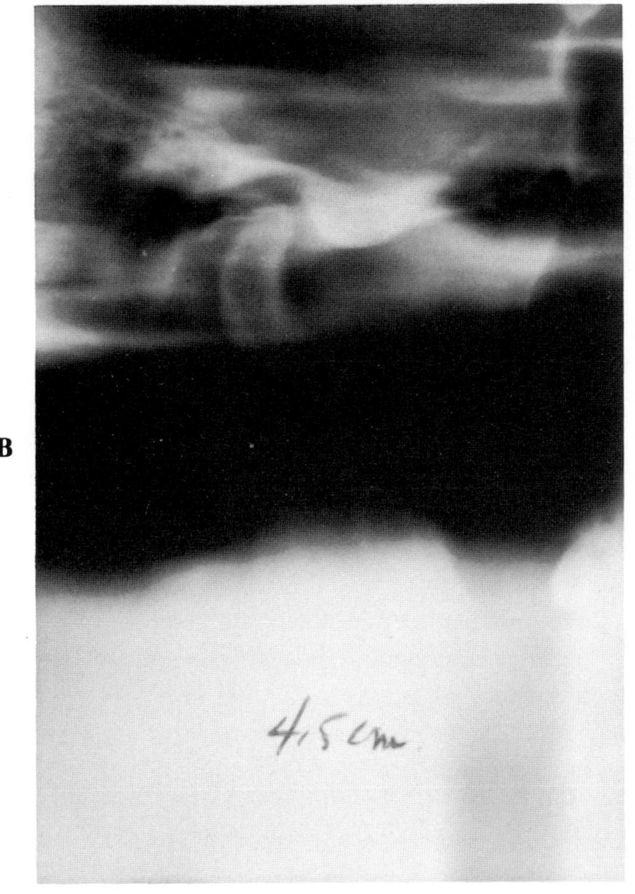

C

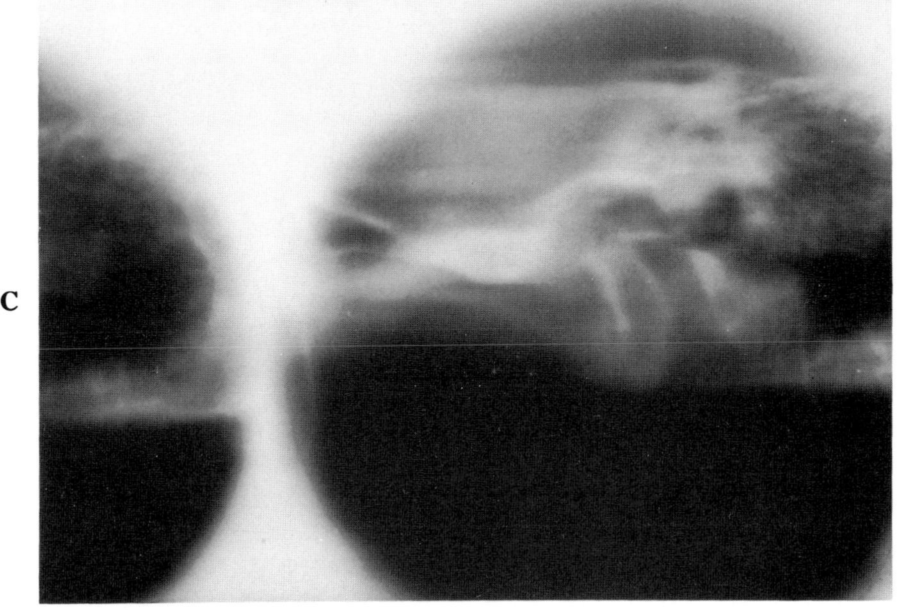

Surgery. Bilateral TMJ arthroplasty with meniscectomies and insertion of Silastic fossa implants were performed.

Surgical findings. On the right side, surgery revealed a grossly thickened meniscus with anteromedial displacement and calcified-appearing deposits in the meniscus that were very inflexible and brittle. There were also superior and inferior compartment adhesions and condylar head changes and morphology, as well as a very protuberant steep slope of the eminence with some arthrotic changes. On the left side, surgery revealed a grossly thickened meniscus with anteromedial displacement, definite arthrosis of the head of the condyle, and superior and inferior compartment adhesions.

Course. The patient had an uneventful postoperative recovery. Subsequent to the surgery and several weeks of progressive physical therapy, the orthotic appliance was gradually thinned to reestablish occlusal contact. Typically these patients demonstrate contact only in the incisor regions. The maxillary incisors were flaired by adding springs in the orthotic appliance lingual to the maxillary four incisors. After 10 weeks of adjusting these springs, there was sufficient clearance of the incisors so that the occlusion could be equilibrated sufficiently to reestablish optimal interdigitation. This was completed first on articulated mounted models to confirm the degree of occlusal reduction necessary in specific areas before actually performing the procedures in the mouth.

Once the equilibration procedures were completed, there was excellent, balanced occlusal contact and coupling in all functional movements. As this was established, the need for the orthotic appliance was eliminated and its wear was discontinued.

D and **E** Excellent balanced occlusion after surgery will help stabilize the joint healing.

It is now 2 years after surgery and the patient has no pain, good mandibular opening, and excellent function. She reports great satisfaction with the procedure.*

*Noninvasive therapy done by Dr. Duane Grummons, Marina del Rey, California.

D

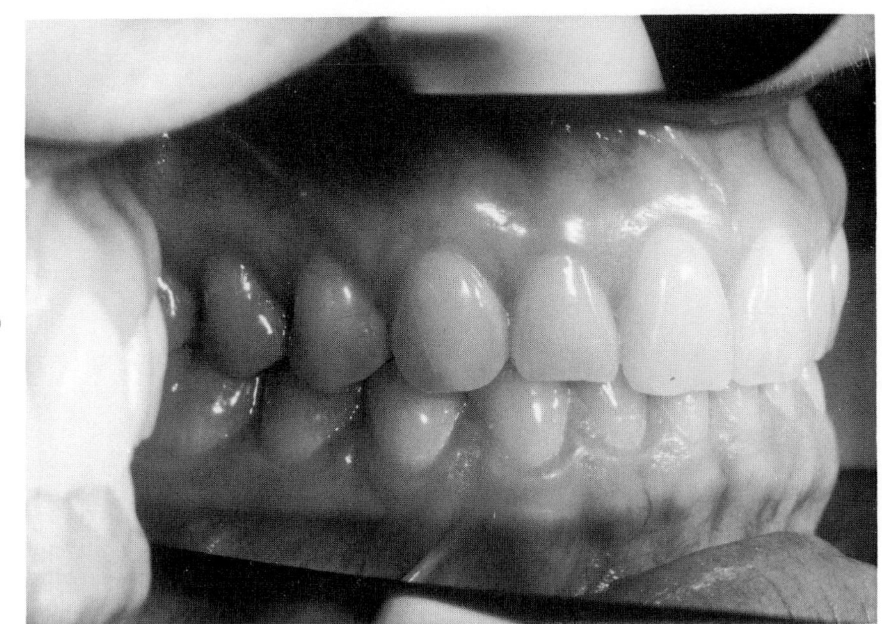

E

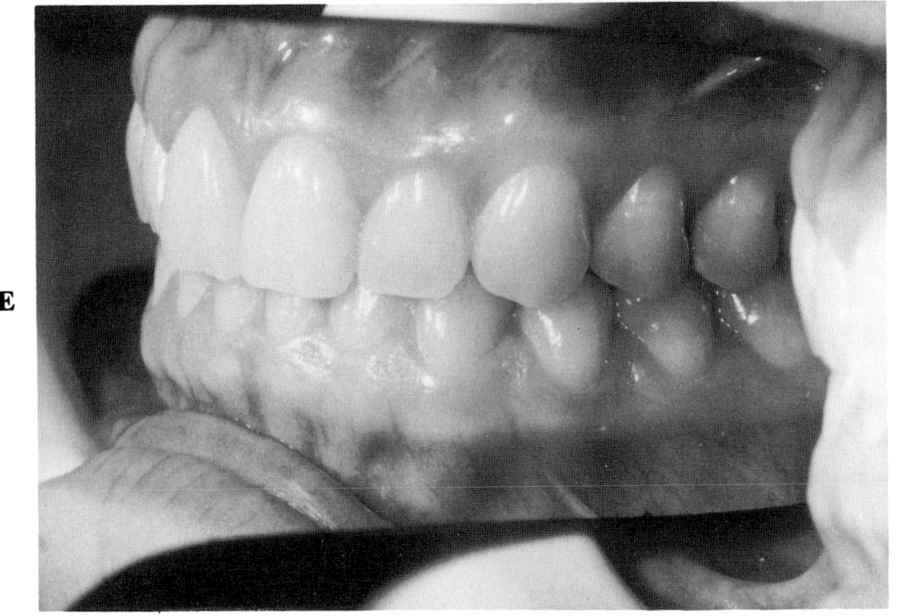

CASE 10

PLATE 8-9

Chief complaint and history of present illness. The patient was a 59-year-old woman who reported a history of left TMJ pain of 1 year's duration following trauma. The patient reported specific preauricular pain when she opened the jaw and when she attempted to chew. She had significant limitation of opening, and reported crepitation and cracking noises in the left TMJ. She reported the pain as an intense, deep ache in the bony aspect of the TMJ.

Past medical history and review of systems. The patient fell in a parking lot 1 year previously and struck her face; she developed extensive ecchymoses and edema. She had radiographs taken that ruled out fracture. She had persistent pain in the left TMJ and associated areas. She underwent extensive noninvasive therapy, including splint therapy for 6 months, and she took ibuprofen (Motrin) consistently. She had extensive physical therapy, and steroid injections into the joints were done without alleviation of symptoms. In addition, she had ethyl chloride spray and stretch, moist heat, hydrocolator therapy, and arthrograms. She reported the symptoms to be worse when she became tired or the weather grew cold. She denied any previous history of severe cardiovascular, pulmonary, hepatic, or renal disorder; diabetes mellitus; anemia; neoplastic disease; severe infectious disease; gastric disorder; ulcers; colitis; hypertension; stroke; rheumatic fever; rheumatic heart disease; heart murmur; chest pain; bronchitis; emphysema; persistent cough; shortness of breath; thyroid disorder; or seizure disorder. She did not smoke and only occasionally drank wine. Otologic examinations and workups were negative.

She reported difficulty in opening the jaw widely, said it was painful to do so, and noted closed lock with clicking and crepitation noises in the joint. She had left ear and left TMJ pain; the pain behind the left orbit she associated with her jaw pain. She reported muscle fatigue in the jaw and an uncomfortable bite.

Examination. Physical examination showed a well-developed, well-nourished, very pleasant 59-year-old woman in moderate distress as a result of left TMJ pain. The maximum interincisal opening was only 22 mm, with discrete pain in the preauricular region. Auscultation with the stethoscope revealed loud, coarse crepitation in the left TMJ, and when the patient opened the jaw there was immediate deviation to the left. There was tenderness to palpation in the left lateral portion and anterior wall of the ear canal areas, indicating adhesive capsulitis. There was no tenderness of the muscles of mastication on palpation. The maxillomandibular relationship revealed a deep bite with Class II, Division II occlusion, and there was occlusal interference present.

A to **C** Preoperative occlusion showing Class II, Division II deep-bite malocclusion. The associated heavy muscular forces could adversely affect the surgery.

A
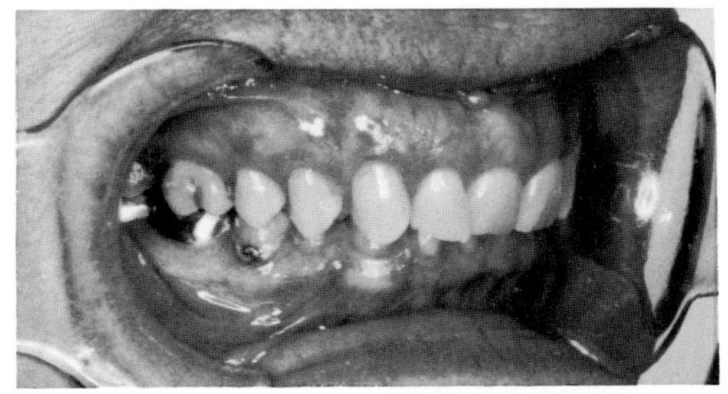

B
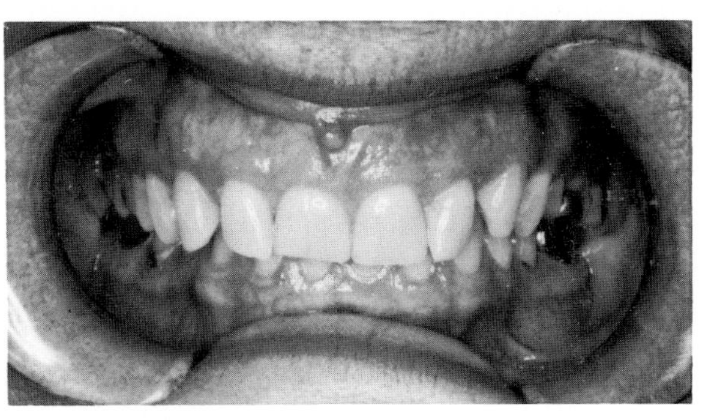

C
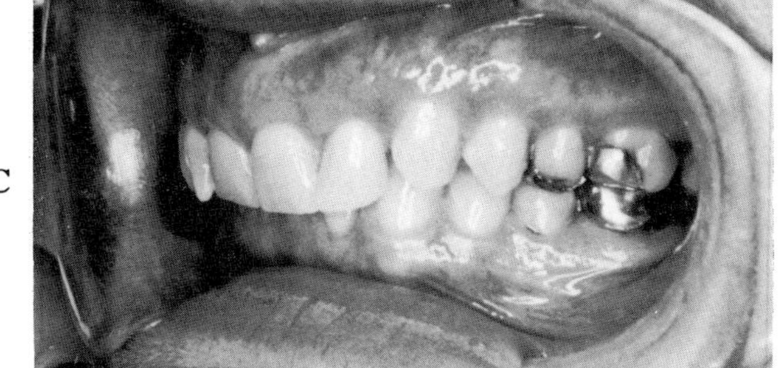

Radiographic findings. Arthrograms revealed a relatively normal right TMJ, but the left TMJ indicated severe degenerative changes and a *perforated meniscus.*

Diagnosis. Left TMJ degenerative disease, which is severe, and adhesive capsulitis.

Recommendation. Since all noninvasive therapy had been exhausted and the patient still had severe symptoms, a left TMJ arthroplasty with meniscectomy and insertion of implant was recommended. All details of surgery, alternatives of therapy, and complications were explained to the patient on multiple occasions.

Surgery. Left TMJ arthroplasty with condylar recontouring and meniscectomy with insertion of Silastic fossa implant.

Surgical findings. Advanced arthrosis of the left TMJ and osteophyte of the head of the condyle were found, as was a large perforation of the disc.

D to **F** The patient's malocclusion was stablilzed postoperatively with an occlusal splint.

Course. At 1½ years after surgery the patient has little or no pain and good mandibular function and mastication. She avoids specific hard and chewy foods such as whole carrots or large pieces of steak. Due to the patient's severe deep bite and brachyfacial muscular pattern, a splint must be worn long-term. Her prognosis is good.*

*Arthrography and noninvasive therapy done by Dr. John Ross, West Los Angeles, California.

D
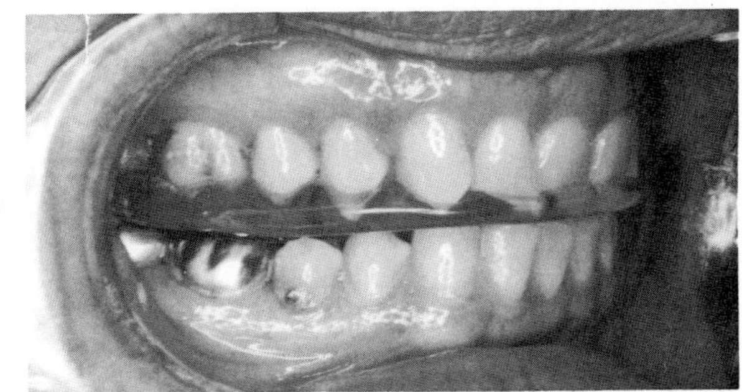

E
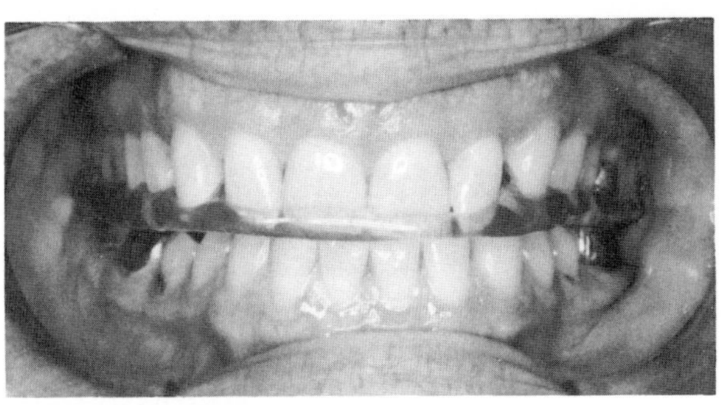

F
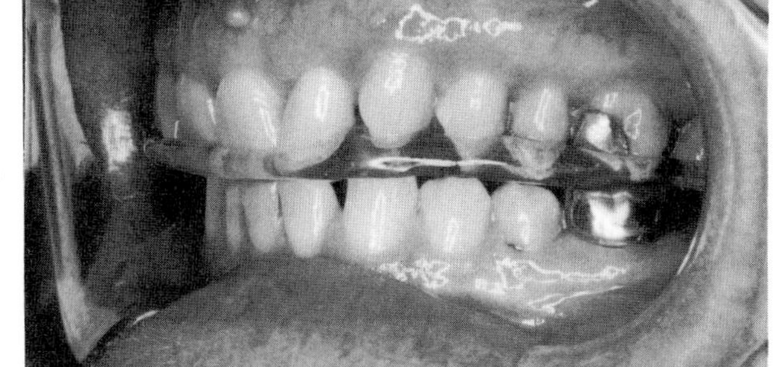

CASE 11

PLATE 8-10

Chief complaint and history of present illness. This 47-year-old woman reported constant pain in the right facial region over a period of 2 years. She indicated the area of pain as the preauricular area on the right and secondarily the region of the right zygoma and coronoid area. The pain was characterized as sharp and severe and hurting much more with jaw use and jaw opening. She had a persistent closed-lock with a history of popping and clicking, but currently there was just persistent lock.

A Preoperative appearance showing painful limited opening.
B to **D** Preoperative open-bite malocclusion.

A

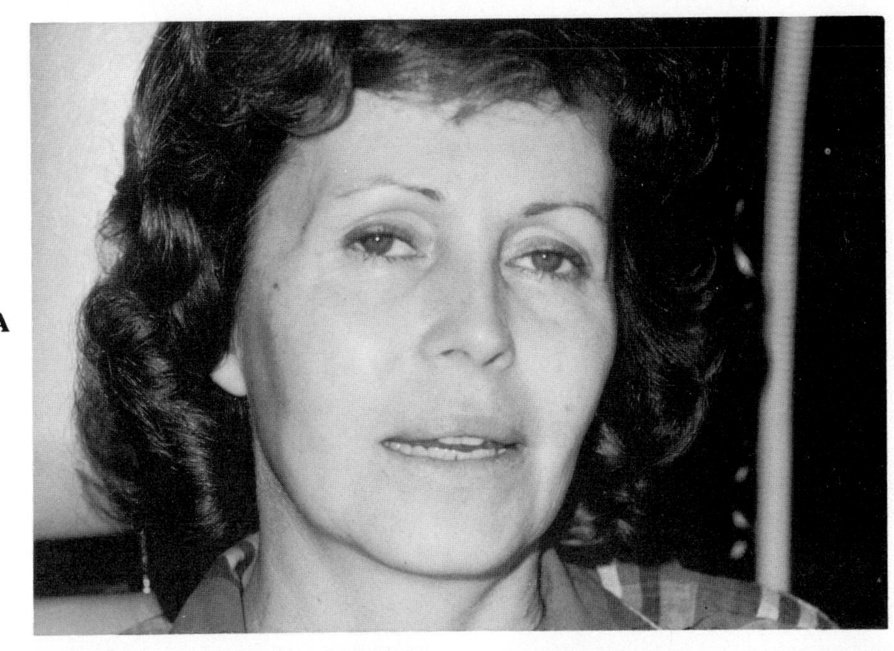

B

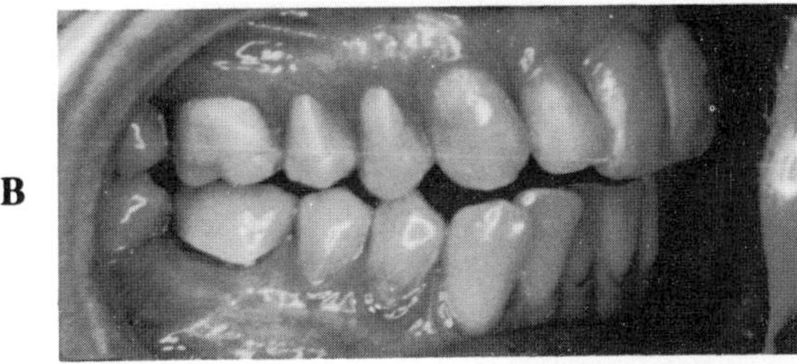

C

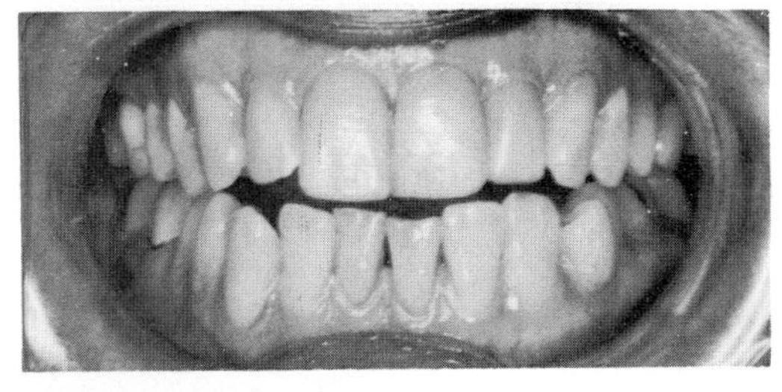

D

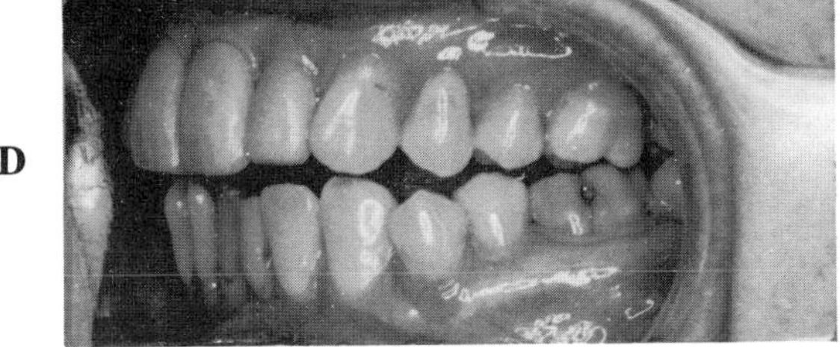

Past medical history and review of systems. Relating to the TMJ, the patient denied any history of trauma to the jaw. She stated that her wisdom teeth were removed 18 years previously without any known complications. She had no orthodontic treatment. Two years before the onset of symptoms, she had an upper respiratory infection with a great deal of severe, exaggerated sneezing, to which she related her jaw complaint. She reported difficulty opening her jaw widely and experienced great pain in doing so. She was in a persistent closed-lock state. She reported pain in the right TMJ, right ear, right cheek, and coronoid area; jaw muscle fatigue; and an uncomfortable bite. She had had pain in other joints, including the neck and hands. There was a familial history of arthritis. She had a history of cervical arthritis as well as beginning degenerative arthritis in her hands. She was examined by an otolaryngologist to rule out any ear problems, and the examination was reportedly negative. She was seen by several dentists and orthodontists. Treatment to date included splint therapy and antiinflammatory nonsteroidal medication. She had psychologic evaluations, physical therapy, diagnostic blocks, and steroid injections into the joint and coronoid area. The diagnostic blocks in the right TMJ and coronoid process eliminated the pain, but movement remained markedly restricted. The patient underwent mandibular manipulation while under general anesthesia in an attempt to relocate the disc and eliminate the closed-lock. The attempt was unsuccessful.

E and **F** Preoperative splint stabilizing occlusion; the splint will also be used postoperatively.

G Maximum preoperative mandibular opening.

E

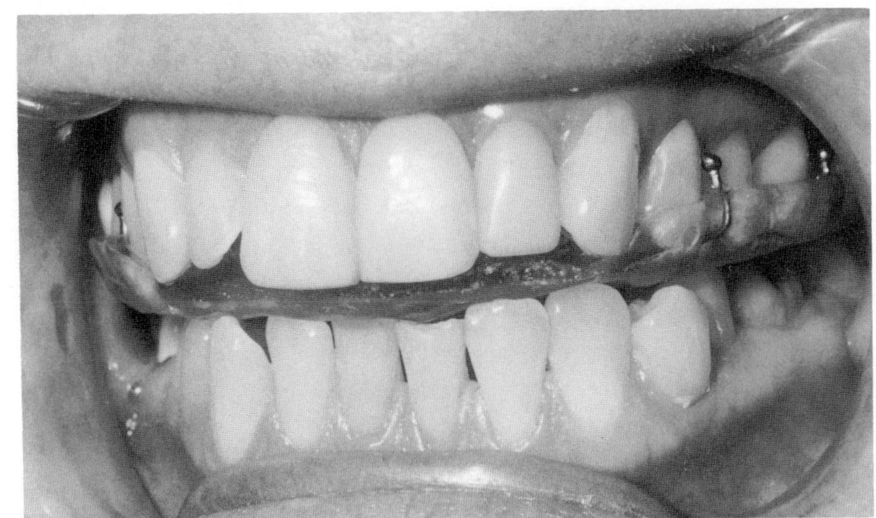

F

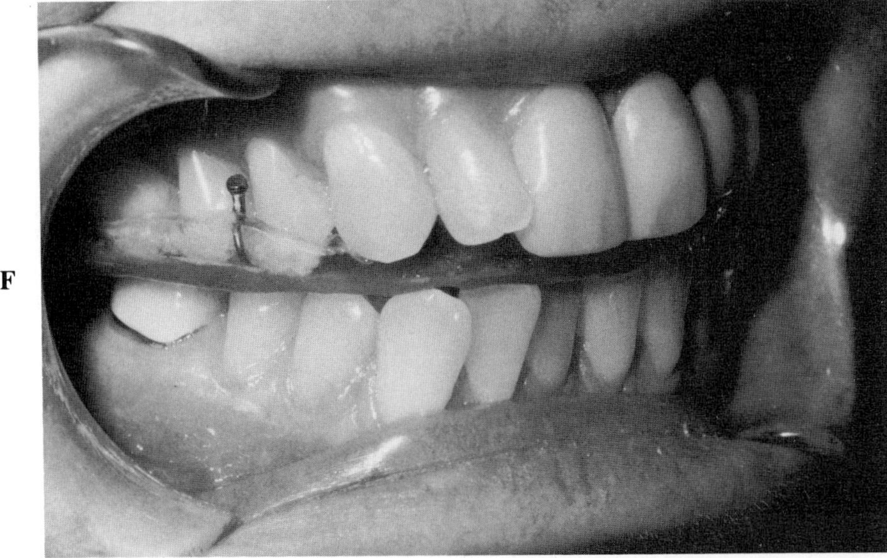

G

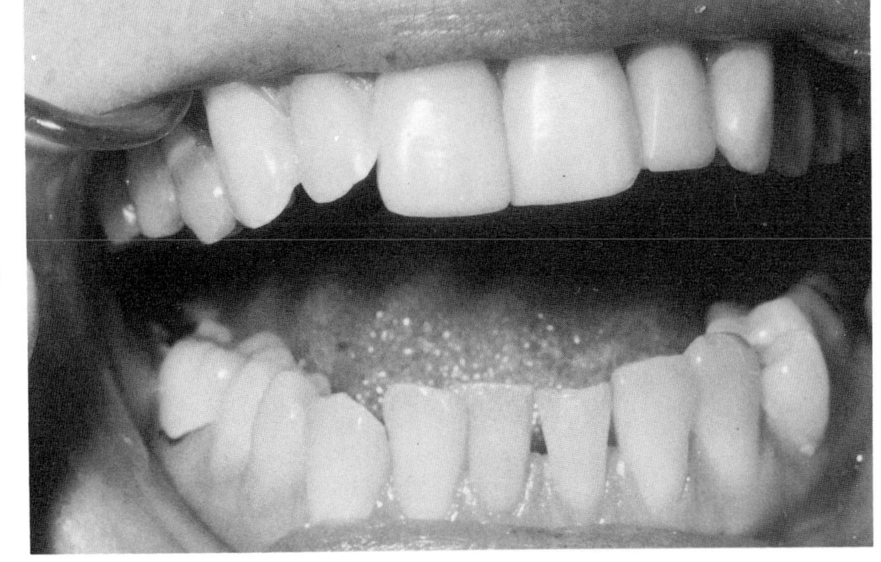

Examination. Examination showed a maximal interincisal opening of 20 mm. Auscultation with the stethoscope of the joints was negative, but this was considered to be the result of the very limited oral opening. The patient's jaw deviated to the right on opening. On initial examination tenderness to palpation was negative. However, on subsequent examinations intraoral and extraoral palpation of the coronoid process and the preauricular area was positive. The patient had a slight open bite and mandibular asymmetry. There were occlusal interferences.

H and **I** Preoperative arthrogram showing disc displacement without reduction.

Radiographic findings. The arthrogram showed an anteriorly displaced disc without reduction. There was no communication observed between the inferior compartment and the superior compartment. There was a severe reduction in the size of the superior compartment and obliteration of the superior compartment resulting from adhesions. The inferior compartment was difficult to infuse, indicating adhesions. The condylar translation view was extremely limited.

Diagnosis. Persistent closed-lock caused by right TMJ internal derangement, displaced disc without reduction and adhesions, coronoid impingement, and temporal tendonitis.

Recommendation. The patient had had all conservative therapy exhausted; therefore surgery was indicated.

H

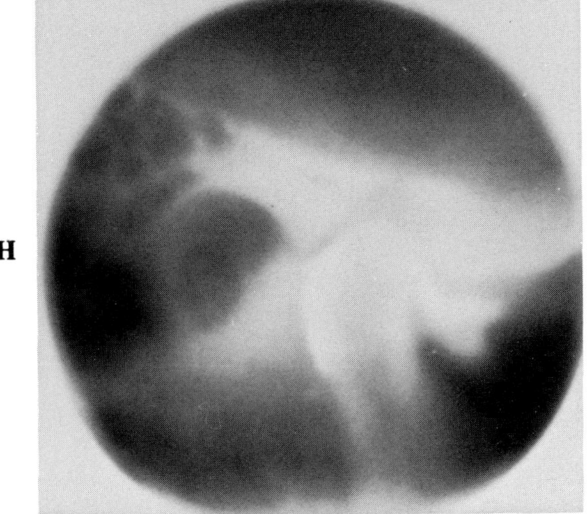

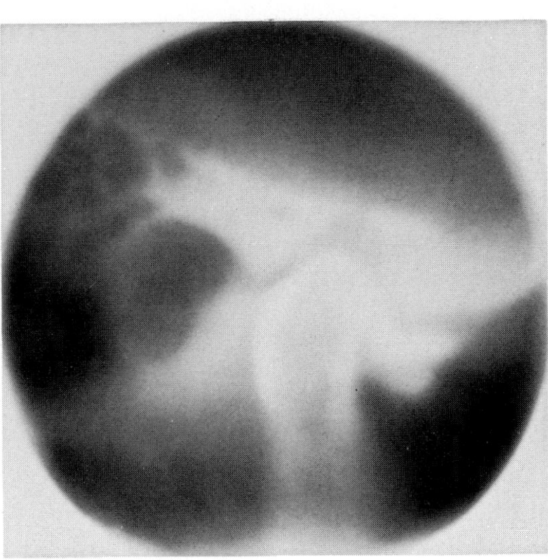

I

Surgery. Right TMJ arthroplasty with meniscectomy and insertion of Silastic fossa implant and right coronoidectomy was performed.

Surgical findings. The superior compartment adhesions were severe and the inferior compartment adhesions moderate. The meniscus was anteromedially displaced without reduction and had gross adhesions, gross thickening, and dystrophic changes. There was a bulbous condylar head with no joint space after meniscectomy. The coronoid process was irregular, with a dense, fibrous connective tissue attachment to the surrounding musculature and an inflexible temporalis tendon.

J to **M** Definitive fixed prosthetic reconstruction.

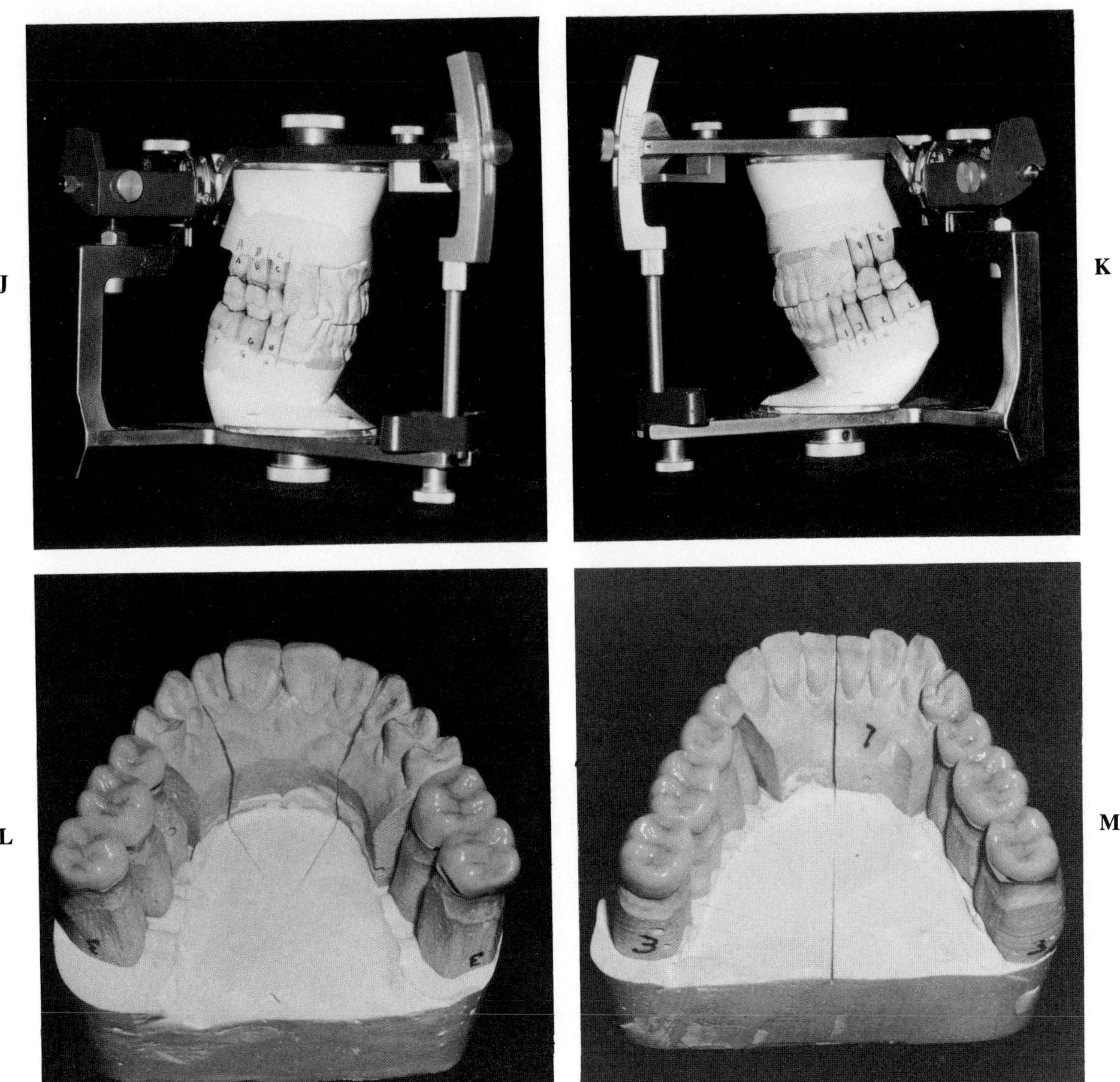
J
K
L
M

N to **P** Stable posttreatment occlusion.
Q One and one-half years after surgery the patient is doing well.

Course. The patient underwent extensive postoperative physical therapy. A postoperative occlusal splint was maintained for 6 months. Following this period, the patient was asymptomatic. Only then was definitive dental reconstruction carried out.*

*Preoperative and postoperative noninvasive TMJ therapy and fixed prosthodontics done by Dr. Greg Arnett, Encino, California.

N

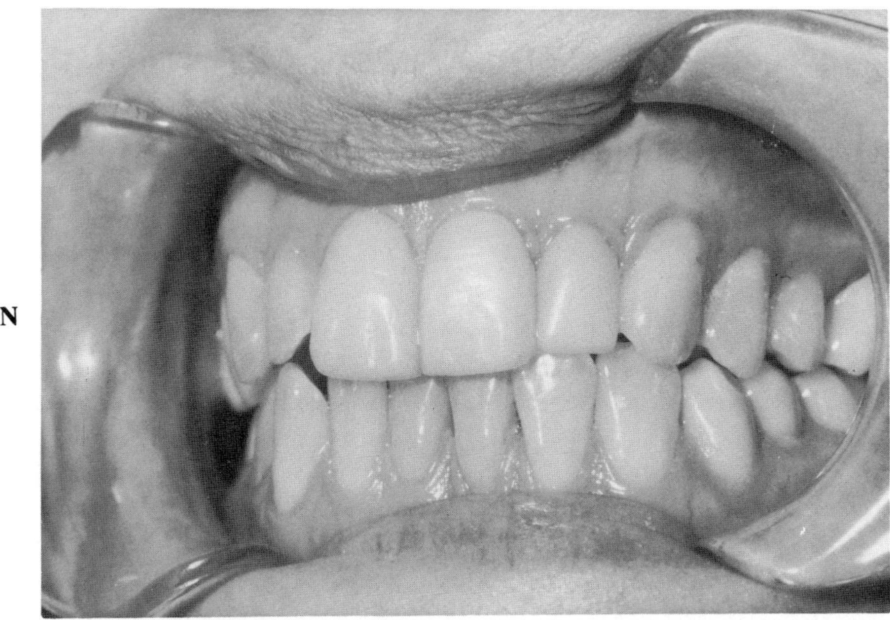

O

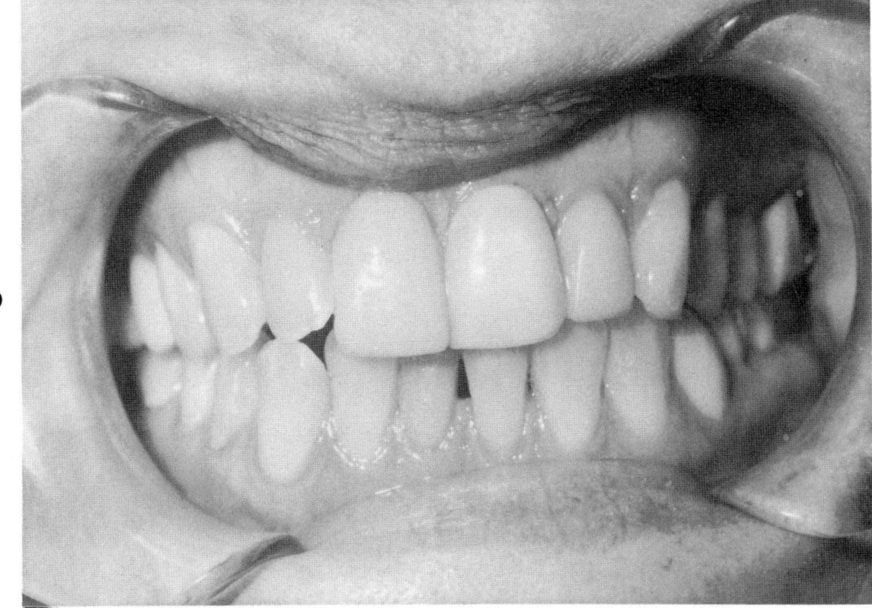

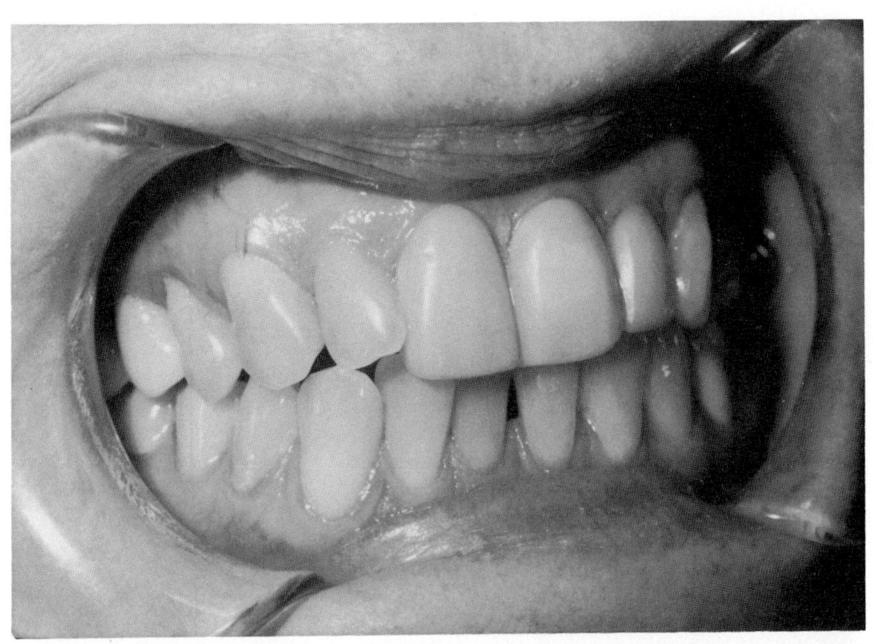

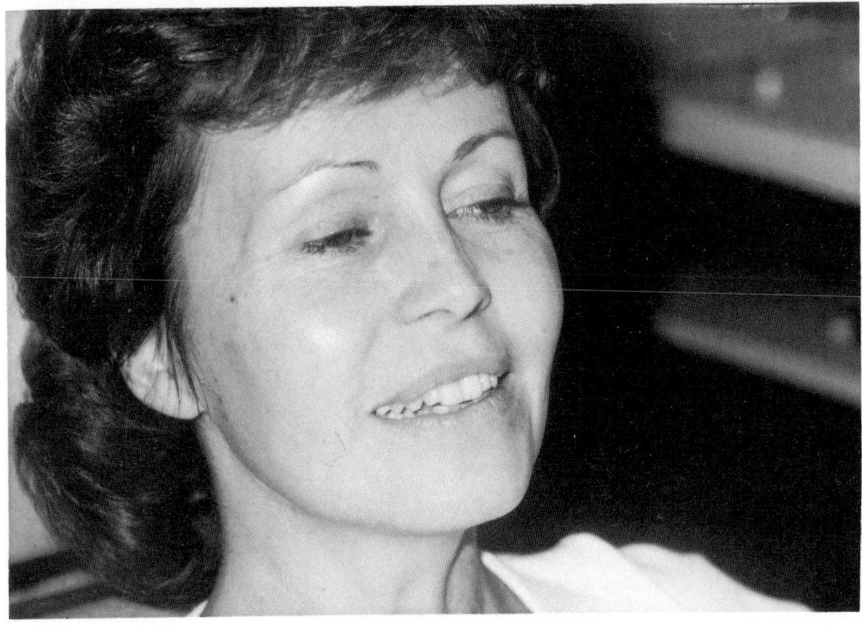

Q

References

Chapter 1 ANATOMY

Anson BJ, Donaldson JA, Warpela RL, et al: Surgical anatomy of the facial nerve. Arch Otolaryngol **97:**201, 1973.

Boyer CC, Williams TW, Stevens FH: Blood supply of the temporomandibular joint. J Dent Res **43:**224, 1964.

Dolwick MF, Lipton JS, Warner MR, et al: Sagittal anatomy of the human temporomandibular joint spaces: Normal and abnormal findings. J Oral Maxillofac Surg **41:**86, 1983.

DuBrul EL: The craniomandibular articulation, in Sicher H (ed): Oral Anatomy, ed 7. St. Louis, The CV Mosby Co, 1980.

Griffin CJ, Hawthorn R, Harris R: Anatomy and histology of the human temporomandibular joint. Monogr Oral Sci **4:**1, 1975.

McNamara JA Jr: The independent functions of the two heads of the lateral pterygoid muscle. Am J Anat **138:**197, 1973.

Mohn ND: Functional anatomy of the temporomandibular joint, in The President's Conference on the Examination, Diagnosis and Management of Temporomandibular Disorders. Chicago, American Dental Association, 1982.

Rees LA: The structure and function of the mandibular joint: Br Dent J **96:**125, 1954.

Sicher H: Functional anatomy of the temporomandibular joint, in Sarnat BG (ed): Temporomandibular Joint. Springfield, Ill, Charles C Thomas Publisher, 1951.

Yale SH, Allison BD, Haupfuehrer JD: An epidemiological assessment of mandibular condyle morphology. Oral Surg **21:**169, 1966.

Chapter 2 PATHOLOGY

Blackwood JHH: Pathology of the temporomandibular joint. J Am Dent Assoc **79:**118, 1969.

Buckley S, Dolwick MF: Prevalence and historical characteristics of muscle disorder and internal derangement patients. AADR Abstracts, 303, 1985.

Dolwick, MF, Aufdemorte TB, Cornelius JD: Histological findings in TMJ internal derangements. J Dent Res **63:**267, 1984.

Dolwick MF, Katzbery RW, Helms CA: Internal derangement of the temporomandibular joint: Fact or Fiction? J Prosthet Dent **49:**415, 1983.

Dolwick MF, Lipton JS, Warner MR: Sagittal anatomy of the human temporomandibular joint spaces: Normal and abnormal findings. J Oral Maxillofac Surg **41:**86, 1983.

Hall MB, Brown RW, Baughman RA: Histologic appearance of the bilaminar zone in internal derangement of the temporomandibular joint. Oral Surg **58:**375, 1984.

Hanson TL, Solberg WK, Penn MD: Temporomandibular joint changes in young adults. J Dent Res **58:**267, 1979.

Katzberg RW, Anderson QN, Manzione JV, et al: Dislocation of jaws. Skeletal Radiol **11**(1):38, 1984.

McCarty WL Jr, Farrar W: Surgery for internal derangements of the temporomandibular joint. J Prosthet Dent **42:**2, 1979.

McCoy M, Gotcher J, Chase D: Histologic characteristics of pathology in TMJ internal derangements, abstracted. J Dent Res **63:**228, 1984.

Scapino RP: Histopathology associated with malposition of the human temporomandibular joint disc. Oral Surg **55:**382, 1983.

Solberg W, Hanson T, Nordstrom B: Morphologic evaluation of young adult TMJs at autopsy, abstracted. J Dent Res **63:**228 1984.

Westesson PL, Rohlin M: Internal derangement related to osteoarthrosis in temporomandibular joint autopsy specimens. Oral Surg **57:**17, 1984.

Zarb GA, Carlsson GE: Temporomandibular Joint Function and Dysfunction. St. Louis, The CV Mosby Co, 1979.

Chapter 3 DIAGNOSIS

Bell WE: Orofascial pains, in Differential Diagnosis, ed 2. Chicago, Year Book Medical Publishers Inc, 1982.

Bell WE: Clinical Management of Temporomandibular Disorders. Chicago, Year Book Medical Publishers Inc, 1983.

Dolwick MF: Diagnosis and etiology, in Helms CA, Katzberg RW, Dolwick, MF (eds): Internal Derangements of the Temporomandibular Joint. San Francisco, Radiology and Research Foundation, 1983.

Dolwick MF, Riggs RR: Diagnosis and treatment of internal derangements of the temporomandibular joint. Dent Clin North Am **27:**561, 1983.

Farrar WB, McCarty WL Jr: A clinical outline of temporomandibular joint diagnosis and treatment, ed 7. Montgomery Normandie Publications, 1983.

McCarty WB: Diagnosis and treatment of internal derangements of the articular disk and mandibular condyle, in Solberg WK, Clark GT (eds): Temporomandibular Joint Problems. Chicago, Quintessence Publishing Co Inc, 1980.

Moffett B: Classification of temporomandibular joint disturbances, in Solberg WK, Clark GT (eds): Tempormandibular Joint Problems. Chicago, Quintessence Publishing Co Inc, 1980.

Rugh JD: A behavioral approach to diagnosis and treatment of functional oral disorders: Biofeedback and self control techniques, in Rugh JD, Perlis DB, Disraeli RJ (eds): Biofeedback in Dentistry: Research and Clinical Applications. Phoenix, Semantodontics, 1977.

Sanders B, Frey N, McReynolds J: Anatomical, radiographic, and clinical evaluation of temporomandibular articular eminence reduction as a treatment for recurrent dislocation and chronic subluxation. Ann Dent **37:**33, 1978.

Zarb GA, Carlsson GE: Temporomandibular Joint Function and Dysfunction. St. Louis, The CV Mosby Co, 1979.

Chapter 4 ARTHROGRAPHY

Blaschke DD, Solberg WK, Sanders B: Arthrography of the temporomandibular joint: Review of current status. J Am Dent Assoc **100:**388, 1980.

Bronstein, SL, Tomasetti BJ, Ryan DE: Internal derangements of the temporomandibular joint: Correlation of arthrography with surgical findings. J Oral Surg **39:**572, 1981.

Dolwick MF, Katzberg RW, Helms CA, et al: Arthrotomographic evaluation of the temporomandibular joint. J Oral Surg **37:**793, 1979.

Farrar WB: Diagnosis and treatment of anterior dislocation of the articular disc. NY J Dent **41:**348, 1971.

Farrar W, McCarty WL Jr: Interior joint space arthrography and characteristics of condylar paths in internal derangements of the TMJ. J Prosthet Dent **41:**548, 1979.

Helms CA, Katzberg RW, Dolwick MF, et al: Arthrotomographic diagnosis of meniscus perforations in the temporomandibular joint. Br J Radiol **53:**283, 1980.

Helms CA, Morrish RB, Kircos LT, et al: Computed tomography of the meniscus of the temporomandibular joint: Preliminary observations. Radiology **145:**719, 1982.

Katzberg RW, Dolwick MF, Bales DJ, et al: Arthrotomography of the temporomandibular joint: New technique and preliminary observations. AJR **132:**949, 1979.

Katzberg RW, Dolwick MF, Helms CA, et al: Arthrotomography of the temporomandibular joint, in Dalinka MK (ed): Arthrography. New York, Springer Publishing Co Inc, 1980.

Katzberg RW, Dolwick MF, Helms CA, et al: Arthrotomography of the temporomandibular joint. AJR **134:**995, 1980.

Katzberg RW, Dolwick MF, Keith DA, et al: New observations with routine and CT-assisted arthrography in suspected internal derangements of the temporomandibular joint. Oral Surg **51:**569, 1981.

Katzberg RW, Keith DA, Guralnick WC, et al: Internal derangements of the temporomandibular joint and arthritis. Radiology **146:**107, 1983.

Manzione JV, Seltzer SE, Katzberg RW, et al: Direct sagittal computed tomography of the temporomandibular joint. AJNR **3:**677, 1982.

Murphy WA: Arthrography of the temporomandibular joint. Radiol Clin North Am **19:**365, 1981.

Wilkes C: Structural and functional alteration of the temporomandibular joint. North West Dent **57:**287, 1978.

Wilkes CH: Arthrography of the temporomandibular joint in patients with the TMJ pain-dysfunction syndrome. Minn Med **61:**645, 1978.

Chapter 5 SURGERY
Chapter 6 POSTOPERATIVE MANAGEMENT AND RESULTS
Chapter 7 TEMPOROMANDIBULAR JOINT SURGERY: COMPLICATIONS AND FAILURE

Agerberg G, Lundberg M: Changes in the temporomandibular joint after surgical treatment. A radiologic follow-up study. Oral Surg **32:**865, 1971.

Al-Kayat A, Bramley P: A modified pre-auricular approach to the temporomandibular joint and malar arch. Br J Oral Surg **17:**91, 1979-80.

Annandale T: On displacement of the interarticular cartilage of the lower jaw and its treatment by operation. Lancet **1:**411, 1887.

Ashhurst A: Recurrent unilateral subluxation of the mandible excision of the interarticular cartilage in cases of snapping jaw. Ann Surg **73:**712, 1921.

Bartlett EJ, Gatto DJ: A restrospective study of TMJ implant arthroplasties, AADR Abstracts, 1003, 1983.

Behan R: Loose cartilage in the temporomaxillar joint: subluxation of the inferior maxilla. Ann Surg **67:**536, 1938.

Bellinger DH: Present status of arthrosis of the temporomandibular joint. J Oral Surg **6:**9, 1948.

Bellinger DH: Internal derangements of the temporomandibular joint. J Oral Surg **10:**47, 1952.

Bowman K: Temporomandibular joint arthrosis and its treatment by extirpation of the disc. Acta Chir Scand **95**(suppl):118, 1947.

Bowman K: A new operation for luxation in the temporomandibular joint. Acta Chir Scand **99:**96, 1949-50.

Bowman K: Surgical treatment of recurrent dislocation of the jaw. Acta Chir Scand **136:**191, 1970.

Bronstein SL: Closure of temporomandibular joint meniscoplasty with figure-of-eight vertical mattress suture. J Oral Maxillofac Surg **40:**248, 1982.

Bronstein SL, Tomasetti BJ, Ryan DE: Internal derangements of the temporomandibular joint: correlation of arthrography with surgical findings. J Oral Surg **39:**572, 1981.

Brown WA: Internal derangement of the temporomandibular joint: review of 214 patients following meniscectomy. Can J Surg **23:**1, 1980.

Carlsson GE, Kopp S, Lindstrom J, et al: Surgical treatment of temporomandibular joint disorders: a review. Swed Dent J **5:**41, 1981.

Cook HP: Teflon implantation in temporomandibular joint arthroplasty. J Oral Surg **33:**706, 1972.

Dingman RO: Supplemental report on meniscectomy in treating lesions of the temporomandibular joint. J Oral Surg **10:**141, 1952.

Dingman RO: Surgical correction of lesions of the temporomandibular joints. Plast Reconstr Surg **55:**335, 1975.

Dingman RO, Constant E: A fifteen year experience with temporomandibular joint disorders. Evaluation of 140 cases. Plast Reconstr Surg **44:**119, 1969.

Dingman RO, Grabb WC: Intra-capsular temporomandibular joint arthroplasty. Plast Reconstr Surg **38:**179, 1966.

Dingman RO, Moorman WC: Meniscectomy in the treatment of lesions of the temporomandibular joint. J Oral Surg **9:**214, 1951.

Dingman RO, Moorman WC: Meniscectomy in the treatment of lesions of the temporomandibular joint. J Oral Surg **10:**141, 1952.

Dolwick MF, Kretzschmar DP: Morbidity associated with the preauricular and perimeatal approaches to the temporomandibular joint. J Oral Maxillofac Surg **40:**699, 1982.

Dunn MJ, Benza R, Moan D, et al: Temporomandibular joint condylectomy: A technique and postoperative follow-up. Oral Surg **51:**363, 1981.

Fitzpatrick B: Indications for surgery on the painful temporomandibular joint. Aust Dent J 1971.

Gallagher DM, Wolford LM: Comparison of silastic and proplast implants in the temporomandibular joint after condylectomy for osteoarthritis. J Oral Maxillofac Surg **40:**627, 1982.

Georgiade N: The surgical correction of temporomandibular joint dysfunction by means of autogenous dermal grafts. Plast Reconstr Surg **30:**68, 1962.

Georgiade N: The surgical correction of chronic luxation of the mandibular condyle. Plast Reconstr Surg **36:**339, 1965.

Gerogiade N, Altany F, Pickrell K: An experimental and clinical evaluation of autogenous dermal grafts used in the treatment of temporomandibular joint ankylosis. Plast Reconstr Surg **19:**321, 1957.

Hansen WC, Deshazo BW: Silastic reconstruction of temporomandibular joint meniscus. Plast Reconstr Surg **43:**4, 1969.

Henny FA, Baldridge OL: Condylectomy for the persistently painful tempormandibular joint. J Oral Surg **15:**214, 1957.

Henny FA: Surgical treatment of the painful temporomandibular joint. J Am Dent Assoc **79:**171, 1969.

James P: The surgical treatment of mandibular joint disorders. Ann R Coll Surg Engl **49:**310, 1971.

Kiehn CL: Meniscectomy for internal derangement of temporomandibular joint. Am J Surg **83:**364, 1952.

Kiehn CL, Des Prez JD: Meniscectomy for internal derangement temporomandibular joint. Br J Plast Surg **15:**199, 1962.

Kreutziger KL: Microsurgical approach to the temporomandibular joint. A new horizon. Arch Otolaryngol **108:**422, 1982.

Laskin DM, Wheat PN, Evaskus DS: Effects of temporomandibular joint meniscectomy in adult and juvenile primates. AADR Abstracts, 350, 1977.

Marciana RD, Ziegler RC: Temporomandibular joint surgery: a review of 51 operations. Oral Surg **56:**5, 1983.

McCarty WL Jr, Farrar W: Surgery for internal derangements of the temporomandibular joint. J Prosthet Dent **42:**2, 1979.

Mercuri LG, Campbell RL, Shanaskin RG: Intra-articular meniscus dysfunction surgery—a preliminary report. Oral Surg **54:**6, 1982.

Merrill RG, Henny FA: Articular pathologic changes in patients with mandibular condylectomy. Abstract presented at the forty-fourth meeting of the IADR, 1966.

Middleton DS: Clinical approach to derangement of the mandibular joint. First Annie McNeil Lecture delivered at College of the Royal Infirmary, Edinburgh, Mar 20, 1970.

Murnane TW, Doku HC: Noninterpositional intracapsular anthroplasty of rabbit temporomandibular joints. J Oral Surg **29:**268, 1971.

Nalbandian RM, Swanson AB, Maupin BK: Long term silicone implant arthroplasty. JAMA **9:**250, 1983.

Nespeca JA, Griffin JM: Temporomandibular joint surgery—a 3 year study. J Haw Dent Assoc **14:**9, 1983.

Poswillo D: The late effects of mandibular condylectomy. Oral Surg **33:**500, 1972.

Poswillo D: Experimental reconstruction of the mandibular joint. Int J Oral Surg **3:**400, 1974.

Poswillo D: Surgery of the temporomandibular joint. Oral Sci Rev **6:**96, 1974.

Pringle J: Displacement of the mandibular meniscus and its treatment. Br J Surg **6:**385, 1918.

Rankow R: Transmeatal condylectomy and meniscectomy. AMA Arch Otolaryngol **70:**703, 1959.

Rongetti JR: Meniscectomy—a new approach to the temporomandibular joint. AMA Arch Otolaryngol **60:**566, 1954.

Rowe NL: Surgery of the temporomandibular joint. Proc R Soc Med **65:**383, 1972.

Sanders B, Brady F, Adams D: Silastic cap TMJ prosthesis. J Oral Surg **35:**933, 1977.

Sanders B, McKelvey B: Osteochondromatous exostosis of the condyle causing severe TMJ pain and clicking. JADA **95:**1151, 1977.

Sanders B, McKelvey D, Adams D: Asceptic osteomyelitis and necrosis of the mandibular condylar head following intracapsular fracture. Oral Surg **43:**665, 1977.

Sanders B, Neuman R: Surgical treatment for recurrent dislocation or chronic subluxation of the TMJ. Int J Oral Surg **4:**1, 1975.

Sanders B, Schneider J, Given J: Chronic dislocation of the mandibular condyle. J Oral Surg **37:**346, 1979.

Saunderson JR, Dolwick MF: Increased hemostasis in temporomandibular joint surgery with H. DeBakey clamp. J Oral Maxillofac Surg **41:**271, 1983.

Schultz LW: Twenty years experience in treating hypermobility of the temporomandibular joints. Am J Surg **92:**925, 1956.

Silver CM, Simon SD: Meniscus injuries of the temporomandibular joint. J Bone Joint Surg **38A:**541, 1956.

Silver CM, Simon SD: Operative treatment for recurrent dislocation of the temporomandibular joint. J Bone Joint Surg **43A:**211, 1961.

Silver CM, et al: The surgical treatment of the arthritic temporomandibular joint. Surg Gynecol Obstet **136:**251, 1973.

Smith AE, Robinson M: Mandibular function after condylectomy. J Am Dent Assoc **46:**304, 1953.

Sprinz R: The role of the meniscus in the healing process following excision of the articular surfaces of the mandibular joint in rabbits. J Anat **97:**345, 1963.

Steinhardt G: Untersuchungen uber die beanspruchung der kiefergelenke und ibre gewebliche folgen. Deutsche Zahneilkunde, 91, 1934.

Steinhardt G: Are plastic operations of temporomandibular arthrosis indicated today? Presented at the First International Congress of Plastic Surgery, Stockholm, 1955.

Steinhardt G: Surgery of the temporomandibular joint. Int Dent J **18:**59, 1968.

Stevenson JR, Evaskus DS, Laskin DM: Role of meniscus in temporomandibular joint ankylosis. IADR Abstracts, 1078, 1978.

Thoma KH: Arthrosis of temporomandibular joint. Oral Surg **2:**651, 1969.

Toller PA: Temporomandibular capsular rearrangement, Br J Oral Surg **11:**207, 1974.

Wallace D, Laskin DM: Healing of surgical defects in retrodiscal tissue of rabbit temporomandibular joint. IADR Abstracts, 866, 1984.

Wakeley C: The causation and treatment of displaced mandibular cartilage. Lancet **2:**543, 1929.

Wakeley C: Surgery of the temporomandibular joint. Surgery **5:**697, 1959.

Walters PJ, Geist ET: Correction of temporomandibular joint internal derangements by post auricular approach. J Oral Maxillofac Surg **41:**616, 1983.

Ward TG: Surgery of the mandibular joint. Ann R Coll Surg Engl **18:**139, 1961.

Wilkes CH: Structural and functional alterations of the temporomandibular joint. North West Dent **57:**287, 1978.

Yaillen DM, Shapiro PA, Luschei ES, et al: TMJ meniscectomy effects on joint structure and masticatory function in macaca fascicularis. J Oral Maxillofac Surg **7:**255, 1979.

Zemla J, Kraszewski J: Extra-articular surgical treatment of luxations and subluxations of the TMJ. Czas. Stom. **23:**1354, 1970.